£24.75

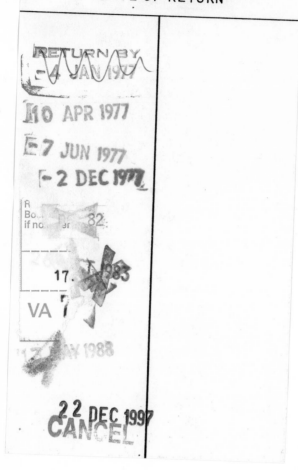

Chapter on Angiography of the Small Bowel

by

STANLEY BAUM, M.D.

Professor and Chairman, Department of Radiology,
University of Pennsylvania School of Medicine, Philadelphia

Chapter on Uncommon Lesions of the Small Intestine

by

ARTHUR CLEMETT, M.D.

Clinical Professor of Radiology,
New York University School of Medicine, New York

Chapter on Patterns of Spread of Malignancy to the Small Bowel

by

MORTON MEYERS, M.D.

Professor of Radiology,
Cornell University Medical College, New York

Chapter on The Small Bowel in Infants and Children

by

JACK G. RABINOWITZ, M.D.

Professor and Chairman of Diagnostic Radiology,
The University of Tennessee (College of Medicine), Memphis

and

JOHN E. MOSELEY, M.D.

Associate Clinical Professor of Radiology,
Mount Sinai School of Medicine, New York

With the assistance of

DANIEL MAKLANSKY, M.D.

Assistant Clinical Professor of Radiology,
Mount Sinai School of Medicine, New York

Radiology
of the
Small Intestine

RICHARD H. MARSHAK, M.D.

Clinical Professor of Radiology,
Mount Sinai School of Medicine, New York

and

ARTHUR E. LINDNER, M.D.

Associate Professor of Medicine,
New York University School of Medicine, New York

—————— *Second Edition* ——————

1976

W. B. SAUNDERS COMPANY / Philadelphia / London / Toronto

W. B. Saunders Company: West Washington Square
Philadelphia, PA 19105

12 Dyott Street
London, WC1A 1DB

833 Oxford Street
Toronto, Ontario M8Z 5T9, Canada

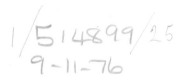

Radiology of the Small Intestine   ISBN 0-7216-6127-0

Last digit is the print number: 9   8   7   6   5   4   3   2   1

Foreword

This monograph needs no foreword but I have wanted to write one to state my belief that this volume will be a radiographic classic. Its virtues are clear: a readable text with superb pictures, an encyclopedic coverage based on firsthand material. There is no hearsay here.

Two explicable factors have contributed greatly. First, this is a text on *clinical* radiology. As the authors have indicated in their own introduction, the experiences condensed in this volume arose in the midst of an active clinical setting: a day-to-day partnership with gastroenterology. Second, this text is based on close pathological correlation. One need only attend one of Dr. Richard Marshak's x-ray conferences to observe how tenaciously these correlations are pursued. The inexplicable factor is, of course, the senior author's talent for "pattern recognition." I do not believe that he himself could explain this gift, but it has enabled him to recognize and define toxic dilatation in ulcerative colitis, dilatation and intussusception in sprue, Crohn's disease of the colon, vascular insufficiency of the small bowel, and so forth.

If there is one section of the present volume I could call attention to, it is the area on malabsorption. The recent explosion of methods for studying small bowel absorptive function and columnar cell morphology has presented clinicians with techniques of considerable complexity. A careful reading of the section on malabsorption will show how far the differential diagnosis of malabsorptive syndromes can be carried on purely radiologic grounds.

While clinical entities involving the small bowel undoubtedly remain to be described, it is hard to see how small bowel radiology in the future can go beyond the morphologic basis of the present volume (although the future of vascular radiology of the gut remains to be explored). The authors' studies of the effect of anticholinergic drugs on the colon, and anticholinesterases on the small bowel, hint that the future of small bowel radiographic analysis will be in a functional direction. This foreword, however, is not intended to speculate about the future (whither radiology?) but to introduce this solid accomplishment of the present, which I confidently predict will have a great future.

HENRY D. JANOWITZ, M.D.

Preface
to the Second Edition

Advances in radiological technique and interpretation as well as rapid progress in our understanding of the diseases that involve the small bowel have required a second edition of Radiology of the Small Intestine five years after the appearance of the first.

The text has been updated and three new chapters have been added. Doctor Morton Meyers, of Cornell University Medical College, has contributed a chapter on the patterns of metastatic cancer seen in the small bowel. Doctor Stanley Baum, of the University of Pennsylvania School of Medicine, has provided a thorough discussion of the applications of angiography to the study of the small bowel and its diseases. Finally, with the assistance of Dr. Charles Hazzi, of New York University School of Medicine, we have added a chapter on the small bowel in the immunoglobulin deficiency syndromes. Immunoglobulin disorders have proved to have important relationships to malabsorption and to malignancy. Increasing knowledge of immunological mechanisms will undoubtedly expand our understanding of other small bowel diseases in the years to come.

In the preparation of this second edition we have been aided by our colleague, Dr. Daniel Maklansky, to whom we are most grateful. We want also to thank our editor, Mr. John Hanley, and the W. B. Saunders Company for their cooperation, their suggestions, and their support.

RICHARD H. MARSHAK

ARTHUR E. LINDNER

Preface to the First Edition

The origins of this book can be traced to the early association of the senior author with Dr. Burrill Crohn. At a time when little was known about the small bowel and its diseases, large numbers of patients were referred to Dr. Crohn for diagnosis and management of regional enteritis. Not all of these patients proved to have regional enteritis, and in the course of studying them some of the differential roentgen features of lymphosarcoma and sprue, in particular, became better understood. From these beginnings the authors extended their interest in the radiologic aspects of the small bowel by studying both well established diseases, such as benign tumors and carcinoma, and new entities as they were described, such as the Zollinger-Ellison syndrome and vasculitis.

The upper gastrointestinal series and the barium enema became routine studies because the examinations could be done easily and disease was often discovered. The small bowel, however, was neglected, probably because so much time was necessary for its examination and there seemed to be a low incidence of disease. In recent years there has been new interest in the small bowel and an awareness that many diseases involve this organ, diseases which can be diagnosed quite accurately by careful attention to their roentgen features.

We have tried to present a systematic study of the diseases of the small bowel from a radiologic point of view. Some unevenness was inevitable, since we have emphasized the diseases with which we are most familiar. The chapters on regional enteritis, lymphosarcoma, sprue, carcinoma, and vascular disease are detailed, for example, while sections on tuberculosis and some of the parasitic diseases are brief. A chapter on granulomatous colitis, which might seem out of place in a volume on the small bowel, has been included because of the authors' special interest in this disease and because the small bowel is always of concern and is often involved in it.

We want to thank Dr. Bernard Wolf, Chairman of the Department of Radiology, Mount Sinai School of Medicine, and the other members of the Department who collaborated on several of the articles which form the basis of this volume; Dr. Burrill Crohn, who provided much of the initial material; and Dr. Henry Janowitz, who supplied more recent cases and offered many helpful and stimulating suggestions.

We believe the illustrations in this book are of unusually fine quality and we are grateful to Mr. Robert Carlin for his excellent photography. The careful typing of the manuscript was the work of Miss Linda Dubester, to whom we express our thanks. Finally we want to note our sincere appreciation to the W. B. Saunders Company for their enthusiasm and encouragement at each step in the preparation of this book. We found that with their help, work that might have been just a chore became a challenging project.

RICHARD H. MARSHAK

ARTHUR E. LINDNER

Contents

1

Roentgen Examination of the Small Bowel

It is impractical to perform a complete small bowel examination on every patient with abdominal complaints; however, at least one small bowel film should be obtained as part of the routine upper gastrointestinal series. This can readily be accomplished as a delayed film at the conclusion of the examination. This film not only permits visualization of part of the small bowel but also provides an emptying film of the stomach. The chance that this single film may reveal a previously unsuspected lesion in the visualized small intestine is great enough to warrant its inclusion in the routine upper gastrointestinal series.

The *indications* for a complete small bowel examination include the following:

1. Gastrointestinal bleeding which cannot be localized to the esophagus, stomach, duodenal bulb, or colon.
2. Diarrhea or steatorrhea.
3. Unexplained abdominal pain.
4. Fever of unknown origin.
5. Retardation of growth and development.
6. Findings of ulcerative or granulomatous colitis on barium enema examination.

It is important to remember that an abnormality discovered in an upper gastrointestinal series or barium enema examination does not necessarily explain a patient's clinical findings and does not rule out a small bowel lesion. Clinical judgment and an awareness of the diseases that involve the small bowel provide additional indications for a small bowel examination.

TECHNIQUE

Patients are examined after an overnight fast, and whenever possible all medications are discontinued the day before the examination. Anticholinergics and ganglionic blocking agents tend to cause dilatation and mimic the sprue pattern, and narcotics affect both the motility and the appearance of the folds of the small bowel.

The most important characteristic of a proper contrast material for the small bowel study is a barium which suspends easily and does not flocculate, precipitate, or settle in the presence of intestinal secretions. These aims can be accomplished by micropulverization of the barium sulfate and addition of a suspending agent. Most modern barium preparations, fortunately, contain adequate suspending agents and are sufficiently micropulverized for small bowel studies. Thus there is no longer need, in describing contrast media, to specify such terms as "flocculating" or "nonflocculating" barium. Plain USP barium, which may flocculate in the small bowel, should not be used for this examination.

A preliminary film of the abdomen prior to the administration of barium is often helpful. In adults the small bowel may contain scattered amounts of gas, but visualization of an entire segment or a loop is an abnormal finding. Large amounts indicate an ileus or obstruction. Gas can serve as a contrast medium on a plain film and demonstrate very effectively an area of pathology within the small bowel. The total absence of gas in the small bowel is abnormal.

The esophagus and stomach should be examined whenever a small bowel series is performed. Since considerable amounts of barium are used in a small bowel series, the examination of the upper gastrointestinal tract does not interfere with the small bowel study.

The small bowel is examined following administration of a mixture which is half barium sulfate, by volume, and half water. At least 16 oz. of the mixture is used, and at times 20 oz. or more may be required. Use of smaller amounts of barium may cause incomplete filling of loops and simulate a small bowel abnormality. The large volume of barium is especially valuable in the interpretation of diffuse lesions in the small bowel. Many intestinal loops may be visualized in continuity at the same time and the relationship of one segment to another is better evaluated (Figs. 1-1 to 1-3).

Compression studies are used whenever necessary for better delineation of a lesion, and they are routinely employed in demonstrating the terminal ileum. There is a tendency for barium to flood ileal loops in the pelvis, but compression studies and appropriate timing of films will usually permit visualization of all segments (Fig. 1-4).

The patient is initially examined fluoroscopically in 15 minutes, and if the barium meal has progressed sufficiently a film is taken. It is desirable to see the entire jejunum on the first film. This initial film may be taken in the supine position if adequate visualization of the ligament of Treitz has not previously been obtained during the upper gastrointestinal series. Subsequent films are all taken in the prone position. Further filming depends upon the rate of passage of the barium meal and usually consists of a film every 30 to 60 minutes until the barium has reached the colon. The later exposures provide evacuation films of the proximal loops of bowel and may better delineate tumors or ulcers of this area. Evacuation films, in fact, often serve the same purpose as compression films.

There is wide variation among subjects in the time of transit of barium through the small bowel. In normal persons the head of the barium column may take from 2 hours to as long as 5 to 6 hours to reach the colon. The range is so

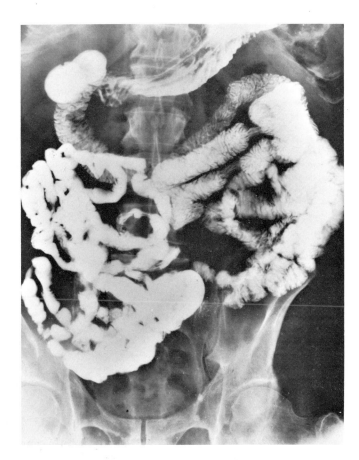

Figure 1-1 *Normal small intestine.* This film was taken thirty minutes after the ingestion of 20 fluid ounces of a barium mixture.

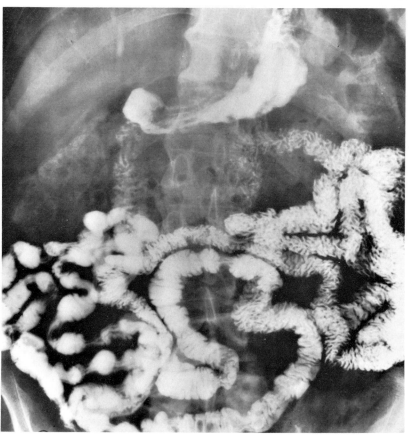

Figure 1-2 *Normal small intestine.* Note that the column of barium is continuous and that the loops have an undulating, serpentine configuration.

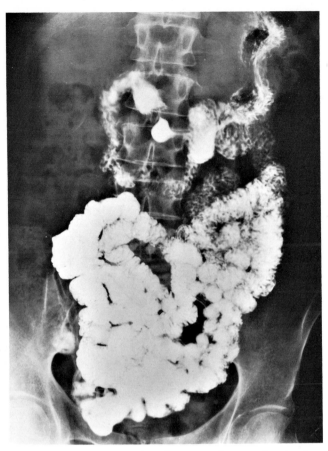

Figure 1-3 Normal small intestine. This film was made immediately after the upper gastrointestinal study was completed. The barium column has reached the distal ileum with visualization of most of the small bowel.

great that it is difficult to make a definite statement about transit time in a given patient. Moreover, the type of barium influences transit time. The examiner should be familiar with the motility pattern of the barium he employs. In general, appearance of barium in the colon less than an hour after the start of the examination suggests rapid transit and may warrant appropriate diagnostic studies for such systemic diseases as hyperthyroidism and carcinoid syndrome.

Often it is worthwhile to extend the small bowel examination to include the entire colon. This procedure is especially indicated in patients with inflammatory bowel disease, for films of the colon visualized from above may detect areas of inflammation not seen after distention of the colon with barium or air during the barium enema study. Conversely, especially in the presence of small bowel obstruction, the terminal ileum may be better visualized by reflux during a barium enema examination than by a small bowel series.

In some instances, when transit is slow, the patient is allowed to eat a small meal to stimulate motility and hasten the barium through the distal bowel. Feeding is permitted only when the proximal loops have been adequately studied.

Neostigmine is helpful in increasing motility and shortening the time of the small bowel examination (Fig. 1-5). A subcutaneous or intramuscular injection of 0.5 mg. will speed the passage of barium through the small bowel, and

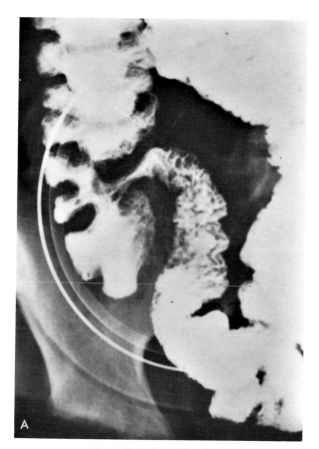
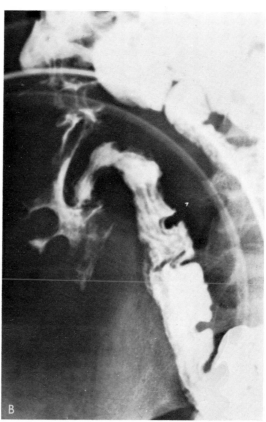

Figure 1-4 *Spot film of a normal terminal ileum.* This is readily accomplished in most cases by the use of an inflated rubber balloon or by compression with a cone.

in most cases the barium column will reach the colon in 30 to 45 minutes. Although use of the drug in this dosage is generally quite safe, it should not be employed in the elderly or in patients with heart disease, asthma, or complete mechanical intestinal or urinary tract obstruction. Atropine should be readily available in case a reaction occurs. It should be noted that neostigmine does not significantly alter the small bowel pattern, although the intestinal hurry may produce areas of narrowing which on occasion can be confusing.

In patients with incomplete small bowel obstruction, prostigmine may be a useful and safe adjuvant. In regional enteritis, for example, prostigmine frequently aids in visualization of stenotic segments of bowel by propelling barium into those areas.

Cholecystokinin (cholecystokinin-pancreozymin; CCK-PZ) is a hormone derived from the duodenal mucosa. Among its other actions is stimulation of propulsive activity in the mesenteric small bowel. Investigators have taken advantage of this property by using commercially prepared CCK-PZ to shorten the duration of the small bowel roentgen study. With this method, 40 units of CCK-PZ is injected intravenously one-half hour after ingestion of the barium suspension (to allow time for gastric emptying). Films are routinely exposed 1,3,5,7 and 10 minutes after the drug has been given. In most patients barium reaches the cecum in less than 15 minutes. Although adequate visualization of the small bowel may be obtained by this method, abdominal cramps and nausea occur as unpleasant side effects in many patients. The drug seems to us to offer

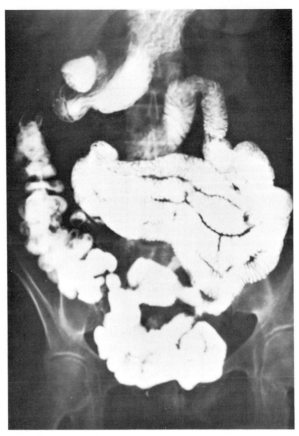

Figure 1-5 Normal small intestine. One-half milligram of neostigmine was administered at the conclusion of the upper gastrointestinal examination. The entire small bowel was visualized in 15 minutes.

little advantage over neostigmine and we do not employ it. At present, CCK-PZ is probably of more value in investigative studies than in the clinical small bowel examination.

In performing as well as in interpreting the small bowel series, the clinical features and the indications for the study should always be kept in mind. The technique must be modified as the examination proceeds, if necessary, and an optimal study may not be achieved if the examination is simply done in a routine fashion with routine filming. The technique for studying the patient with sprue, for example, with principal findings in the jejunum, may be very different from that of studying the patient with regional enteritis whose major findings are in the terminal ileum. The small bowel examination must be performed with an understanding of small bowel physiology and with knowledge of the clinical features of each patient's illness.

Examination of the Small Bowel in the Presence of Obstruction

In most patients with chronic or incomplete small bowel obstruction barium sulfate mixtures may safely be used for the small bowel examination. These may be administered either by mouth or through an indwelling small bowel tube (e.g., Miller-Abbott or Cantor tube). Spot films are taken to identify the point of obstruction. Barium does not inspissate in the fluid-filled small bowel, and there is no evidence that barium will convert an incomplete small intestinal obstruction into a complete one. The advantage of barium over iodinated water-soluble media is that far better visualization of small bowel loops and of the lesion is obtained. Barium should not be employed, however, in acute or in closed loop obstruction when surgical intervention is imminent.

Although the iodinated water-soluble compounds would seem of value in patients with obstruction, they are hypertonic and their use may complicate the patient's clinical course. These substances cause an increase in fluid within the small bowel, decrease circulating volume and may cause fluid shifts leading to shock. Such profound effects are especially likely to occur in children. Even in the absence of clinical complications, dilution of these media by fluid in the bowel renders the films very difficult to interpret.

In acute or closed-loop obstructions or in suspected perforation, small amounts of the iodinated water-soluble media may be helpful in identifying a lesion, but often the plain abdominal film, upright and recumbent, will be of great value and no contrast material at all may be required to decide upon management. Moreover, as previously noted, in the presence of an obstructive lesion in the terminal ileum the barium enema examination with reflux through the ileocecal valve provides a more rapid diagnosis (Fig. 1-6).

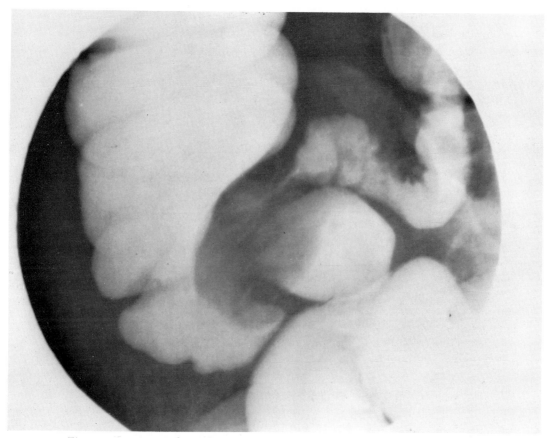

Figure 1-6 *Retrograde examination of a normal terminal ileum.* The ileocecal valve is prominent, but the contours are smooth. The narrowing of the terminal ileum at the entrance into the ileocecal valve is a normal finding.

Hypotonic Duodenography

Hypotonic duodenography is a technique to improve visualization of the duodenal sweep. The method involves relaxing the duodenum by means of a parenteral anticholinergic agent or glucagon and then instilling into the duodenum barium and air to outline the duodenal lumen. The procedure is often useful in defining inflammatory and neoplastic lesions of the duodenal sweep.

One method in current use requires passage of a nasogastric tube either into the stomach or through the pylorus into the duodenum. Sixty mg. of propantheline (Pro-Banthine) is then injected intramuscularly. Three or four ounces of barium is instilled through the tube into the stomach or duodenum, and the patient is placed in the prone, right anterior oblique position. Spot films are taken as barium fills the hypotonic duodenal sweep. The patient is then turned into a supine position and 100 to 200 ml. of air is instilled through the tube. Air flows into the duodenum and spot films are taken as the patient is moved into appropriate oblique positions. These films provide air contrast studies of the sweep.

The authors have found that a simpler technique is often effective and does not require passage of a nasogastric tube or instillation of air. In this method, 5 mg. of propantheline is injected intravenously after barium has been administered by mouth and the second portion of the duodenum has been initially visualized. Barium now fills the relaxed duodenal sweep. Films are taken in the prone and then in the supine position, the latter providing sufficient air for contrast study. Some radiologists also administer gas-producing substances by mouth in order to obtain more air for contrast studies.

Glucagon, administered as a 1 mg. dose intravenously, induces excellent relaxation of the duodenal sweep without the sometimes unpleasant anticholinergic side effects of propantheline.

THE NORMAL SMALL BOWEL

In almost all patients the jejunum is located in the left upper quadrant and the ileum in the right lower quadrant. Occasionally, as in congenital malrotations and in paraduodenal hernias, the relationship may be altered. The valvulae conniventes are quite well developed in the jejunum and therefore appear as prominent folds, which persist even in the presence of distal obstruction (Fig. 1-7). In the ileum the valvulae are smaller, and less prominent, and tend to be obliterated in the presence of obstruction. The caliber of the jejunum (2 to 3 cm.) is slightly greater than that of the ileum (1.5 to 2.5 cm.). The normal small intestine has an undulating, coiled appearance. The loops of bowel touch one another and there is no persistent separation of loops (Figs. 1-1, 1-2, 1-3, and 1-5). The barium column in the normal small bowel is continuous, but identification of an occasional area of segmentation or of some fragmentation does not indicate disease. Such findings may relate to the characteristics of the barium used or to the presence of somewhat more fluid in the bowel lumen than is usually seen.

Peristaltic activity in the small bowel, as visualized fluoroscopically or

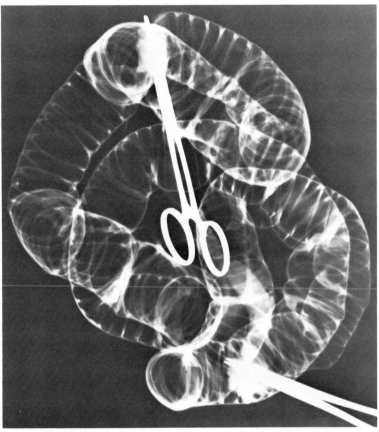

Figure 1-7 *Specimen of jejunum coated with barium and filled with air.* Despite distention, the valvulae conniventes are still present.

demonstrated on serial films, varies considerably. In some patients the bowel is active with peristaltic movements, but in others it is quiet radiologically. The significance of such variations in observed activity has not been established.

The terminal ileum must always be compressed. This segment of bowel tends to be hidden by overlapping loops in the pelvis, and because it so often is the site of disease, special study during the small bowel examination is required. Compression is often simplified because the terminal ileum commonly rises from the pelvis to join the cecum at the iliac crest. Sometimes, especially in the presence of adhesions, the terminal ileum cannot be properly separated from the adjacent loops of bowel.

2

Malabsorption Syndrome: Sprue

The term "malabsorption syndrome" refers to a heterogeneous group of diseases which have in common defective absorption of the main foodstuffs—carbohydrate, protein and fat—from the small intestine. As a rule, this results in the passage of stools which are bulky, fatty, and foul-smelling. Besides this steatorrhea, there may occur such clinical features as weight loss, abdominal distention, skin pigmentation, retarded growth and development, and various deficiency states, including lack of folic acid, vitamin B_{12}, iron, B complex vitamins, vitamin K, calcium, or magnesium.

The causes of malabsorption syndrome may be broadly grouped as indicated in Table 2-1. This somewhat arbitrary classification has proved to be useful in considering malabsorption from a roentgen viewpoint. It includes sprue, constitutional diseases, primary diseases of the small bowel, surgical operations on the gastrointestinal tract, and conditions leading to faulty digestion of food.

PHYSIOLOGY OF ABSORPTION

The small intestine is remarkably adapted to its function of absorption by means of several devices which serve to increase the surface area of its mucosa: (1) The mucosa is thrown into folds, called the valvulae conniventes. (2) The villi, finger-like mucosal processes about 1 mm. in length, project into the lumen. (3) The microvilli, about 1 micron in length and seen by electron microscopy, form the luminal border of the columnar absorbing cell. Wilson[1] has estimated that these devices may increase the small bowel surface area for absorption some 600-fold in comparison with the area of a simple tube.

The villi are lined by columnar absorbing cells and mucus-producing goblet cells and contain smooth muscle fibers, blood capillaries, and lymphatics. Substances absorbed via the blood capillaries ultimately enter the portal vein; those absorbed via the lymphatic vessels enter the thoracic duct. Between the bases of the villi are the glandlike crypts of Lieberkühn, from which the cells lining the villi are generated. Radioautographic studies have demon-

Table 2-1.* *Causes of Malabsorption Syndrome

1. "Sprue group"
    Celiac disease
    Nontropical sprue
    Tropical sprue
2. Constitutional diseases
    Whipple's disease
    Scleroderma
    Lymphosarcoma
    Amyloidosis
    Diabetes
    Carcinoid syndrome
    Systemic mastocytosis
    A-betalipoproteinemia
    Dermatitis herpetiformis
    Hypogammaglobulinemia
    Hyperthyroidism
3. Small bowel diseases
    Intestinal lymphangiectasia
    Parasitic infection
    Diverticula, blind loops, strictures
    Regional enteritis
    Tuberculosis
    Mesenteric vascular insufficiency
    Disaccharidase deficiency
    Radiation injury
    Eosinophilic gastroenteritis
4. Surgical operations on the gastrointestinal tract
    Small bowel resections
    Gastroileostomy
    Total or subtotal gastrectomy
5. Faulty preparation of food
    Diseases of the liver and biliary tract
    Zollinger-Ellison syndrome
    Pancreatic insufficiency

strated that intestinal epithelial cells originate in the crypts of Lieberkühn and migrate upward along the villus as sheets of cells to the apex, where they are extruded into the lumen. The intestinal epithelium is completely renewed within two or three days in rodents and the commonly studied mammals, but probably in five or six days in man. As the epithelial cells move upward, they become progressively more differentiated for absorptive functions. These functions are at their peak at the tip of the villus where the most mature cells are located just prior to their extrusion.[2, 3]

At least three processes of general physiology are thought to be involved in absorption from the small intestine. *Passive diffusion* is movement of a substance across a membrane in accordance with concentration gradient and electrical charge. *Active transport* is movement of a substance across a membrane against an electrochemical gradient. Such a process requires energy which is supplied by cellular metabolism. *Facilitated diffusion* is movement of a substance across a membrane without direct expenditure of energy but at a rate greater than would be expected by simple diffusion. A carrier mechanism has been postulated to account for this phenomenon. Unlike active transport, movement is not against a concentration gradient.

Carbohydrates are digested by salivary and pancreatic amylase and by the disaccharidases of the intestinal mucosa to the monosaccharides glucose, galactose, and fructose. Glucose and galactose are absorbed largely in the proximal jejunum by mechanisms of active transport. Fructose is absorbed in the same area by facilitated diffusion. Protein is hydrolyzed to amino acids, which are absorbed by active transport, largely in the proximal jejunum.

Fats are emulsified and hydrolyzed by action of pancreatic lipase and bile salts. Most fat is absorbed in the upper jejunum. Fat droplets enter the absorbing cell by diffusion through the lipid membrane of the cell. Fatty acids and some monoglycerides are the end products absorbed. Normally, almost all the dietary fat is absorbed; about 5 gm. of fat is excreted in the stool each day, but this is derived largely from desquamated intestinal cells and bacterial bodies.

In man most fluid and electrolytes are absorbed from the jejunum. Relatively little net fluid absorption occurs in the duodenum where intestinal contents are equlibrated and made isotonic.

SPRUE

The name "sprue" is given to a group of three diseases of the small bowel which have a close clinical relationship. This group comprises celiac disease of children, nontropical sprue or idiopathic steatorrhea of the adult, and tropical sprue. All available evidence now indicates that celiac disease and nontropical sprue are the same entity, occurring at different times of life. Whether tropical sprue is a distinct disease or a variant of nontropical sprue is not yet established.

All three members of the "sprue group" demonstrate similar findings on small bowel biopsy. There is a flattening, broadening, and coalescence of villi and sometimes complete loss of villi. The crypts of Lieberkühn become elongated, so the overall thickness of the mucosa may not be much different from the normal. The lamina propria is infiltrated with lymphocytes, plasma cells, and occasionally eosinophils. The epithelial cells of the villi are flattened and cuboidal, and the nuclei, instead of maintaining a regular basal orientation, present at irregular levels. These mucosal abnormalities in sprue tend to be more marked in the jejunum than in the ileum. Histochemical evidence suggests that in sprue the tip of the villus, physiologically the most active site of absorption, is not formed but instead is replaced by an abnormal epithelium which has both morphologic and chemical defects.[2, 3]

Patients with sprue present the classic clinical expressions of malabsorption. Diarrhea and steatorrhea are commonly present, with passage of bulky, fatty, foul-smelling stools. Other clinical features of sprue include weight loss, weakness, abdominal distention, skin pigmentation, retarded growth and development, and the manifestation of a variety of mineral and vitamin deficiency states.

Celiac disease and nontropical sprue have in common a peculiar relationship to diet; this is a feature that separates them from tropical sprue. In 1950 Dicke, in Holland, demonstrated that in children with celiac disease, removal of wheat from the diet caused the signs and symptoms of the disease to disappear and that reintroduction of wheat caused recurrence. Subsequently, workers extended the list of offending cereals to include wheat, rye, oats, and barley, and they showed that a rigorous diet avoiding these grains brought dramatic remissions to children with celiac disease and to adults with nontropical sprue.

The toxicity of the cereal grains to the sprue patient lies in the water-insoluble protein fraction which is called gluten, but the specific cause of the toxicity remains elusive.[4] It has been suggested that sprue patients, because of an inborn or acquired error of metabolism, may lack an enzyme in the small bowel mucosa which can inactivate the deleterious agent in gluten.

The nature of the relationship between gluten and the intestinal lesion is obscure. The lesion may improve or disappear in young patients with celiac disease on a gluten-free diet within three months to a year. In adults, some improvement may be noted but the lesion persists in the great majority of cases. The fact that complete clinical remission may occur even though the small bowel mucosal lesion persists without change suggests that the morphologic changes are secondary effects rather than the cause of sprue. Moreover, the severity of the histologic lesion does not correlate with the clinical state or with the degree of absorptive impairment.

When a patient is in clinical remission on a gluten-free diet, reintroduction of gluten into the diet increases the fecal fat excretion to abnormal levels and causes a clinical exacerbation. The time needed for these changes to occur varies from several days to several weeks.

Tropical sprue is probably distinct from nontropical sprue and celiac disease, although the clinical manifestations are similar and the intestinal mucosal lesion appears to be the same. The principal difference clinically seems to be that tropical sprue often responds dramatically to folic acid,[5] antibiotic therapy,[6] or both, whereas celiac disease and nontropical sprue do not. On the other hand, celiac disease and nontropical sprue usually respond to a gluten-free diet, which is without effect in tropical sprue. Severe deficiencies of folic acid and of vitamin B_{12} occur frequently in tropical sprue but are uncommon in nontropical sprue. Nontropical sprue appears to be widespread in its geographic incidence, but tropical sprue is remarkably localized. It occurs, for example, in India and the Far East but not in Africa; it is common in Puerto Rico but not in Jamaica.

Recent studies indicate that folic acid rapidly improves the clinical status in tropical sprue but fails to improve intestinal function or heal the mucosal lesion so quickly. In one study about half the patients with the disease eventually recovered from the initial episode with healing of the mucosal lesion and return of biochemical tests to normal. Those who failed to enter a full remission remained relatively asymptomatic but showed persistent biochemical and histologic evidence of disease.[5]

Roentgen Findings in Sprue

The roentgen findings to be described are similar in celiac disease, nontropical sprue, and tropical sprue, and they are present in virtually all patients in the active phase of their disease. In clinical remissions the roentgen findings, like the small bowel lesion, may improve or may remain unchanged.

Inflammatory changes are not seen in sprue. Rarely, however, single or multiple ulcers have been reported in this disease.[7a,b] Almost every patient with sprue exhibits in varying degrees the small intestinal changes of dilatation, segmentation, fragmentation and scattering of the barium column, and hypersecretion.[8,9] The fold pattern may appear thickened or thinned, depending on the degree of dilatation and the amount of secretion. Transit time of barium through the small bowel is usually normal but in severe cases can be prolonged. Transient intussusceptions may be seen.

There are some micropulverized barium mixtures with suspending agents which diminish the degree of segmentation and flocculation, but the characteristic dilatation of the small intestine persists and the increased fluid, although less prominent, is still apparent within the lumen.

Dilatation

Dilatation of the lumen of the small intestine is one of the most important and constant findings in sprue. Some of the individual features of the sprue pattern are seen in other disorders, but in none is dilatation more striking or constant than in sprue (Figs. 2-1 to 2-5). It is usually best visualized in the mid- and distal jejunum. Dilatation of the distal ileum is not as common as elsewhere in the small intestine, but diffuse dilatation of the entire intestine may occur. The dilated loops are generally long and tortuous with pliable walls. The degree of dilatation is exceedingly variable, and often a single intestinal segment may manifest varying degrees of dilatation during the course of a single roentgen study. In general, dilatation appears to be related to the severity of the disease and is most marked in the advanced cases. The large intestine may also show dilatation.

Fluoroscopic observations of the altered contractility of the dilated small

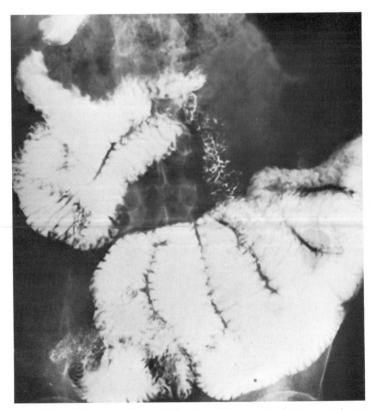

Figure 2-1 Sprue. There is moderate dilatation of the proximal jejunum. The intestinal loops are pliable and flaccid.

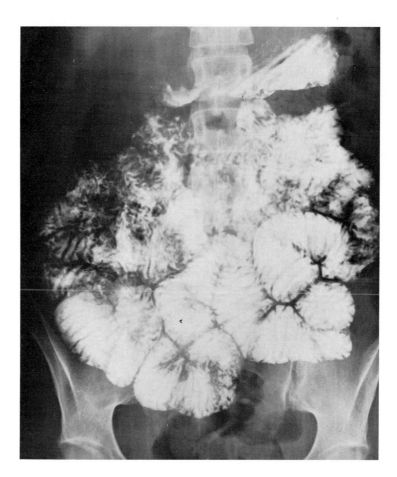

Figure 2-2 Sprue. The dilatation is best seen in the mid- and distal jejunum. The valvulae conniventes in this area are less prominent. Again note the pliable and flaccid intestinal loops.

intestinal loops are of some interest. In many patients, barium flows more freely than usual through the dilated intestinal loops, apparently unhindered by intestinal contraction. When secretions are encountered, progress is slowed and the column segmented. In those patients with marked dilatation, there is prolonged transit time, which appears to be due to ineffective peristaltic activity. These findings suggest that in sprue the tonicity of the small intestine is altered, so that there is little resistance to dilatation by ingested substances and that once the lumen is dilated, peristalsis becomes disordered and ineffective. Decompensation of the bowel wall may occur in severe cases of sprue with marked small intestinal dilatation.

The dilatation of sprue may superficially resemble that of mechanical intestinal obstruction. In sprue, however, the dilated loops of bowel are flaccid, contract poorly, and do not have the erectile configuration seen in mechanical obstruction. This observation is important when micropulverized barium mixtures are used with suspending agents, for these may modify the associated findings in sprue of segmentation and fragmentation.

Intestinal fluid does not appear to be a factor in the production of dilatation. Dilatation is generally most marked in the jejunum where fluid is least, and minimal in the ileum where excessive fluid is most often found.

The cause of dilatation remains unknown. At autopsy, the only gross finding may be thinning of the small intestinal wall. Whether this finding is the cause of the dilatation or its sequela has been subject to speculation.

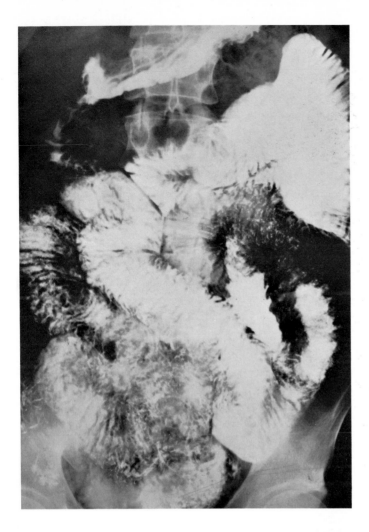

Figure 2-3 Sprue. The entire jejunum is moderately dilated, with increased fluid distally. Minimal contractions are noted.

Figure 2-4 Sprue. There is moderate dilatation of the entire jejunum, with thinning of the valvulae conniventes, minimal fragmentation, and increased fluid. Nonobstructive intussusception is noted in the distal jejunum.

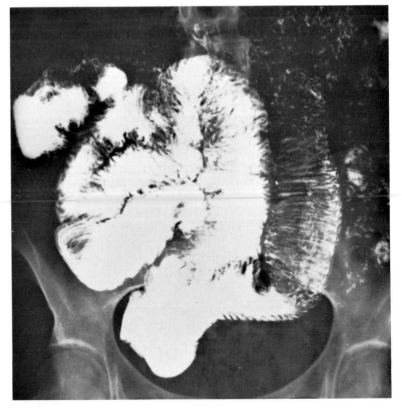

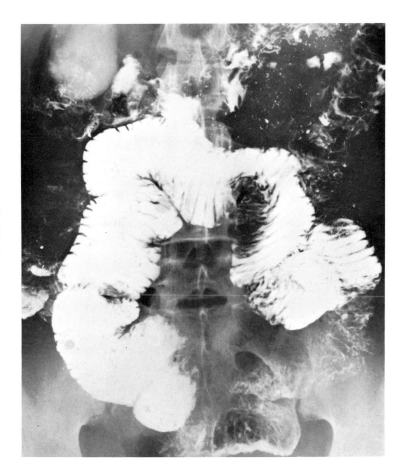

Figure 2-5 *Sprue.* There is considerable dilatation of the mid-jejunum, associated with thinning of the valvulae conniventes. The intestinal loops are flaccid and pliable, and differ from the erectile loops usually noted in intestinal obstruction.

Segmentation

We restrict use of the term segmentation to indicate those masses of barium which are moderately large, definitely separated from adjacent clumps, and usually in dilated loops which contain excessive fluid. The small, contracted, barium-filled segments of small intestine connected by strands of barium seen in association with spasm are not included in this definition.

Segmentation is most pronounced in the distal jejunum and ileum and is best seen in the more advanced cases. Two forms are noted, delayed and immediate. The more common form is delayed segmentation, i.e., segmentation that occurs in those intestinal segments that are in the process of evacuation. The less common immediate segmentation is noted as soon as the barium enters the small intestine and persists throughout the study (Fig. 2-6). In a mild or moderately severe case of sprue, diffuse dilatation of the jejunum and proximal ileum is noted, followed by segmentation of the barium column (Figs. 2-7 to 2-11). The phenomenon of segmentation is probably caused by excessive fluid within the intestinal tract.

Between the segmented clumps of barium, wormlike or stringlike strands of barium are often noted. These seemingly collapsed intestinal loops are usually associated with segmentation. They are inconstant and vary from film to film, possibly because of altered motor activity of the bowel segment or incomplete filling and emptying. Since these seemingly collapsed segments occur only in the presence of segmentation (which is always associated with

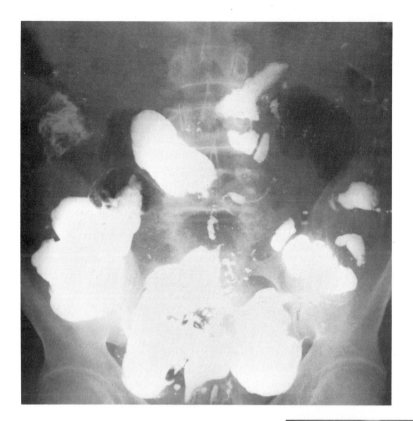

Figure 2-6 *Sprue.* There is immediate persistent and marked segmentation. The segmental loops are dilated and contain a considerable amount of fluid. The absence of valvulae conniventes is secondary to this increased fluid content and has been termed the moulage sign. It is a late feature of sprue and is rarely seen at the present time, probably because the diagnosis of sprue is made earlier.

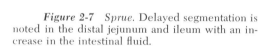

Figure 2-7 *Sprue.* Delayed segmentation is noted in the distal jejunum and ileum with an increase in the intestinal fluid.

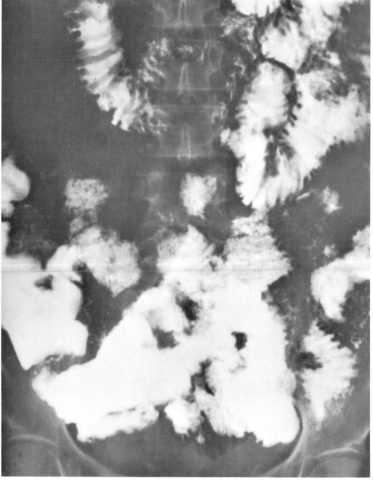

hypersecretion), they may actually represent only the barium stream as it passes through a secretion-filled loop (Figs. 2-10 and 2-11).

As the barium leaves the small intestine, a faint, irregular stippling of residual barium may be seen along the course of the jejunum. This is a normal finding. However, in sprue, the mottling is coarser and more amorphous, resembling snowflakes. This is called fragmentation and is usually associated with segmentation and increased fluid (Figs. 2-12 to 2-15).

Hypersecretion

An excessive amount of fluid in the intestinal tract is a constant phenomenon in most cases showing the sprue pattern and especially in those with marked segmentation.[10, 11] Air-fluid levels may be seen occasionally during the course of study. The usual homogeneous appearance of the barium in the normal small intestine is replaced by barium which presents a coarse granular appearance, with areas of flocculation dispersed irregularly in the barium-filled loops. Flocculation is best visualized at the periphery of the segment.

Fold Pattern

When dilatation of the jejunum occurs, whether due to mechanical or functional changes, the mucosal folds appear straightened and less prominent and thinned. When secretions are abundant, the folds may appear to be thickened rather than thinned, and an associated hypoalbuminemia may contribute to some prominence of the fold pattern. Consistent thickening of the folds, as seen (for example) in lymphosarcoma or Whipple's disease, is not present.

The term "moulage sign" has been utilized to describe the roentgen appearance of the jejunum in sprue, in which the folds appear to be completely effaced and the barium-filled lumen resembles a tube into which "wax has been poured and allowed to harden" (Figs. 2-6, 2-9, and 2-10). It is most frequently noted in association with hypersecretion and segmentation. In these cases the secretions probably obscure the mucosal markings. In a few cases, no mucosal markings are seen, even when there is no dilatation and no hypersecretion. The bowel wall appears flaccid. The cause of the moulage sign in these cases is not clear.

Intussusception

Intussusception is not an uncommon finding in patients with sprue, and, when present, it is a useful roentgen manifestation which helps to support the diagnosis of the sprue pattern. The intussusceptions are characteristically non-obstructive with a typical coiled-spring appearance and they usually extend over a short distance (Figs. 2-4, 2-16 to 2-19). They are transient and therefore can easily be missed during the course of a single examination. Only rarely have they been associated with abdominal pain or other clinical manifestations. The cause of the intussusceptions is not known[12] but is probably related to the dilated, flaccid bowel and the secretions.

Transit time

Transit time refers to the interval during which the barium traverses the small intestine and enters the cecum. The average time in adults has been found to be approximately three hours. However, there is a wide range of normal variation. In most of the patients with sprue, transit time varies from three to five hours. In a few it is less, diminishing to as little as 30 minutes. In occasional patients, it is as long as six and seven hours. Rarely is there marked

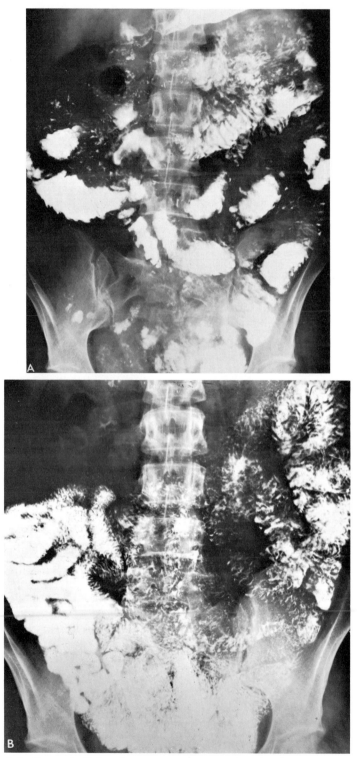

Figure 2-8 Sprue. A, Delayed segmentation is noted in the distal jejunum and proximal ileum. *B*, The same patient after treatment with a gluten-free diet. There remain minimal alterations in the small bowel.

(Illustration continued on opposite page.)

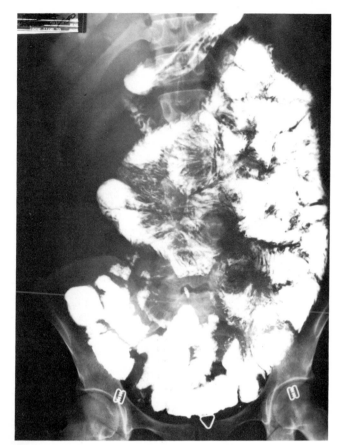

Figure 2-8 C *Nontropical sprue.* The typical roentgen alterations of dilatation, fragmentation, segmentation, and increased secretions are identified.

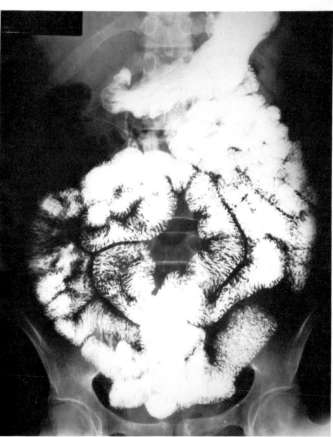

Figure 2-8 D Same patient as Figure 2-8 C, after two months of treatment with a gluten-free diet. There has been a marked improvement. Only minimal dilatation is seen.

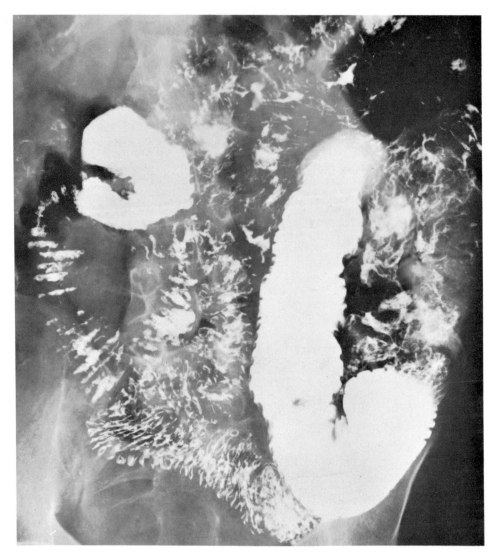

Figure 2-9   Sprue. There is segmentation, fragmentation, and increased fluid.

prolongation of transit time. This may be accounted for by the fact that we use larger quantities of barium (20 fluid ounces) than are often employed, and thereby tend to overcome the effect of puddling of barium in a single dilated segment.

Differentiation from Lymphosarcoma

When lymphosarcoma of the small bowel occurs with malabsorption and steatorrhea, differentiation from sprue can be very difficult.[13] If there is enlargement of extra-abdominal lymph nodes, or if abdominal masses are palpable, a diagnosis of lymphosarcoma may be suspected and confirmed on biopsy. In the absence of such findings, differentiation from sprue rests largely on the shorter and more fulminant course of lymphosarcoma, on bowel complications, such as perforation and ulceration in lymphosarcoma, and on failure of the patient to respond to a gluten-free diet, folic acid, or antibiotics.

(*Text continued on page 30*.)

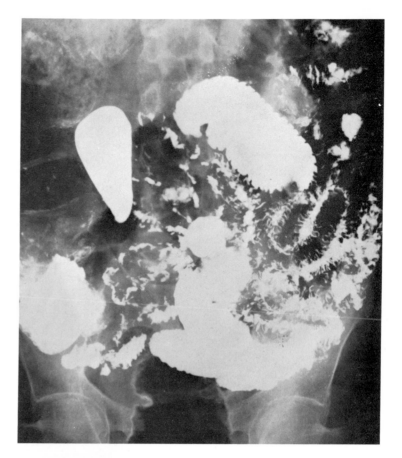

Figure 2-10 *Sprue*. There is segmentation and moulage phenomenon with stringlike strands of barium between these segmented loops. The contracted loops of bowel probably represent barium within a fluid-filled intestinal loop.

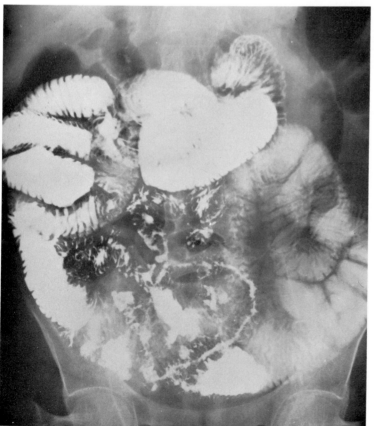

Figure 2-11 *Sprue*. Same patient as in Figure 2-10. A special barium was employed and has produced less segmentation and a continuous dilated column of barium. The administration of this type of barium mixture permits better visualization of the intestinal wall, but the segmentation characteristic of sprue may not be seen.

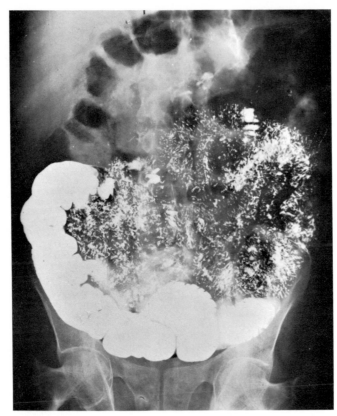

Figure 2-12　Sprue. There is marked fragmentation associated with slight dilatation and segmentation.

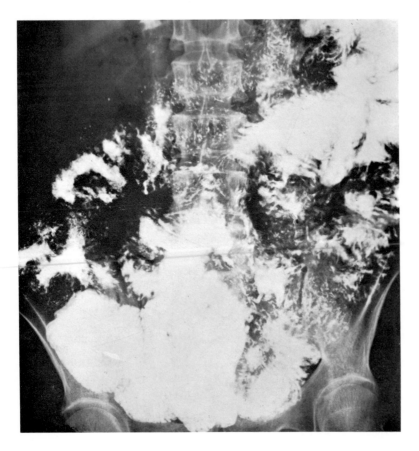

Figure 2-13　Sprue. There is marked fragmentation and segmentation, producing a disorganized appearance of the entire small bowel. The folds appear to be thickened, probably because secretions are abundant.

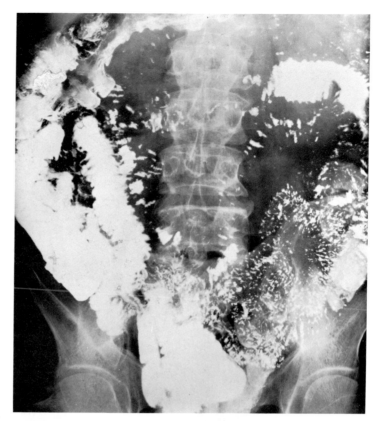

Figure 2-14 *Sprue.* Fragmentation and segmentation.

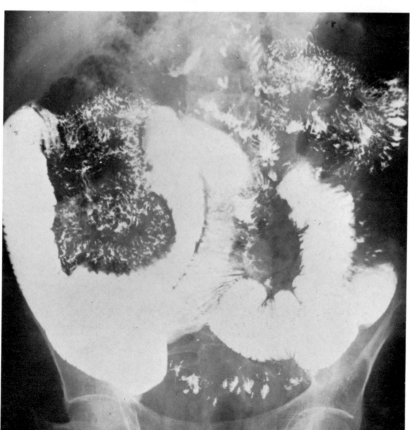

Figure 2-15 *Sprue.* Fragmentation is seen in the evacuated loops of jejunum. Evacuation films are helpful not only in sprue but in many other conditions. They may demonstrate pathology not otherwise identified.

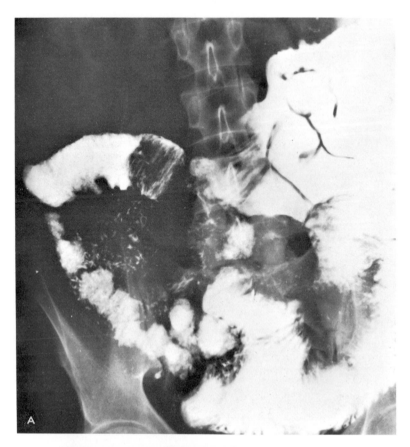

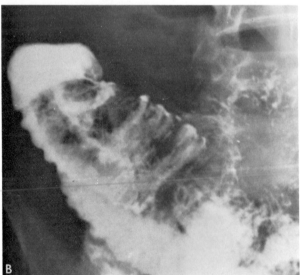

Figure 2-16 *Sprue. A,* There is slight dilatation and increased fluid. An area of nonobstructive intussusception is noted in the midportion of the abdomen on the right side. *B,* Spot film of the area of intussusception.

(*Illustration continued on opposite page.*)

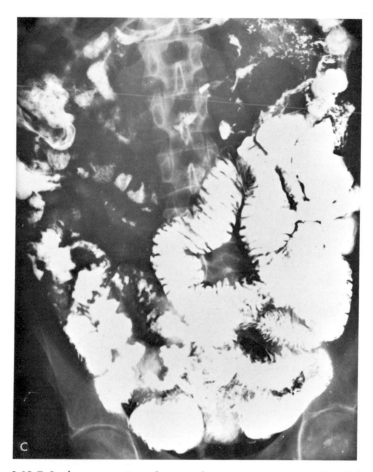

Figure 2-16 C, In the same patient, the area of intussusception is not identified. The characteristic dilatation of the mid- and distal jejunum associated with thinning of the folds is noted.

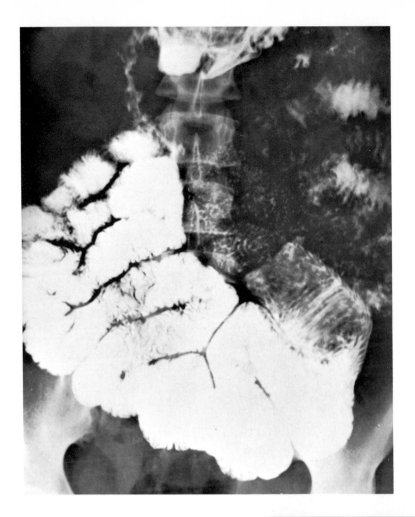

Figure 2-17 *Sprue*. An area of nonobstructive intussusception is seen in the left lower quadrant.

Figure 2-18 *Sprue*. An area of nonobstructive intussusception is identified in the right lower quadrant.

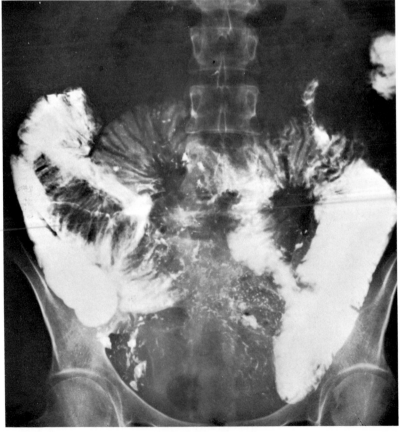

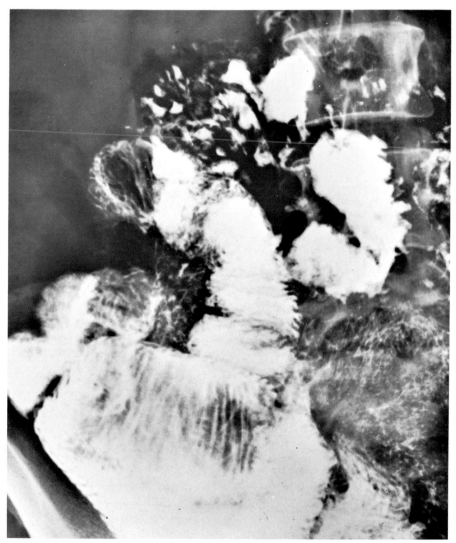

Figure 2-19 *Sprue.* Intussusception associated with the sprue pattern is noted in the right lower quadrant.

The distinction between the two diseases is further confused by reported cases of the development of lymphosarcoma in patients with sprue.[14] Carcinoma elsewhere also appears to occur with increased frequency in sprue patients. It is more likely that in these cases lymphosarcoma develops as a complication of longstanding sprue than that it has been responsible for the entire course of the disease. The complication of lymphosarcoma should be considered when a patient with sprue develops fever, bowel perforation, or hemorrhage, or shows exacerbation of sprue symptoms despite maintenance treatment.

Just as clinical and laboratory findings of malabsorption can occur in lymphosarcoma of the small bowel and mesentery, roentgen alterations simulating sprue may also be found. In some cases of lymphosarcoma dilatation of small intestinal loops, hypersecretion, and segmentation of the barium column are seen. Often the dilatation is less extensive than it would be in sprue alone, and the intestinal folds appear to be coarsened, thickened, and sometimes nodular (Figs. 2-20, 2-21, and 18-19). At times there may be obvious evidence of lymphosarcoma with extraluminal masses, thickening of the bowel wall, and displacement and invasion of the small bowel loops, superimposed upon the sprue pattern.

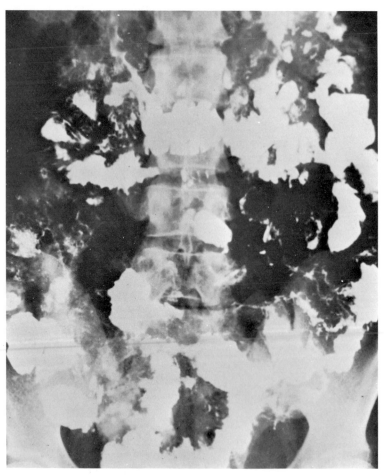

Figure 2-20   Lymphosarcoma. In this patient the clinical picture of sprue was simulated. At autopsy there was diffuse lymphosarcoma of the mesentery and retroperitoneum. The roentgen manifestations of segmentation, hypersecretion, and flocculation of the barium column mimic the sprue pattern. The lack of significant dilatation may be a clue to the correct diagnosis.

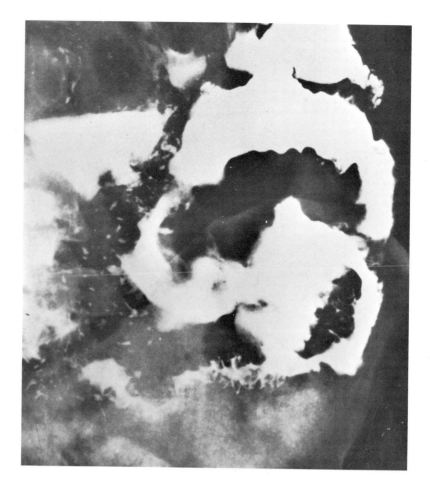

Figure 2-21 *Lymphosarcoma mimicking the sprue pattern.* There is segmentation, fragmentation, increased fluid, and irregularity of contour. The separation of the loops of bowel is due to infiltration of the wall of lymphosarcoma.

Extensive involvement of the small bowel with lymphosarcoma may occur with little clinical or roentgen evidence of malabsorption.

Differentiation from Regional Enteritis

Rarely, multiple strictures confined to the jejunum in regional enteritis may be obscured by the intervening dilated segments of bowel. Because of the associated malabsorption, an erroneous diagnosis of sprue may be made in these cases. A lateral or oblique film is helpful to visualize better the stenotic segments (Figs. 13-46, 13-47).

References

1. Wilson, T. H.: Intestinal Absorption. Philadelphia, W. B. Saunders Co., 1962.
2. Gardner, J. D., Brown, M. S., and Laster, L.: The columnar epithelial cell of the small intestine: digestion and transport. New Eng. J. Med., 283:1196-1202, 1970.
3. Pearse, A. G. E., and Riecken, E. O.: Histology and cytochemistry of the cells of the small intestine, in relation to absorption. *Brit. Med. Bull.*, 23:217-222, 1967.
4. Stewart, J. S.: Clinical and morphologic response to gluten withdrawal. *In* Coeliac Disease. Clinics in Gastroenterology 3:109-126, 1974.
5. Sheehy, T. W., Baggs, B., Perez-Santiago, E., and Floch, M. H.: Prognosis of tropical sprue. A

study of the effect of folic acid on the intestinal aspect of acute and chronic sprue. *Ann. Intern. Med.*, 57:892-908, 1962.

6. Rickles, F. R., et al.: Long-term follow-up of antibiotic-treated tropical sprue. *Ann. Intern. Med.*, 76:203-210, 1972.

7a. Bayless, T. M., Kapelowitz, R. F., Shelley, W. M., et al.: Intestinal ulceration—a complication of celiac disease. New Eng. J. Med., 276:996-1002, 1967.

7b. Blau, J. S., Stolzenberg, J., and Toffler, R. B.: Small bowel ulcerations—an unusual complication of celiac disease. *J. Canad. Assoc. Radiol.*, 25:77-78, 1974.

8. Marshak, R. H., Wolf, B. S., and Adlersberg, D.: Roentgen studies of the small intestine in sprue. *Amer. J. Roentgen.*, 72:380-400, 1954.

9. Burrows, F. G. O., and Toye, D. K. M.: Barium studies. *In* Coeliac Disease. Clinics in Gastroenterology. 3:91-107, 1974.

10. Frazer, A. C., French, J. M., and Thompson, M. D.: Radiographic studies showing the induction of a segmentation pattern in the small intestine in normal human subjects. *Brit. J. Radiol.*, 22:123-136, 1949.

11. Ardran, G. M., French, J. M., and Mucklow, M. B.: Relationship of the nature of the opaque medium to the small intestine radiographic pattern. *Brit. J. Radiol.*, 23:697-702, 1950.

12. Ruoff, M., Lindner, A. E., and Marshak, R. H.: Intussusception in sprue. *Amer. J. Roentgen.*, 104:525-528, 1968.

13. Sleisenger, M. D., Almy, T. P., and Barr, D. P.: The sprue syndrome secondary to lymphoma of the small bowel. *Amer. J. Med.*, 15:666-674, 1953.

14. Barry, R. E., and Read, A. E.: Celiac disease and malignancy. *Quart. J. Med.*, NS, 42:665-673, 1973.

3

Malabsorption Syndrome: Miscellaneous Causes

Although sprue provides an excellent illustration of malabsorption syndrome, a variety of other illnesses and conditions may also be associated with this entity. Table 2-1 (page 11) classifies some of these causes. Many are discussed in detail in separate chapters or sections of this volume: Whipple's disease, scleroderma, amyloidosis, intestinal lymphangiectasia, Zollinger-Ellison syndrome, parasitic diseases, intestinal ischemia, vasculitis, regional enteritis, radiation enteritis, carcinoid syndrome, lymphosarcoma, abetalipoproteinemia, hypogammaglobulinemia, systemic mastocytosis, and eosinophilic gastroenteritis.

The purpose of this chapter is to review several entities which may be associated with malabsorption syndrome but are not discussed elsewhere in this book.

DIVERTICULA, BLIND LOOPS, AND STRICTURES

Patients with spontaneously occurring or surgically created small bowel diverticula, blind loops, or strictures may develop malabsorption syndrome. The significant feature common to these anatomic abnormalities is local hypomotility, stasis, and overgrowth of intestinal bacteria, especially anerobic organisms. A macrocytic anemia may develop because the bacteria compete with mucosal absorbing cells for supplies of intraluminal vitamin B. Both the macrocytic anemia and the malabsorption syndrome can be corrected by the administration of systemic antibiotics or by surgical revision of the anatomic anomaly. The mechanism by which bacterial overgrowth induces malabsorption is not yet entirely clear. Recent studies have implicated abnormalities in bile salt metabolism as a cause of steatorrhea. Intestinal bacteria have been found to deconjugate bile salts, and the steatorrhea of bacterial overgrowth has been attributed to the toxic effects of unconjugated bile salts on the intestinal mucosa[1] or to a decreased amount of conjugated bile salts available for digestion of fat within the lumen of the bowel.[2]

   The roentgen diagnosis of diverticulosis depends upon the visualization of the multiple sacs, which may appear as oval, circular or flask-shaped projections from the bowel lumen (Fig. 3-1). They can be tiny or very large and are usually smooth in outline with no distinct mucosal folds. Because of the mobility of the intestinal loops they may change in position rapidly. When they are large and numerous the diverticula may simulate the segmentation seen in sprue. An emptying film or lateral projection is useful in differentiating these two entities. The pseudosacculations of scleroderma may produce large sacs which may simulate diverticulosis (Fig. 3-2). The wide, gaping openings and marked hypomotility are distinguishing features of scleroderma. Enteroliths are occasionally noted in small bowel diverticula (Fig. 16-35, page 330).

   Blind loops are frequently associated with a side-to-side intestinal anastomosis (Fig. 3-3), but the same effect may be produced when there are two segments of constriction with an intervening area of dilatation, as is seen in the stenotic phase of regional enteritis (Figs. 3-4 and 3-5). Bleeding occurs more frequently from an erosion in a blind loop than from diverticula (Fig. 3-6), but such erosions are difficult to recognize on roentgen study.

(Text continued on page 38.)

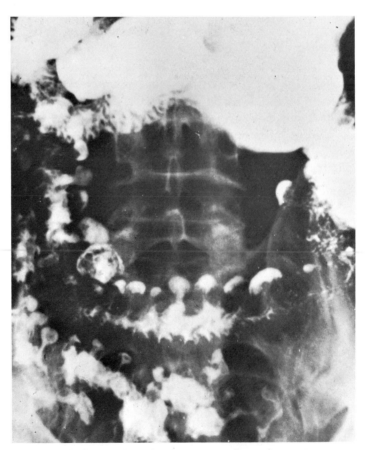

Figure 3-1   Multiple diverticula of the small bowel. The necks are characteristically narrow, and the outpouchings vary in size.

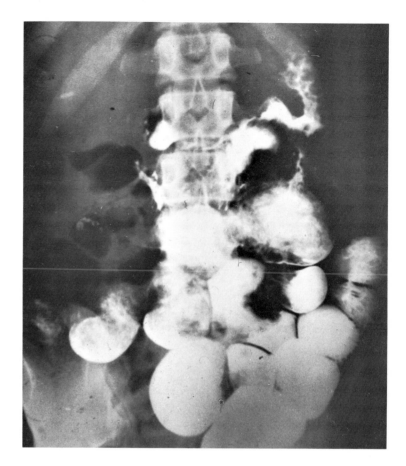

Figure 3-2 Scleroderma. There are multiple large sacs with retained secretions throughout most of the small bowel. The necks are large. The findings are the result of pseudosacculation of scleroderma. Hypomotility was marked.

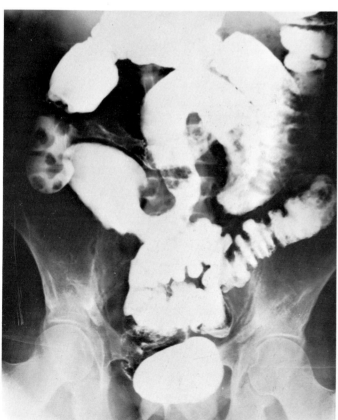

Figure 3-3 Status post-ileosigmoidostomy with side-to-side anastomosis. The procedure was performed for granulomatous disease. A large blind loop is identified on the right side of the abdomen.

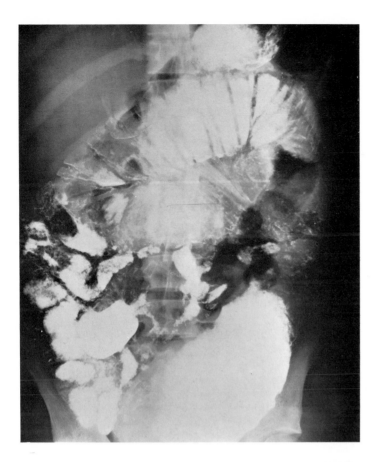

Figure 3-4   Regional enteritis with multiple areas of constriction and dilatation. A markedly dilated segment simulating a blind loop is seen in the pelvis.

Figure 3-5   Status post-resection of a segment of mid-small bowel for regional enteritis, with side-to-side anastomosis. There is a large blind loop, containing increased secretions, on each side of the stoma.

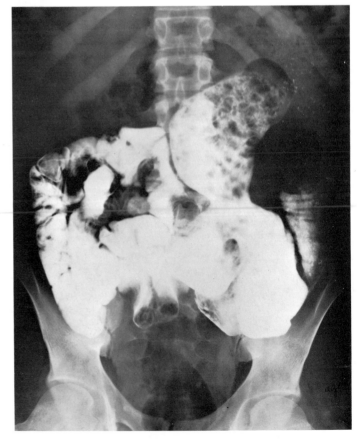

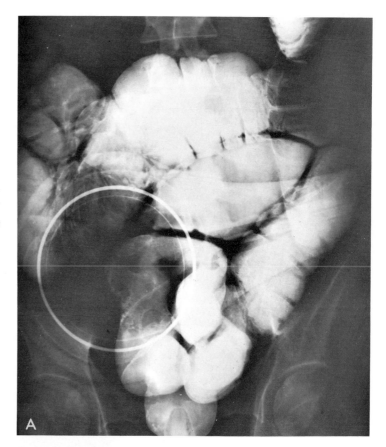

Figure 3-6 *A*, Status post-ileotransverse colostomy for regional enteritis. There is a large blind loop beneath the transverse colon. This patient had several massive hemorrhages which ceased after resection of the loop.

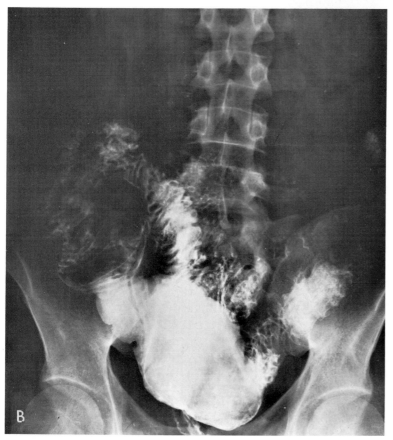

B, Evacuation film of barium enema in the same patient. The blind loop, filled with barium, has changed position and is seen in the pelvis.

SURGICAL PROCEDURES ON THE GASTROINTESTINAL
TRACT

Roentgen examination may contribute to a diagnosis of malabsorption syndrome by documenting or characterizing a postsurgical construction of the gastrointestinal tract. *Partial resection of the small bowel* reduces, and *inadvertent gastroileostomy* (Fig. 3-7) bypasses, the principal areas for absorption in the duodenum and jejunum. Resections involving the terminal ileum interrupt the enterohepatic circulation of bile salts by removing their principal site of absorption in the bowel. The liver is unable to compensate for the loss of bile salts by increased synthesis, and decreased amounts of bile salts become available to the digesting segments of the intestine, resulting in malabsorption.[3, 4]

Following both total and subtotal *gastrectomy,* there is a decrease in the absorption of protein and fat. One of the major complications of gastric resection is failure to gain or maintain weight. Malabsorption after gastrectomy may

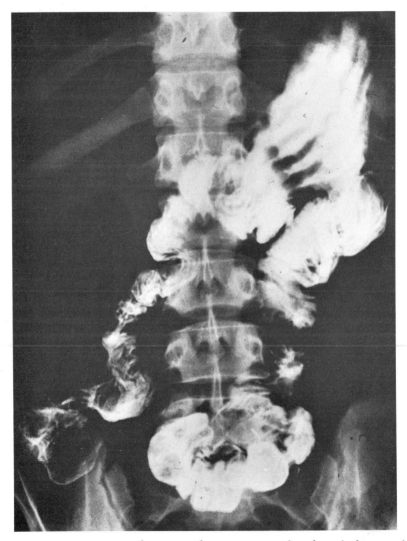

Figure 3-7 Status post-gastroileostomy. This patient manifested marked steatorrhea and malabsorption.

be due to loss of the reservoir function of the stomach, rapid small bowel motility and transit, inadequate stimulation of bile and pancreatic secretions with consequent poor mixing of digestive enzymes and food within the gut, or increases in small bowel bacterial content.

The roentgen appearance of the small bowel in patients with partial gastric resection is in most cases normal. Slight dilatation of the jejunum is frequently identified because of over-filling of these loops, especially when large quantities of barium are employed. The interpretation of minimal degrees of segmentation, hypersecretion, and fragmentation is difficult, especially in patients with diarrhea. In those cases in which the changes are marked, the patients are usually found to have an associated sprue.

PANCREATIC INSUFFICIENCY

Malabsorption may occur in patients with pancreatic disease involving obstruction to the duct system or destruction of acinar tissue. Thus malabsorption may be a manifestation of chronic pancreatitis, carcinoma of the pancreas, or fibrocystic disease. The malabsorption is actually maldigestion, the principal defect being absence of pancreatic bicarbonate and lipase and other enzymes from the intestine. The stool contains neutral fat, and absorption of radioactive oleic acid is normal. Tests of carbohydrate absorption are usually normal. Treatment of pancreatic steatorrhea consists of oral administration of large amounts of commercial pancreatic extracts with meals.

The roentgen findings in the small bowel in pancreatic insufficiency are usually normal. In an occasional patient with severe chronic pancreatitis, segmentation and increased secretions may be seen. Dilatation, such as is identified in sprue, is absent. The presence of a normal small bowel series in a patient with severe steatorrhea suggests that the underlying disease may be pancreatic insufficiency.

DISEASES OF THE LIVER AND BILIARY TRACT

Diseases of the liver and biliary passages which exclude bile from the small bowel may be associated with malabsorption. Absence of bile salts from the intestine results in impaired digestion and absorption of fat. Steatorrhea is therefore a feature of primary and secondary biliary cirrhosis. Small bowel examination is usually normal, although some of the roentgen features associated with sprue may be found in an occasional case. Malabsorption is corrected if liver function improves or biliary obstruction can be relieved.

DIABETES

Severe diarrhea occasionally occurs in patients with diabetes mellitus who have normal exocrine pancreatic function. The diarrhea has been attributed to visceral neuropathy. In some of the patients with diarrhea, steatorrhea has also been described. Such malabsorption may in part reflect a rapid transit time, but small bowel biopsy studies have suggested that the malabsorption

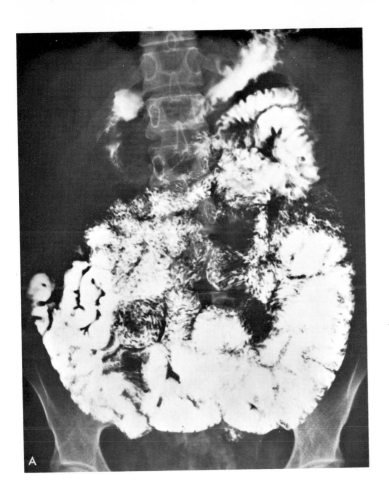

Figure 3-8 *A*, Intestinal lactase deficiency. Small bowel study shows slight thickening of jejunal folds and a slight increase in secretions. Transit time to the cecum was 90 minutes.

B, Intestinal lactase deficiency. In the same patient, following administration of 25 gm. of lactose mixed with barium, there is a considerable increase in secretions and a marked increase in peristaltic activity. Barium appears to race through the small bowel into the colon.

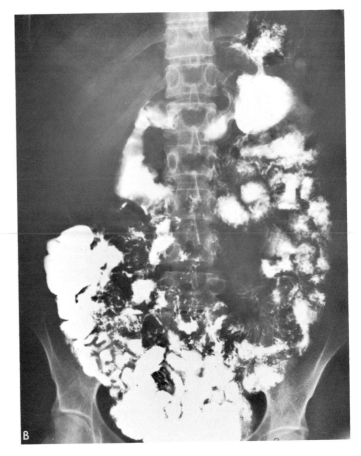

40

may be due to a concomitant sprue.[5] Alternatively diabetes may induce secondary sprue-like changes in the small bowel mucosa, but thus far direct evidence for this is lacking. In some cases diabetic patients with diarrhea and malabsorption have displayed a sprue pattern on small bowel roentgen examination. Usually, except for slight dilatation, the appearance of the small bowel in patients with diabetes is normal.

INTESTINAL LACTASE DEFICIENCY

Enzymes which hydrolyze dietary disaccharides are located in the brush border of the intestinal epithelial cells. Deficiency of these enzymes, either as an isolated finding or secondary to another small bowel disease, may lead to diarrhea and malabsorption. Clinically the most common disaccharidase deficiency encountered is that of lactase, and patients experience diarrhea and abdominal cramps after ingestion of milk but are without symptoms on a milk-free diet.[6]

Patients with isolated lactase deficiency usually abstain from milk, and the small bowel examination is normal. When lactose is added to the barium mixture, however, a marked increase in transit occurs with an increase in the intraluminal fluid[7] (Fig. 3-8A and B).

DERMATITIS HERPETIFORMIS

Several diffuse skin diseases, including exfoliative erythroderma, psoriasis, and especially dermatitis herpetiformis, have been reported to be associated with malabsorption syndrome.[8] On small bowel biopsy a lesion apparently identical to sprue has been found,[9] and the enteropathy usually responds to a gluten-free diet,[10] but the relationship between the skin and small bowel lesion remains unclear. We have not had the opportunity to study the small bowel roentgen pattern in these patients.

References

1. Donaldson, R. M., Jr.: Studies on the pathogenesis of steatorrhea in the blind loop syndrome. *J. Clin. Invest.*, 44:1815-1825, 1965.
2. Kim, V. S., Spritz, N., Blum, M., Terz, J., and Sherlock, P.: The role of altered bile acid metabolism in the steatorrhea of experimental blind loop. *J. Clin. Invest.*, 45:956-962, 1966.
3. Hofmann, A. F.: The syndrome of ileal disease and the broken enterohepatic circulation: cholerheic enteropathy. *Gastroenterology*, 52:752-757, 1967.
4. Hofmann, A. F., and Poley, J. R.: Role of bile acid malabsorption in pathogenesis of diarrhea and steatorrhea in patients with ileal resection. *Gastroenterology*, 62:918-934, 1972.
5. Wruble, L. D., and Kalser, M. H.: Diabetic steatorrhea: a distinct entity. *Am. J. Med.*, 37:118-129, 1964.
6. Bayless, T. M., Rothfeld, B., Massa, C., et al.: Lactose and milk intolerance: Clinical implications. *New Eng. J. Med.*, 292:1156-1159, 1975.
7. Laws, J. W., and Neale, G.: Radiological diagnosis of disaccharidase deficiency. *Lancet*, 2:139-143, 1966.
8. Shuster, S., and Marks, J.: Dermatogenic enteropathy. A new cause for steatorrhea. *Lancet*, 1:1367-1368, 1965.
9. Shuster, S., Watson, A. J., and Marks, J.: Celiac syndrome in dermatitis herpetiformis. *Lancet*, 1:1101-1106, 1968.
10. Soter, N. A.: Dermatitis herpetiformis. *New Eng. J. Med.*, 288:1020-1021, 1973.

4

Whipple's Disease

In 1907 G. H. Whipple reported the first case of the disease which now bears his name. He described a patient with the clinical picture of weight loss, steatorrhea, abdominal signs, and arthritis. At autopsy he found deposits of fat and fatty acids in the intestinal wall and the mesenteric lymph nodes, and in those areas he found large pale macrophages which gave a negative reaction to fat stains. The next case of the disease was not reported until 1923, and it was not until 1949 that it was discovered that the material within the macrophages of the lamina propria of the small bowel and lymph nodes reacts positively to PAS stain, and that this material is a glycoprotein. In recent years more cases of Whipple's disease have been reported, especially with the advent of small bowel biopsy techniques, and although the etiology of the disease remains obscure, much has been learned about the pathology and treatment.

Characteristically, Whipple's disease causes a syndrome of intermittent arthralgia or arthritis, abdominal pain, diarrhea, steatorrhea, and weight loss. Physical findings include evidence of dehydration and weight loss, lymphadenopathy, abdominal distention and diffuse tenderness, and skin pigmentation. Biochemical and hematologic findings resemble those of sprue. Pathologic examination shows polyserositis and generalized lymphadenopathy. The lumen of the small bowel is dilated, and the bowel wall and mesentery are thickened. There is extensive lymphatic distention and intestinal edema.

The hallmark of Whipple's disease is the presence in the lamina propria and in the lymph nodes of macrophages which are Sudan-negative and PAS-positive. The diagnosis of Whipple's disease can be established by demonstrating this specific lesion in material obtained from small bowel biopsy, from abdominal lymph nodes during laparotomy, or from peripheral nodes.

The nature and significance of the PAS-positive material are of great interest. Light and electron microscopic studies in Whipple's disease have been reported, utilizing small bowel biopsy specimens obtained during active disease and during remission.[1] When the disease is active, biopsy specimens show abundant PAS-positive and gram-positive granules within the macrophages and extracellularly in the lamina propria. During treatment there is a decrease in both extracellular and intracellular granules. Electron microscopy and histochemistry show that the PAS-positive and gram-positive rods and granules seen under the light microscope are bacteria and bacterial substances.

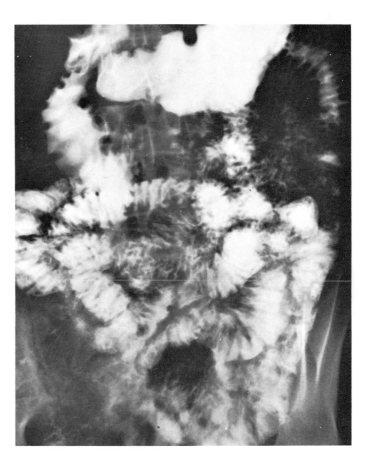

Figure 4-1 *Whipple's disease.* Thickening of the folds of the duodenum and jejunum is noted.

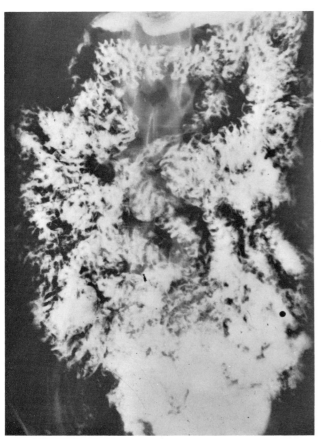

Figure 4-2 *Whipple's disease.* The folds are wild, redundant, thickened, and slightly nodular. Minimal dilatation, fragmentation, and segmentation are identified. The findings are more pronounced in the jejunum than the ileum.

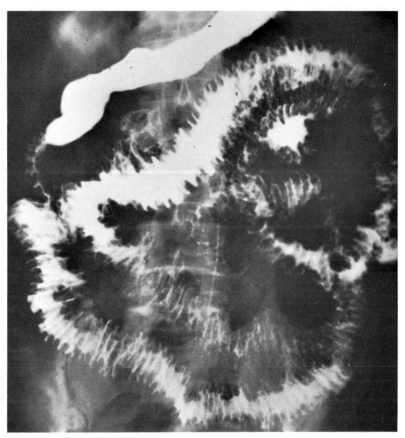

Figure 4-3 *Whipple's disease.* There is thickening of the folds, associated with multiple nodules along the contour of the bowel. Differentiation from lymphosarcoma is difficult in this case. (Courtesy of Dr. G. J. Triano, Harrisburg, Pennsylvania.)

The significance of the bacteria found in the mucosa of patients with Whipple's disease is difficult to evaluate. They tend to disappear or be modified during antibiotic treatment. These organisms may be the cause of the disease, or they may be secondary invaders through a damaged epithelium. Whether their role is primary or secondary, the organisms disappear very slowly during antibiotic therapy, suggesting that prolonged treatment may be required to effect remission or cure.

Adrenocorticotropic hormone and corticosteroids have been used in the treatment of Whipple's disease, and although some prolonged remissions have been reported, results have been variable and often disappointing. The treatment of choice appears to be prolonged administration of antibiotics.[2, 3] The current recommendation is an initial two week course of penicillin and streptomycin, followed by a course of broad spectrum antibiotics, extending for as long as a year. Patients have now been reported with complete clinical, biochemical, radiologic, and histologic recovery.

Roentgen Features

Although a large series of cases of Whipple's disease is difficult to accumulate, enough individual cases have appeared in the literature that a roentgen

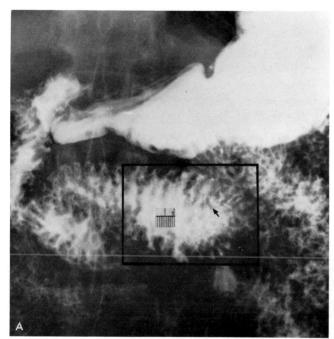

Figure 4-4A *Whipple's disease.* Thickened folds with small punctate filling defects.

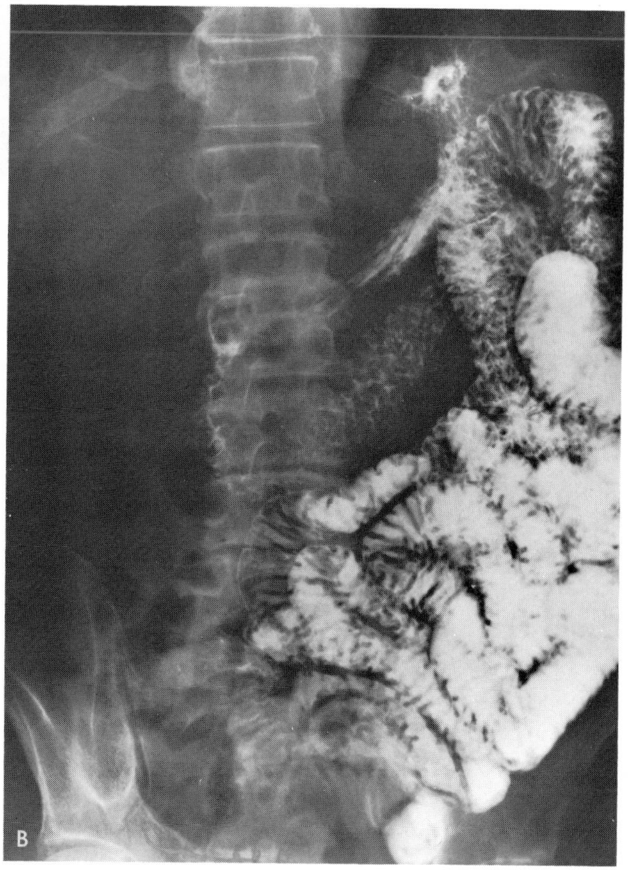

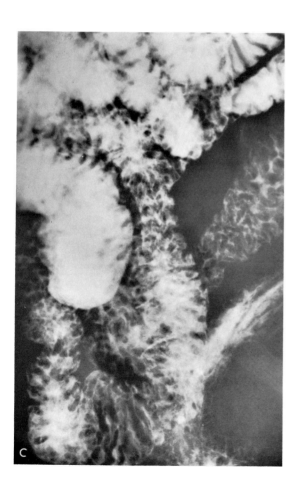

Figure 4-4B *Whipple's disease.* Another case demonstrating thickened folds and small filling defects.

Figure 4-4C Same case as Figure 4B—Magnified view again demonstrating thickened folds and small filling defects.

pattern has emerged.[4] The most prominent radiologic finding in Whipple's disease is the alteration in the appearance of the fold pattern. (Figs. 4-1 and 4-2). The valvulae conniventes are thickened and sometimes appear slightly nodular (Fig. 4-3). The folds may appear to be wild, redundant, and lacking a homogeneous configuration (Fig. 4-2). The intestinal villi may become swollen, bulbous structures which are visible to the naked eye and are sometimes apparent on careful inspection of the films (Figs. 4-4A and 4-5). The thickening of the folds varies with the severity of the disease. Occasionally the thickening is minimal and difficult to recognize (Figs. 4-6 to 4-10). The lumen of the bowel may be normal or slightly dilated. A moderate amount of secretion, segmenta-

(*Text continued on page 50.*)

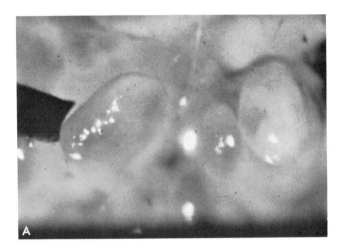

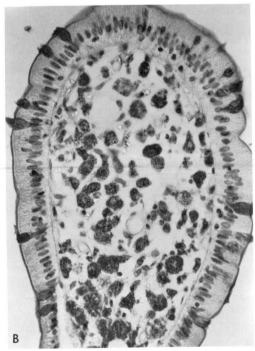

Figure 4-5 A, Bulbous villi are seen in the gross peroral biopsy specimen.
B. Thickened villi infiltrated with PAS-positive macrophages. It is possible that the small lucent defects described above are due to these bulbous villi.

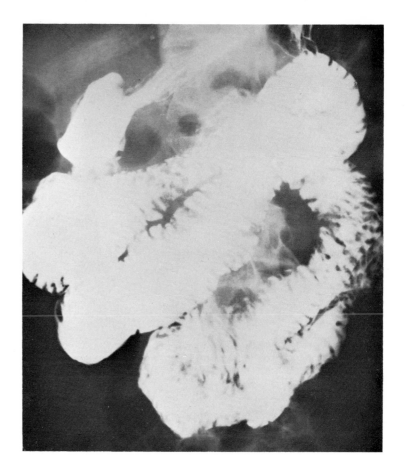

Figure 4-6 *Whipple's disease.* There is slight thickening of the folds of the proximal jejunum.

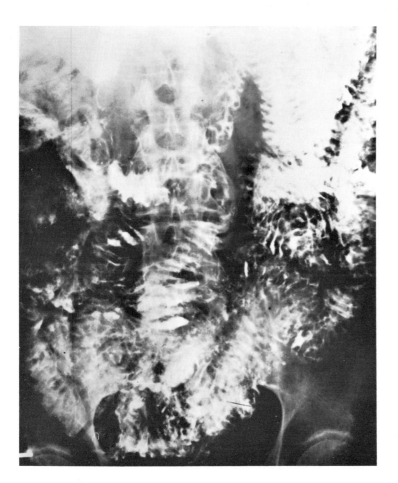

Figure 4-7 *Whipple's disease.* Same case as in Figure 4-6, two years later, when the diagnosis was established. There is more thickening of the folds, fragmentation, and evidence of increased secretions.

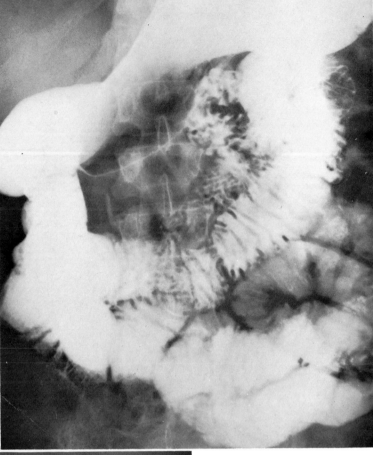

Figure 4-8 The bowel is minimally dilated, and the thickening of the folds is slight. The clinical features were characteristic and the diagnosis was confirmed by biopsy.

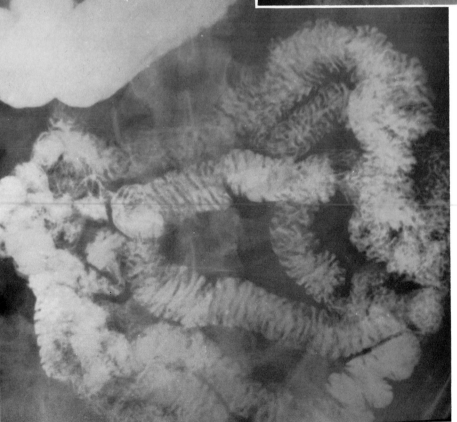

Figure 4-9 Same case as Figure 4-8. Normal small bowel six months after antibiotic therapy resulted in remission of symptoms.

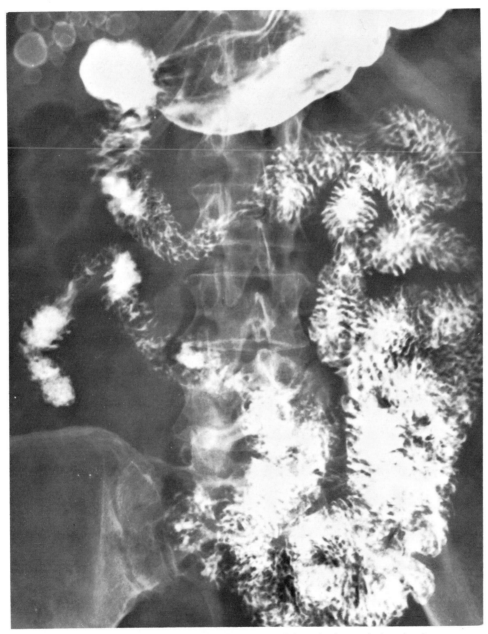

Figure 4-10 *Whipple's disease.* The thickening of the valvulae is slight. The diagnosis was made after exploratory laparotomy. This case is also unusual because the patient is a female.

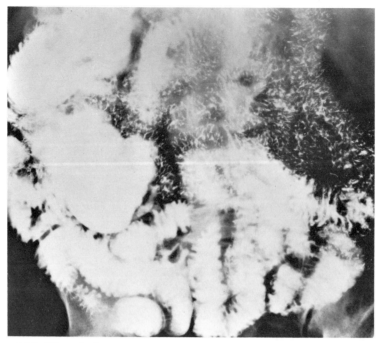

Figure 4-11 The valvulae conniventes are thickened. Several loops of the bowel are dilated. Moderate fragmentation is noted.

tion, and fragmentation may be identified (Figs. 4-11 and 4-12). Rigidity, inflammatory change, or ulceration, such as are noted in regional enteritis, are not seen. Transit time is within normal limits.

The most difficult differential diagnosis is in relation to sprue. However,

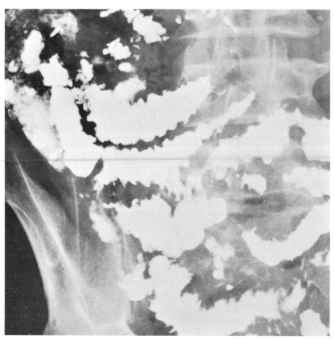

Figure 4-12 Whipple's disease. There is segmentation, fragmentation, increased fluid and thickening of the folds. There is no significant dilatation. The former findings may be a function of the degree of malabsorption.

the thickening of the folds and the less marked dilatation associated with only minimal evidence of segmentation and fragmentation suggest Whipple's disease rather than sprue. Intestinal lymphangiectasia may also simulate the roentgen findings in Whipple's disease, except for the distribution of the thickened folds. In Whipple's disease this finding is more prominent in the jejunum, whereas in intestinal lymphangiectasia it is usually diffuse.

Other lesions which on occasion may mimic Whipple's disease include those of amyloidosis, systemic mastocytosis, hypogammaglobulinemia, and histoplasmosis. In amyloidosis the thickening of the folds tends to be uniform throughout the small bowel, and secretions are minimal or absent. Fortunately, the other conditions are uncommon and the clinical findings helpful.

References

1. Trier, J. S., Phelps, P. C., Eidelman, S., and Rubin, C. E.: Whipple's disease: light and electron microscope correlation of jejunal mucosal histology with antibiotic treatment and clinical status. *Gastroenterology,* 48:684-707, 1965.
2. Davis, T. D., McBee, J. M., Borland, J. L., Jr., Kurtz, S. M., and Ruffin, J. M.: Effects of antibiotics and steroid therapy in Whipple's disease. *Gastroenterology,* 44:112-116. 1963.
3. Meizel, H., Ruffin, J. M., and Dobbins, W. O. III: Whipple's disease: a review of 19 patients from one hospital and a review of the literature since 1950, *Medicine,* 49:175-205, 1970.
4. Rice, R. P., Roufail, W. M., and Reeves, R. J.: The roentgen diagnosis of Whipple's disease (intestinal lipodystrophy). *Radiology,* 88:295-301, 1967.

5

Scleroderma (Progressive Systemic Sclerosis)

Scleroderma is a systemic disease which commonly involves the esophagus but may also involve the small bowel and be associated with malabsorption syndrome.[1] Although the small intestine can become affected at any time in the course of the disease, it is usually preceded by skin changes, Raynaud's phenomenon, or joint symptoms.

On pathologic examination[2] the intestine involved in scleroderma shows atrophy of the muscular layers and replacement by collagen tissue. Both mucosa and submucosa are atrophic. The villi are atrophic, and round cell infiltration of the submucosa has been reported. Mesenteric vascular arteritis has been noted. According to a recent report,[3] biopsy of the mucosa of the duodenum demonstrated considerable fibrosis of the submucosal tissue and fibrosis around Brunner's glands. The mucosa itself was normal. Up to the present time there have been no extensive studies of the mucosa by small bowel biopsy in scleroderma.

The cause of the malabsorption associated with scleroderma is speculative, but several possibilities exist.[4, 5] Replacement of the muscular layers with fibrous tissue may alter peristaltic activity. Arteritis may contribute to alterations in small bowel absorptive capacity. Increases in bacterial flora as a result of changes in motility may be a cause of malabsorption. Long-term administration of broad-spectrum antibiotics has been found to improve absorption from the small bowel involved with scleroderma.

The roentgen findings in the esophagus are atony, hypomotility or absent peristaltic activity, shortening, sliding hiatus hernia, regurgitation, esophagitis, and stricture. The inability of the esophagus to empty in the prone position is a characteristic roentgen finding. Unlike achalasia, the esophagogastric junction is patulous.

The roentgen findings in the remainder of the intestinal tract are similar to those described in the esophagus but occur less frequently. A marked delay in peristaltic activity associated with dilatation is the most conspicuous roentgen feature of scleroderma. The findings in the stomach and the duodenal bulb are usually minimal. The second portion of the duodenum demonstrates varying changes in its caliber, characterized by dilatation and delayed emptying (Figs. 5-1 and 5-2). This dilatation may be marked, suggesting an obstruction at the ligament of Treitz, as from metastasis, extension from carcinoma of the pancreas, regional enteritis, or adhesions. Since many patients are thin, it is possible that compression from the superior mesenteric artery may contribute to the dilatation of the duodenum seen in scleroderma. In one of our cases, the duodenum was so large that it extended into the pelvis. In the jejunum and ileum, the most striking alteration is hypomotility with varying degrees of dilatation. Segmentation, fragmentation, and increased secretions are usually not present. There is no roentgen evidence of an inflammatory process. The fold pattern is usually normal, and there is no disturbance of the architecture of the small bowel. On occasion the valvulae conniventes may appear closer together than normal, presumably secondary to intramural fibrosis (Figs. 5-3 and 5-4). When the hypomotility is marked, a small bowel obstruction may be simulated, and several patients have been operated upon to exclude this possibility. In several patients exploration with removal of the dilated loops has been done in an effort to relieve the marked stasis that was present.[6] Sacculation[7] with the formation of pseudodiverticula may occur where hypomotility is prominent (Fig. 5-5). This finding in association with fecaliths is more frequently seen in the colon (Fig. 5-6).

Pneumatosis cystoides intestinalis has recently been described in small bowel scleroderma,[8] and we have seen one such case (Figs. 5-7 and 5-8). The cause of pneumatosis is not known but presumably is related to partial obstruc-

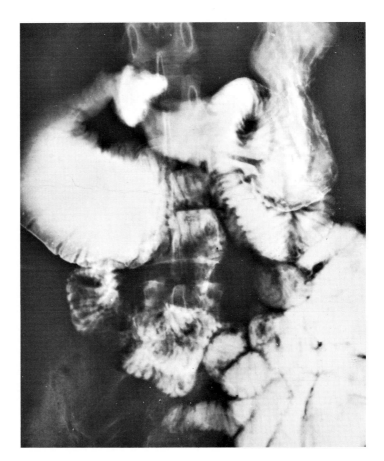

Figure 5-1 *Scleroderma.* There is marked dilatation of the duodenum unassociated with organic obstruction at the ligament of Treitz. Hypomotility of the barium through the small bowel was noted.

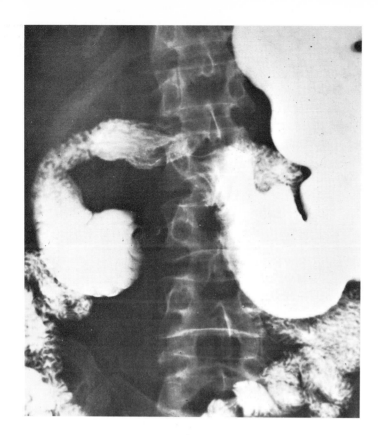

Figure 5-2 Organic obstruction near the ligament of Treitz due to metastatic carcinoma. The dilatation of the second portion of the duodenum in this case simulates the findings in Figure 5-1 and must be differentiated from scleroderma.

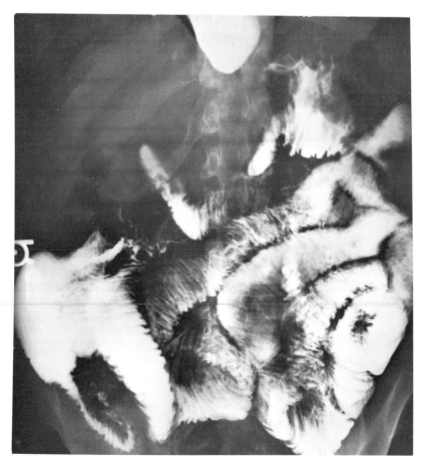

Figure 5-3 *Scleroderma.* A small amount of barium is still noted in a moderately dilated esophagus. The valvulae conniventes are closer together than normal, presumably due to intramural fibrosis. Hypomotility is present.

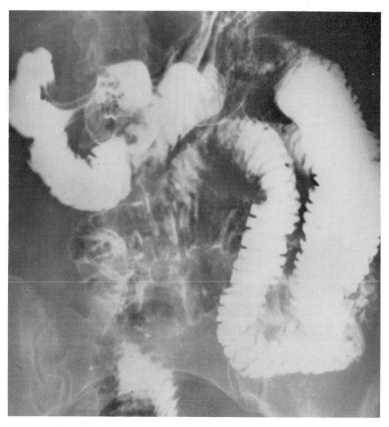

Figure 5-4 *Scleroderma.* This film was taken three hours after the start of a small bowel examination and revealed marked hypomotility. There is minimal dilatation with slight thinning of the valvulae conniventes.

tion and chronic dilatation of the small bowel or to interstitial pulmonary fibrosis and emphysema.

The differential diagnosis from sprue, as a rule, is not difficult because of the lack of increased secretions, segmentation, and fragmentation. Moreover, the dilatation of sprue is most marked in the mid-jejunum and is usually associated with normal motility, whereas in scleroderma the dilatation is more diffuse. The presence of sacculation should also suggest a diagnosis of scleroderma.

The colon exhibits changes similar to those in the small bowel. The degree of dilatation may be enormous and occasionally may simulate adult Hirschsprung's disease. Stercoral ulceration due to retained fecal material may be seen pathologically but is difficult to identify on the roentgen examination.

Dermatomyositis

Dermatomyositis, a systemic connective tissue disorder having many features in common with scleroderma, can also involve the gastrointestinal tract.[9] The clinical and pathologic features resemble those of scleroderma, although the complaint of dysphagia may be related more to involvement of the pharyngeal muscles than to pathologic changes in the esophagus.

(*Text continued on page 61.*)

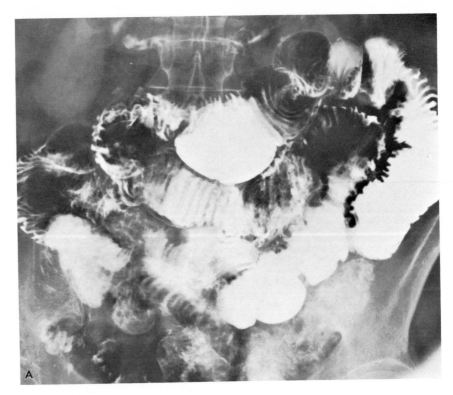

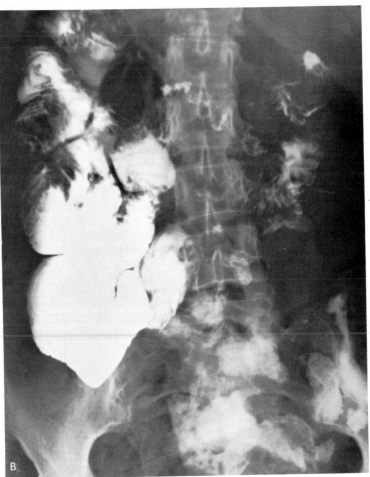

Figure 5-5 *Scleroderma. A,* There is marked hypomotility with pseudosacculation and minimal dilatation. Pleating of the valvulae conniventes is noted. *B,* Marked hypomotility with pseudosacculation.

56

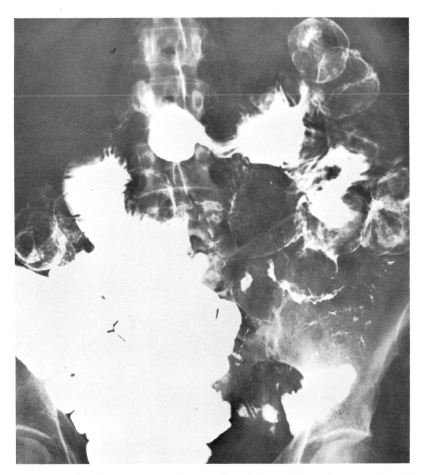

Figure 5-6 *Scleroderma.* There is hypomotility of the small bowel associated with fecaliths in the colon. Slight dilatation of the duodenum is present.

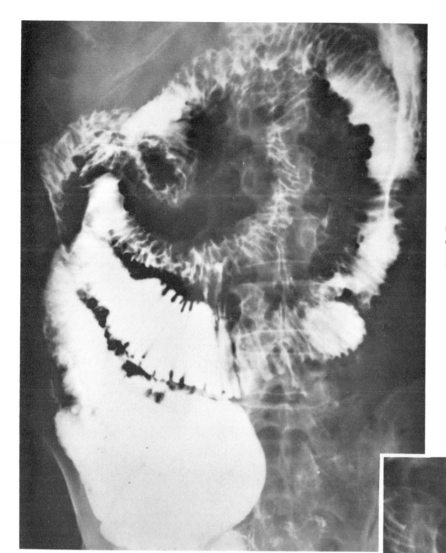

Figure 5-7 Scleroderma. Hypomotility was present, associated with thinning of the valvulae conniventes. An area of pneumatosis intestinalis is seen in the left upper quadrant.

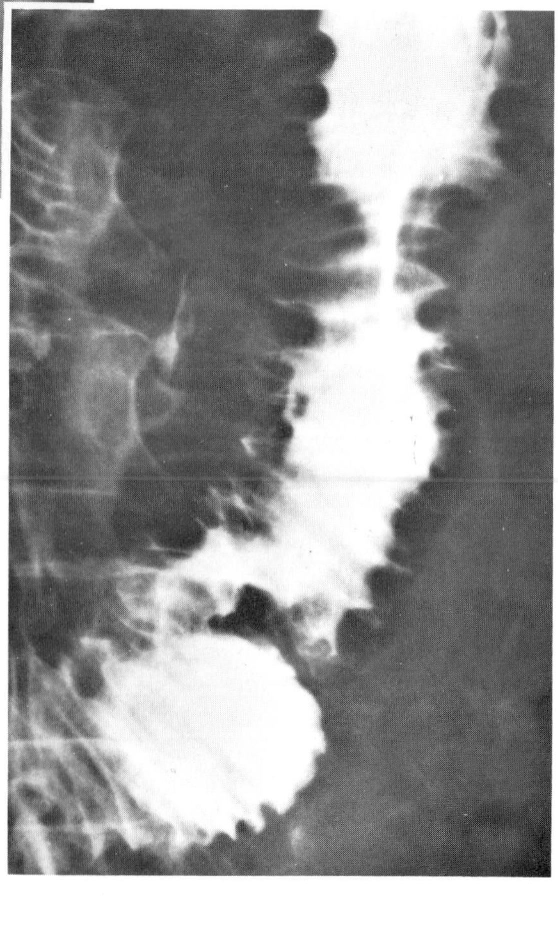

Figure 5-8 Scleroderma. In the same patient (Fig. 5-7) a spot film of the segment of jejunum reveals the pneumatosis intestinalis. (Courtesy of Dr. Alexander Margulis, University of California, San Francisco.)

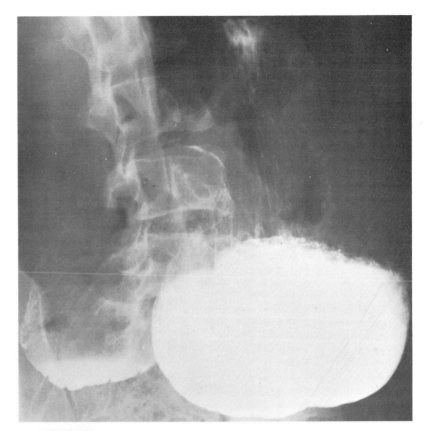

Figure 5-9 Dermatomyositis. There is a large atonic ptotic stomach with retained secretions. The duodenum contains a small amount of barium and appears markedly dilated.

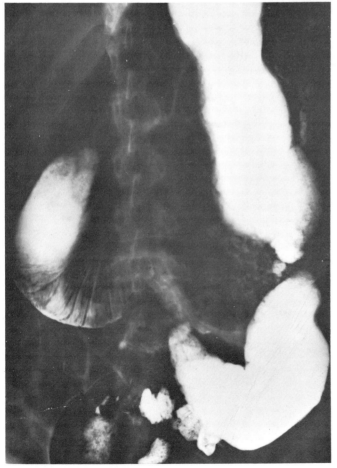

Figure 5-10 Dermatomyositis. Same case as in Figure 5-9. Six hours after ingestion of barium the stomach still contains the major portion of the barium meal. The second and third portions of the duodenum are dilated, and the mucosal folds appear stretched and somewhat effaced. There is clumping and segmentation of the barium distally and dilatation of the loops of proximal jejunum.

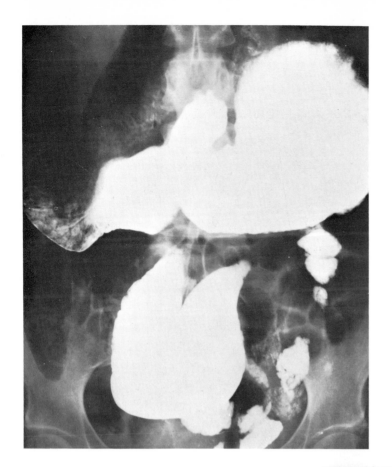

Figure 5-11 Dermatomyositis. Same case in Figs. 5-9 and 5-10. At the end of twenty-four hours there is 90 per cent retention of barium within the stomach. Dilatation of the duodenum and a dilated loop of proximal jejunum associated with segmentation is also noted.

Figure 5-12 Dermatomyositis. Same case as in Figs. 5-9 to 5-11. Barium enema study five days later shows a markedly redundant, slightly dilated colon. There is ptosis of the transverse colon. Residual barium is still seen in the stomach and duodenum.

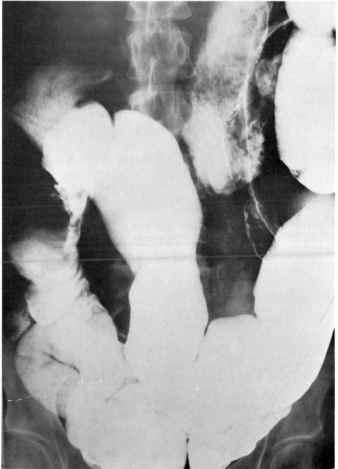

60

Involvement of the small bowel and colon may be associated with crampy abdominal pain, diarrhea, constipation, vomiting, and gastrointestinal bleeding.

Roentgen changes in the small bowel in dermatomyositis resemble those of scleroderma and may be striking. Dilatation is the characteristic feature, and the caliber of the bowel may suggest segmental ileus or small bowel obstruction. Hypomotility prolongs the transit time of a barium meal so that a bolus of barium entering an involved loop may remain for several days (Figs. 5-9 to 5-12).

The colon reveals varying degrees of dilatation and sacculation, and fecaliths may be present. Incomplete evacuation is a frequent finding on barium enema examination.

References

1. Poirier, T., and Rankin, G.: Gastrointestinal manifestations of progressive systemic sclerosis, based on a review of 364 cases. *Am. J. Gastroent.*, 58:30–44, 1972.
2. Hoskins, L. C., Norris, H. T., Gottlieb, L. S., and Zamcheck, N.: Functional and morphologic alterations of the gastrointestinal tract in progressive systemic sclerosis (scleroderma). *Amer. J. Med.*, 33:459-470, 1962.
3. Rosson, R. S., and Yesner, R.: Peroral duodenal biopsy in progressive systemic sclerosis. *New Eng. J. Med.*, 272:391, 1965.
4. Salen, G., Goldstein, F., and Wirts, C. W.: Malabsorption in intestinal scleroderma. *Ann. Int. Med.*, 64:834-841, 1966.
5. Kahn, I. J., Jeffries, G. H., and Sleisenger, M. H.: Malabsorption in intestinal scleroderma. *New Eng. J. Med.*, 274:1339-1344, 1966.
6. Treacy, W. L., Bunting, W. L., Gambill, E. E., and Code, C. F.: Scleroderma presenting as obstruction of the small bowel. *Proc. Mayo Clinic*, 37:607-618, 1962.
7. Queboy, J. M., and Woloshin, H. J.: Sacculation of the small intestine in scleroderma. *Radiology*, 105:513-515, 1972.
8. Meihoff, W. E., Hirschfield, J. S., and Kern, F., Jr.: Small intestinal scleroderma with malabsorption and pneumatosis cystoides intestinalis. *J.A.M.A.*, 204:854-858, 1968.
9. Feldman, F., and Marshak, R. H.: Dermatomyositis with significant involvement of the gastrointestinal tract. *Amer. J. Roentgen.*, 90:746-752, 1963.

6

Amyloidosis

Amyloidosis is a disease in which the tissues of the body are infiltrated by a peculiar amorphous material which, over a century ago, was called "amyloid" by Virchow, because its staining reaction to iodine and sulfuric acid resembled that of starch. The precise chemical nature of amyloid remains unknown, but in the past decade a number of clues have been found to the nature of amyloidosis and its underlying mechanisms.

Traditionally amyloidosis has been classified into three types. *Primary amyloidosis* appears in the absence of underlying disease and may involve diffuse tissues and organs, including the skin and the heart. *Secondary amyloidosis* develops in association with prolonged inflammation or infectious diseases, such as tuberculosis, leprosy, rheumatoid arthritis, and chronic pyelonephritis; the predominant sites of amyloid deposition tend to be the liver, spleen, kidneys, and adrenals. The third form of amyloidosis is that *associated with multiple myeloma;* it has been reported that 10 percent or more of patients with myeloma develop amyloidosis.

Recent clinical and laboratory studies have tended to blur these classifications and to suggest that most if not all cases of amyloidosis represent a neoplasm or a dyscrasia of plasma cells or reticuloendothelial cells.[1,2] Whatever its exact composition, amyloid is composed in large measure of a protein-polysaccharide complex. Fluorescent antibody and other immunological techniques have demonstrated gamma globulin or related moieties, especially the light chains of immunoglobulins (Bence-Jones protein), in amyloid and give support to a hypothesis that amyloid infiltration results from abnormalities of immune mechanisms. It is postulated that so-called primary amyloidosis is a disorder of plasma cells which elaborate the abnormal proteins that are incorporated into amyloid. In this context, secondary amyloidosis results from chronic reticuloendothelial stimulation, as by long-standing inflammation or infection, which under certain conditions—perhaps genetically determined—gives rise to a population of abnormal plasma cells that produce amyloid.

Gastrointestinal involvement in amyloidosis is common,[3] and infiltration occurs at all levels of the bowel. Diagnosis of the disease can usually be made by rectal, small bowel, or gingival biopsy. The early gastrointestinal infiltration

62

may occur only in and about blood vessels of the submucosa. Later amyloid deposits are found throughout the bowel wall, especially in the muscularis mucosae and the muscular coats. The mesentery and omentum may also contain amyloid.

Clinical manifestations of intestinal amyloidosis include diarrhea, protein loss, ulceration, bleeding, obstruction, and malabsorption syndrome. It has been suggested[4] that occlusion of mesenteric vessels by amyloid may cause local vascular insufficiency leading to ulceration and bleeding. Disruption of the mucosa, with consequent ulceration, may also be secondary to infiltration of the bowel wall itself. The diarrhea of amyloidosis has been attributed to infiltration of both enteric nerve plexuses and extrinsic autonomic nerves. Clinical manifestations of mechanical intestinal obstruction in the absence of occlusion of the lumen (pseudo-obstruction) has been reported in association with gastrointestinal involvement of the small bowel in systemic amyloidosis.[5] At times the dilatation is so extreme that laparotomy has been performed. Segments of bowel have been removed in an effort to relieve the profound stasis that may occur.

Malabsorption syndrome may be more common in amyloidosis than has generally been thought. Often the appropriate diagnostic tests are not done, and the course of the illness is frequently too brief and other complications are too severe for attention to be drawn to malabsorption. A retrospective study from the Mayo Clinic[6] yielded findings of malabsorption in five of 59 patients with primary amyloidosis and in one of 44 patients with secondary amyloidosis. In some patients with malabsorption, deposits of amyloid have been demonstrated in the lamina propria and in the tips of the villi.[7] The epithelial cells may appear to be intact, but with more extensive involvement the villi are flattened and in some areas may be destroyed and replaced by bands of amyloid.

There is no specific treatment for amyloidosis. In some patients with so-called secondary amyloidosis, effective treatment of the underlying disease has appeared to lead to regression of amyloid, but direct biopsy proof of this phenomenon has been scant. Rarely, it may be possible to resect localized lesions in the intestinal tract.

Roentgen Findings

The principal roentgenographic finding in amyloidosis is conspicuous thickening of the valvulae conniventes. The enlargement of the folds may be symmetric, producing a uniform appearance throughout the entire intestinal tract. There is no ulceration, tumor nodules, or significant dilatation. Thickening of the folds in the ileum produces an appearance which we have termed jejunization. When ileal folds are prominent and resemble the valvulae conniventes of jejunum, an abnormality should be suspected.

The most difficult differential diagnosis is from Whipple's disease. However, in the latter the process is usually more severe in the jejunum. Slight dilatation is frequently present and increased secretions are more common. At times the diagnosis can be made only by clinical features or by biopsy. In some cases of amyloidosis, large deposits are distributed throughout the intes-

(*Text continued on page 68.*)

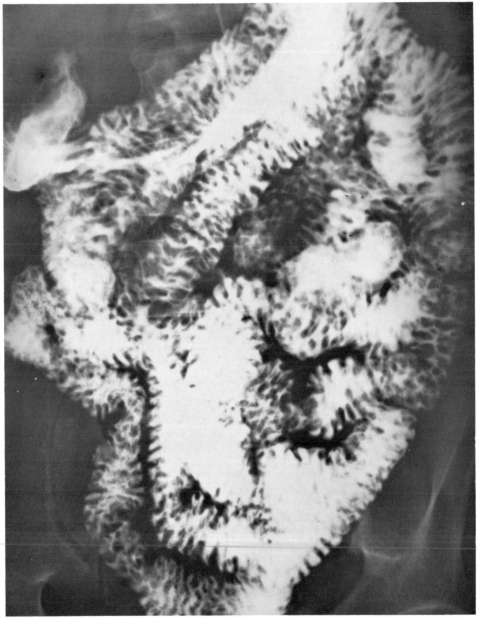

Figure 6-1 *Amyloidosis.* There is striking symmetric, diffuse, sharply demarcated thickening of the valvulae conniventes. Dilatation is minimal and there is no segmentation, fragmentation, or evidence of an inflammatory lesion.

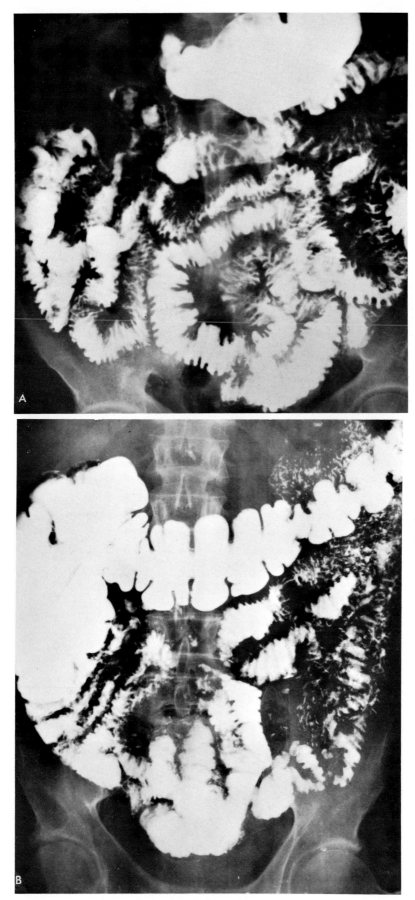

Figure 6-2 *Amyloidosis.* The folds throughout the entire small bowel are thickened. Slight fragmentation is noted but there is no dilatation.

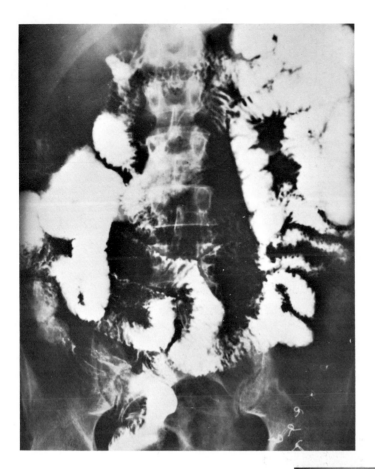

Figure 6-3 *Amyloidosis*. There is diffuse thickening of the folds throughout the small intestine.

Figure 6-4 *Amyloidosis*. The thickening of the folds is uniform throughout the small bowel.

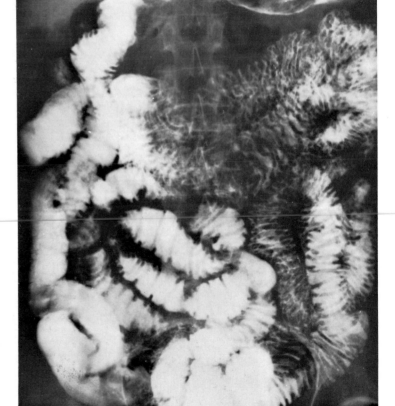

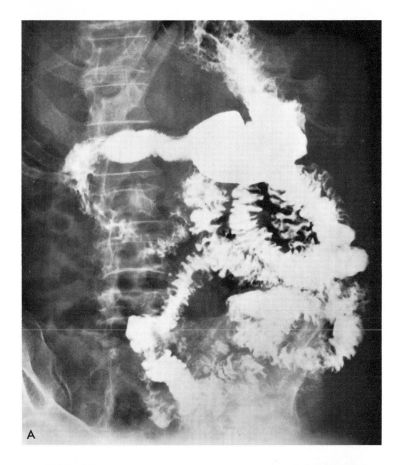

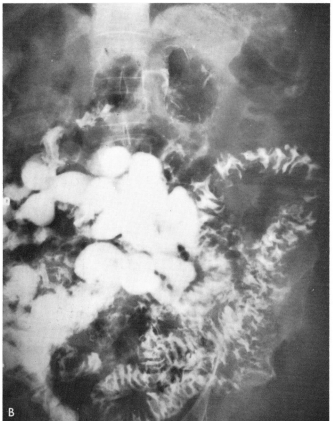

Figure 6-5 *A* and *B*, *Amyloidosis*. There is prominent thickening of the folds throughout the jejunum and proximal ileum. In some areas the large folds simulate nodules which may also suggest a diagnosis of lymphosarcoma.

tinal tract producing tumor-like nodules. Unless the primary cause of the condition is established, it is impossible to make a definite diagnosis.

Occasionally amyloidosis is associated with severe malabsorption. In these cases the roentgenologic pattern is that of the underlying amyloidosis rather than that of the malabsorption syndrome. Segmentation, fragmentation, and dilatation are usually not pronounced.

Other roentgen findings in amyloidosis, such as atony, slight dilatation, and disordered motor activity, occur in so many diseases that they are not useful features in differential diagnosis.

References

1. Glenner, G. G., Terry, W. D., and Isersky, C.: Amyloidosis: its nature and pathogenesis. *Seminars in Hematology,* 10:65-86, 1973.
2. Isobe, T., and Osserman, E. F.: Patterns of amyloidosis and their association with plasma-cell dyscrasia, monoclonal immunoglobulins and Bence-Jones proteins. *New Eng. J. Med.,* 290:473-477, 1974.
3. Cohen, A. S. Medical Progress: Amyloidosis (concluded). *New Eng. J. Med.,* 277:628-638, 1967.
4. Brody, I. A., Wertlake, P. T., and Laster, L.: Causes of intestinal symptoms in primary amyloidosis. *Arch. Intern. Med.,* 113:512-518, 1964.
5. Legge, D. A., Wollzeger, E. E., and Carlson, H. C.: Intestinal pseudo-obstruction in systemic amyloidosis. *Gut,* 11:764-767, 1970.
6. Herskovic, T., Bartholomew, L. G., and Green, P. A.: Amyloidosis and malabsorption syndrome. *Arch. Intern. Med.,* 114:629-633, 1964.
7. Pettersson, T., and Wegelius, O.: Biopsy diagnosis of amyloidosis in rheumatoid arthritis. Malabsorption caused by intestinal amyloid deposits. *Gastroenterology,* 62:22-27, 1972.

7

Intestinal Lymphangiectasia and Intestinal Edema

INTESTINAL LYMPHANGIECTASIA

Intestinal lymphangiectasia, first defined by Waldmann and his associates[1] in 1961, is a distinctive cause of protein loss into the gastrointestinal tract, hypoproteinemia, and in some patients malabsorption and steatorrhea.

Clinically, the condition is manifested by edema, serous effusions, and diarrhea.[2] Laboratory studies demonstrate hypoalbuminemia and hypogamma-globulinemia, increased protein catabolism, and loss of albumin into the gastrointestinal tract.

The pathologic findings in the small bowel are characteristic. The bowel appears edematous, and the serosal surface is dark and congested. The lumen is only slightly dilated, and the valvulae conniventes are swollen and broad. The tips of the villi are enlarged and bleblike. Histologically, the hallmark is dilatation of the lymphatics in the mucosa and submucosa. Within the mucosa are abundant foamy macrophages which stain for fat and are negative to periodic-acid-Schiff (PAS) stain. Studies of the ultrastructure of the intestinal mucosa in lymphangiectasia have suggested a mechanical block to lymphatic outflow.[3]

In some patients, with onset of symptoms in infancy, the condition appears to be congenital; in others onset of symptoms is late in life and is probably an acquired abnormality. Multiple abnormalities of the systemic lymphatics may be present.[4]

It is not clear how protein is lost through the bowel wall in intestinal lymphangiectasia. Waldmann has suggested that dilated lymphatic vessels may rupture and discharge their contents into the lumen of the gut. Alternatively, lymphatic blockage might result in leakage of protein from an intact epithelium.

Studies of the immunologic status of patients with intestinal lymphangiectasia[5] have demonstrated important consequences of leakage of gamma globulin and, presumably, lymphocytes into the intestine, resulting in reduced

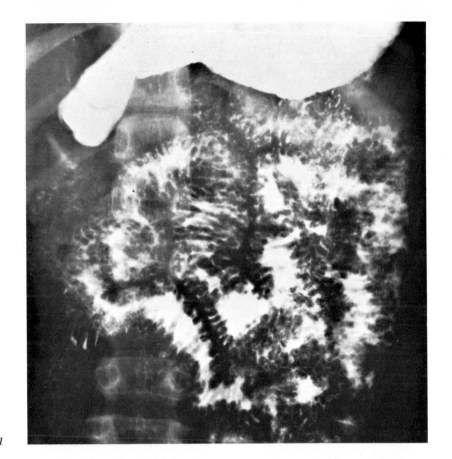

Figure 7-1

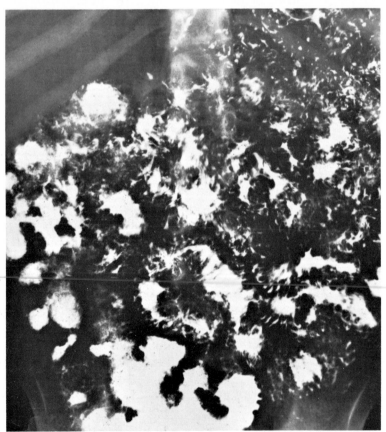

Figure 7-2

Figures 7-1 and 7-2   Intestinal lymphangiectasia. The serum albumin is 1 gram per cent. There is diffuse thickening of the valvulae conniventes associated with excessive secretions and slight dilatation. Blunting of the folds, fragmentation of the barium column and minimal segmentation are noted.

70

serum and total body levels of immunoglobulins, lymphocytopenia, skin anergy, and impaired homograft rejection.

Steatorrhea, which sometimes occurs in intestinal lymphangiectasia, might be due to obstruction of intestinal lymphatics, damage to the mucosal epithelial cells, or chronic leakage of fat-containing lymph into the lumen.

Efforts to treat intestinal lymphangiectasia with steroids, gluten-free diets, and segmental small bowel resection have proved unsuccessful. However, treatment of patients with a low fat diet results in increase in serum proteins, decrease in albumin catabolism, and decrease in intestinal protein loss.[6] It has been suggested that the low fat diet may decrease pressure in obstructed intestinal lymphatics by decreasing lymph production and consequently decreasing leakage of lymph. Availability of synthetic medium-chain triglycerides, which are absorbed via the intestinal capillaries and portal blood rather than by the lymphatics, provides another means of treating intestinal lymphangiectasia.

Roentgen Findings

Thickening of the mucosal folds is an outstanding feature in all of our cases and is usually diffuse. The fold pattern is symmetric. Nodular defects, especially of varying size, are unusual. The folds appear to be redundant and excessive. Increased secretions are invariably present (Figs. 7-1 and 7-2). The combination of marked edema and secretion may produce blunting and fragmentation of the folds (Figs. 7-3 and 7-4). Segmentation is usually minimal. Dilatation is minimal or absent, with slight evidence of rigidity of the folds. No ulceration or separation of the loops of bowel is identified. Differential diagnosis from other lesions producing thickening of the folds can be difficult. In Whipple's disease, there is usually more segmentation and fragmentation,

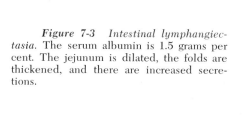
Figure 7-3 Intestinal lymphangiectasia. The serum albumin is 1.5 grams per cent. The jejunum is dilated, the folds are thickened, and there are increased secretions.

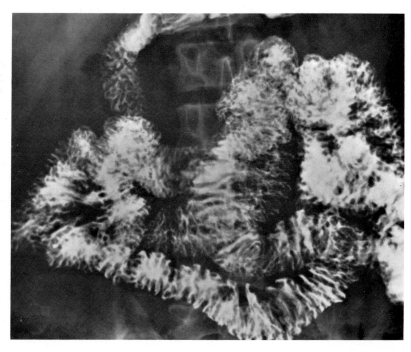

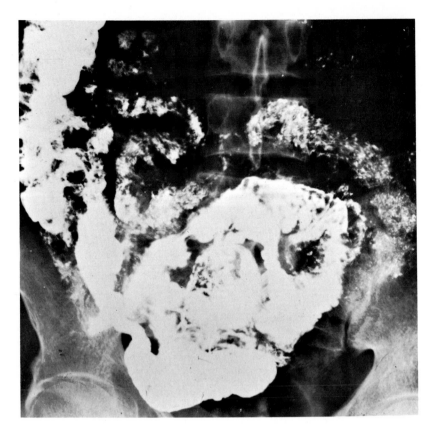

Figure 7-4 Same case as in Figure 7-3. Delayed film. The barium has a granular appearance due to excessive fluid. No segmentation is seen.

and the fold appearance is usually less symmetric and not as diffuse. In amyloidosis, edema and secretions are usually absent. Patients with hypoalbuminemic states, such as nephrosis or cirrhosis, may demonstrate a symmetric diffuse thickening of the folds of the small intestine. In these cases the thickening is usually less marked and the secretions are less prominent.

In an occasional patient with intestinal lymphangiectasia, tiny punctate lucencies can be demonstrated in the small intestine. These may represent droplets of secretion or enlarged villi distended by dilated intestinal lymphatics. When ascites is present, bulging of the flanks with a central configuration of the small intestinal loops is seen.

INTESTINAL EDEMA

Although intestinal lymphangiectasia is a specific clinical and radiologic entity, one of its manifestations, hypoproteinemia, results in pathologic changes in the small bowel. These changes have been termed intestinal edema[7] and occur in a variety of other diseases.

The most common cause of noninflammatory intestinal edema is hypoproteinemia, specifically hypoalbuminemia, resulting from liver or kidney disease or from leakage of protein from the gastrointestinal tract. When the serum albumin level is 1.5 grams per cent or lower, intestinal edema can often be demonstrated radiologically.

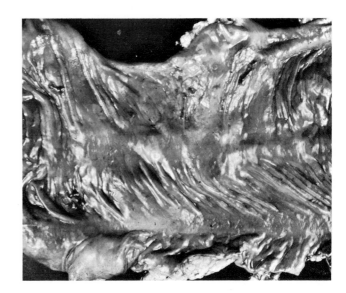

Figure 7-5 *Cirrhosis of the liver with hypoproteinemia;* colonic segment showing thick, boggy, edematous folds.

Protein loss from the gastrointestinal tract in the normal person is small. When the loss is excessive, hypoproteinemia occurs. Such so-called "protein-losing enteropathy" is not a single disease entity. It has been demonstrated in a variety of gastrointestinal disorders, including intestinal lymphangiectasia, Menetrier's disease, regional enteritis, Whipple's disease, lymphosarcoma, carcinoma, and ulcerative colitis.[8, 9] Protein loss from the intestinal tract has also been described in apparently unrelated conditions such as congestive heart failure, constrictive pericarditis, exudative skin conditions, burns, and allergy.[10]

Patients who display intestinal mucosal edema may have no gastrointestinal symptoms; their complaints are related to the primary disease or to the peripheral edema resulting from hypoproteinemia.

Pathologically, hypoalbuminemia causes an accumulation of cell-free, noninflammatory fluid within the wall of the intestinal tract, producing uniform thickening of the mucosal folds (Figs. 7-5 to 7-7). The bowel lumen may be slightly dilated. Presumably as a result of the fluid accumulation, there are anatomic and motor alterations in the intestine which are reflected in the roentgenogram.

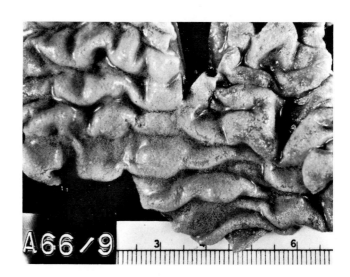

Figure 7-6 *Cirrhosis of the liver with hypoproteinemia;* edema of the small intestine.

The roentgen changes of intestinal edema are often present throughout the gastrointestinal tract but are best appreciated in the jejunum. The entire small intestine is usually slightly dilated. Loops of bowel are slightly separated and uncoiled due to edema of the bowel wall and intervening soft tissues. The mucosal folds are uniformly and symmetrically thickened (Figs. 7-8 to 7-15). Occasionally the thickening may be so pronounced that the appearance resembles a stack of coins, as has been described in intramural hemorrhage.[11] The stacked-coin appearance is a feature of several entities and is presumably the result of intramural fluid accumulation. The intramural fluid alters the motor activity of the bowel, and contractions are irregular and incomplete, producing a bizarre pattern which can mimic intramural hemorrhage, inflammatory disease, or lymphoma (Figs. 7-13, 7-14A, and 7-15). However, there are no nodules or ulcerations. The barium column is continuous and neither segmentation nor flocculation is present. In many patients ascites is found. Ascites itself due to causes other than cirrhosis does not produce thickening of the mucosal folds, but in cirrhosis with ascites, even without marked hypoproteinemia, there may be some thickening. In this instance, portal hypertension with resultant venous stasis may be responsible for the roentgen changes (Fig. 7-16).

In our patients, only the right side of the colon has been involved. The reason for this localization is obscure. There is some limitation of distensibility of the bowel wall, and evacuation is usually incomplete because of the thickened wall and altered motor function. A conspicuous feature is absence of normal longitudinal shortening following evacuation (Figs. 7-17 to 7-20). The anatomic configuration of the colon remains the same on both the barium-filled and postevacuation roentgenograms. Multiple irregular contractions are seen, which may be persistent. If the edema is marked, the haustra may be deformed

(*Text continued on page 88.*)

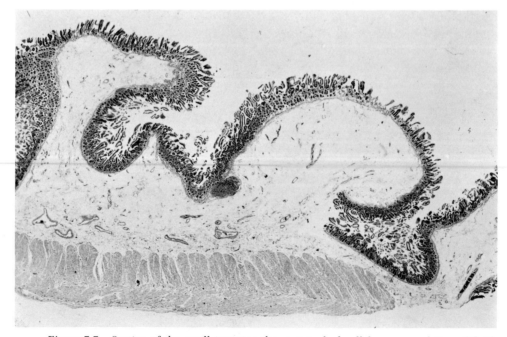

Figure 7-7   Section of the small intestine showing marked cell-free accumulation of fluid in the submucosa in a patient with cirrhosis of the liver.

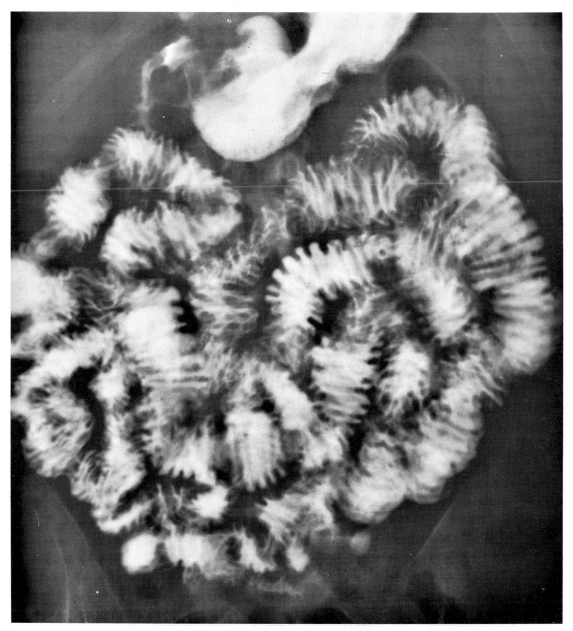

Figure 7-8 *Cirrhosis of the liver.* Serum albumin is 2 grams per cent. Minimal dilatation of the lumen with symmetric thickened folds suggesting a stacked coin configuration is seen. Contractions are present but incomplete. The loops are separated and uncoiled as soft tissue edema intervenes.

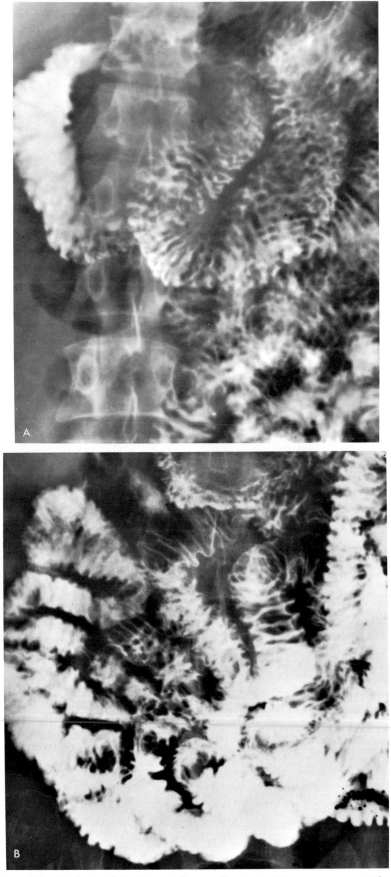

Figure 7-9 *Cirrhosis of the liver.* A, Serum albumin is 1.8 grams per cent. There is symmetric thickening of the folds associated with slight dilatation. B, Two months later the changes persist but to a lesser degree. Many of the individual folds have a biconvex appearance.

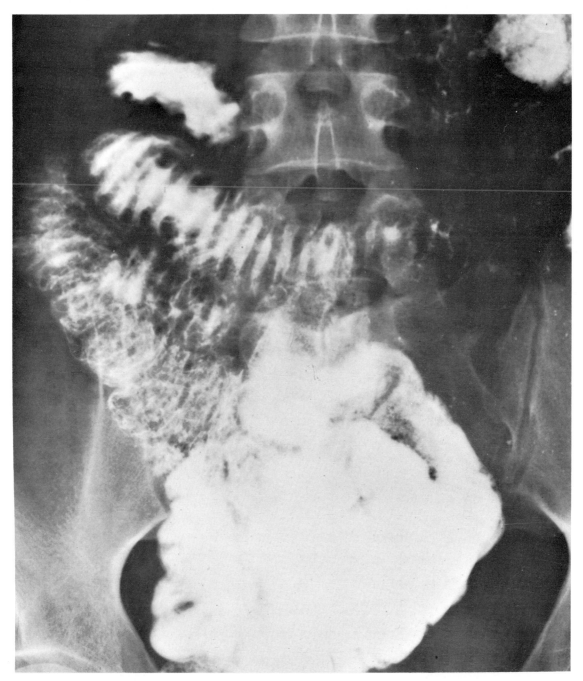

Figure 7-10　*Ulcerative colitis with hypoproteinemia.* Serum albumin is 1.7 grams per cent. The typical thickening of the folds of hypoproteinemia is seen.

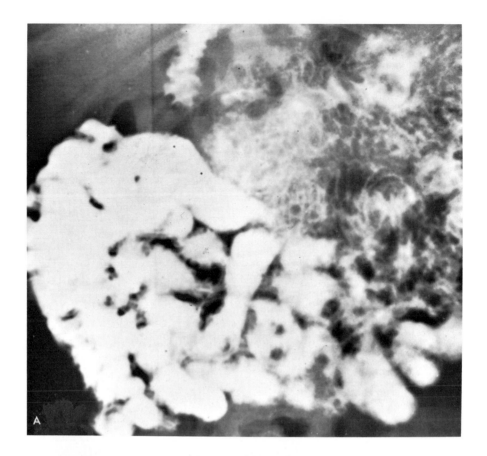

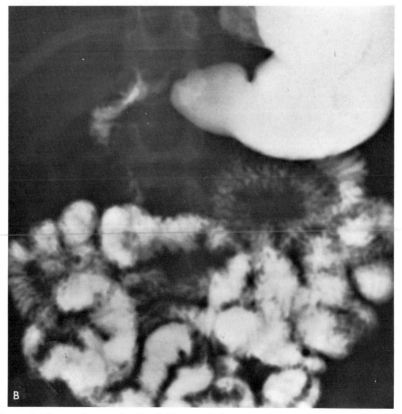

Figure 7-11   *Nephrosis.* A, The folds are thickened and hazy. Abnormal motor activity is demonstrated. *B,* Two months previously the small bowel was normal.

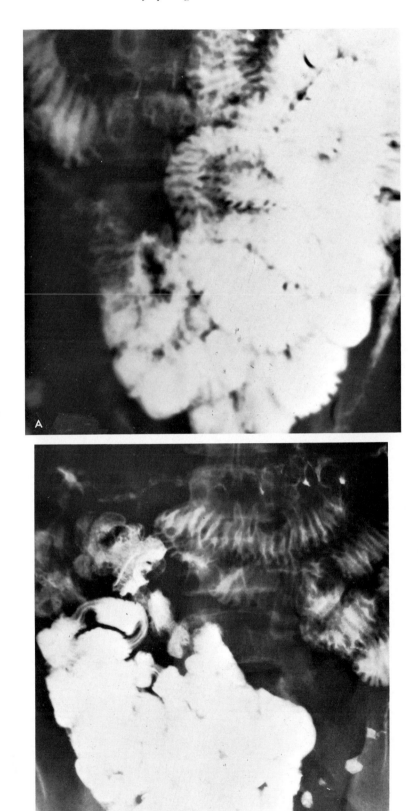

Figure 7-12   *Nephrosis. A,* The serum albumin is 1 gram per cent. Intestinal edema. *B,*
Two hours later; the changes appear to be limited to the jejunum. The ileum is normal.

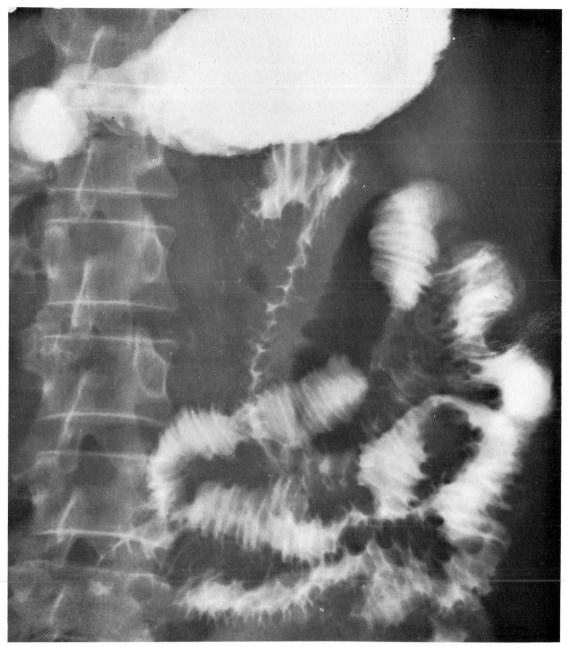

Figure 7-13   *Nephrosis.* Incomplete contractions are prominent in the proximal small intestine. The appearance is transient. Thickened, edematous folds are seen throughout. The stomach wall shows changes of edema.

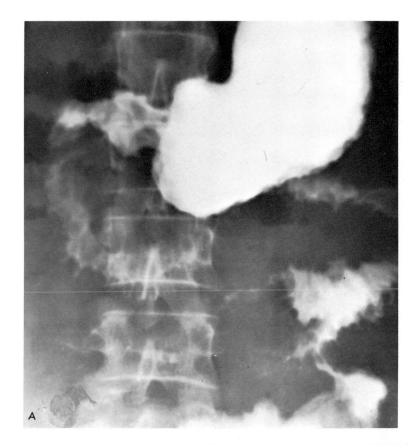

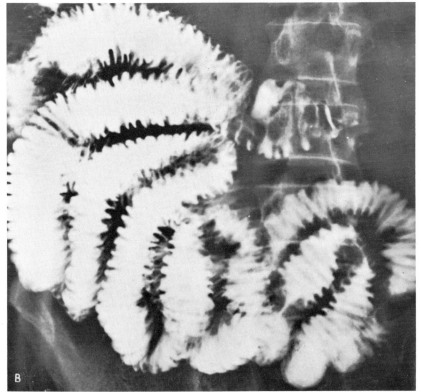

Figure 7-14   Nephrosis. Serum albumin 1 gram per cent. The stomach is slightly dilated and atonic. The folds along the greater curvature are flattened, irregular, and indistinct. These changes are due to edema of the gastric wall. Abnormal motor activity and thickened mucosal folds are seen in the jejunum. In a later study, *B,* typical changes of intestinal edema are present.

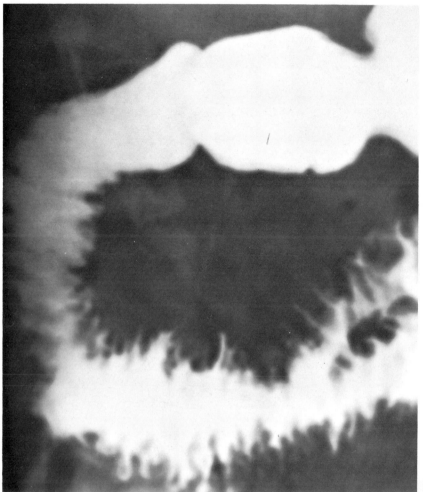

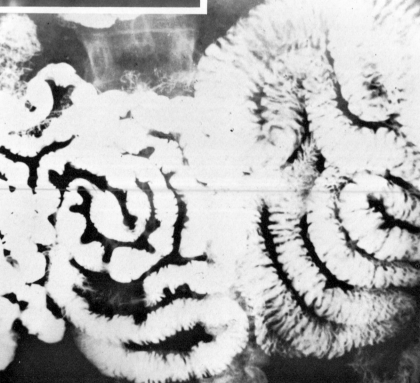

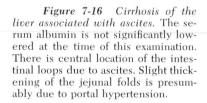

Figure 7-15   Cirrhosis of the liver. Serum albumin is 2 grams per cent. The duodenal loop is dilated and the folds are thickened. The irregularity of the folds and nodular defects along the contour were transient and due to abnormal motor activity. This appearance also resembles Henoch's purpura.

Figure 7-16   Cirrhosis of the liver associated with ascites. The serum albumin is not significantly lowered at the time of this examination. There is central location of the intestinal loops due to ascites. Slight thickening of the jejunal folds is presumably due to portal hypertension.

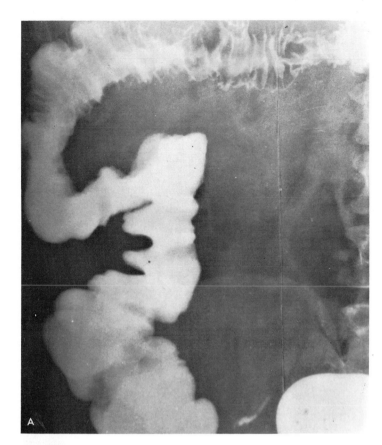

Figure 7-17   Chronic congestive heart failure. A, Hypoalbuminemia. The right side of the colon has an irregular caliber and haustrations. Despite filling, the folds are still visible and appear thickened.

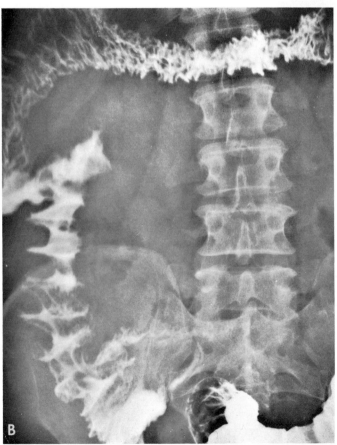

Figure 7-17   B, Following evacuation, the arrangement of boggy, thickened folds is maintained. This is due to incomplete contractility secondary to intramural edema. The normal longitudinal shortening is absent and the right side of the colon retains the same anatomic configuration as seen in A. Repeat examination three years later showed no abnormality.

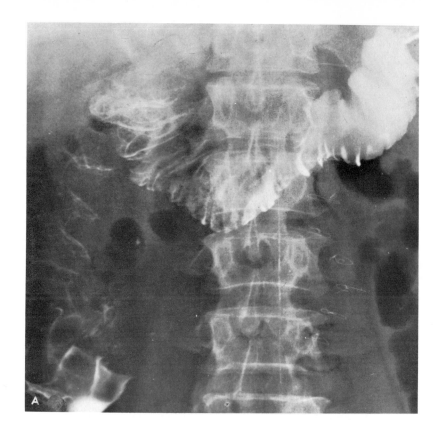

Figure 7-18 A, *Cirrhosis of the liver.* Serum albumin is 1.8 grams per cent. The mucosal folds are markedly swollen and indistinct. The colon does not contract adequately, and there is an over all haziness due to an associated ascites.

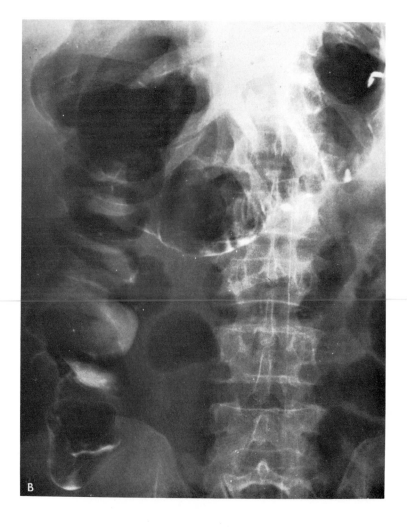

Figure 7-18 B, Air study of the same case. The right side of the colon does not distend completely. The haustra are deformed as the result of swollen mucosa.

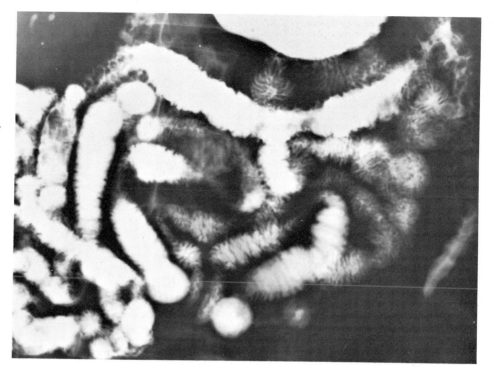

Figure 7-19 *Cirrhosis of the liver with ascites.* Hypo-albuminemia. A striking demonstration of multiple nodular defects in the transverse colon as a result of edema of the bowel. The colon is visualized following barium meal examination. Two months earlier, the colon was normal.

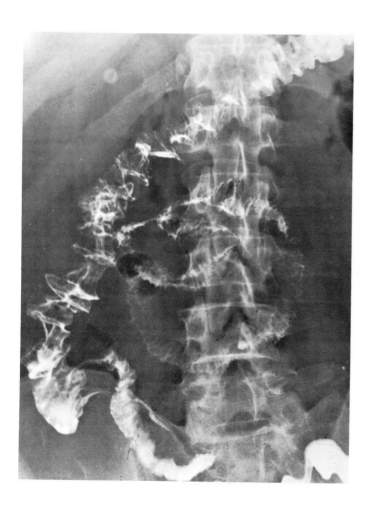

Figure 7-20 *Budd-Chiari syndrome.* The serum albumin is 2 grams per cent. Thickening of the mucosa involves the distal ileum and the right side of the colon. Ascites and a calcified gall stone are present.

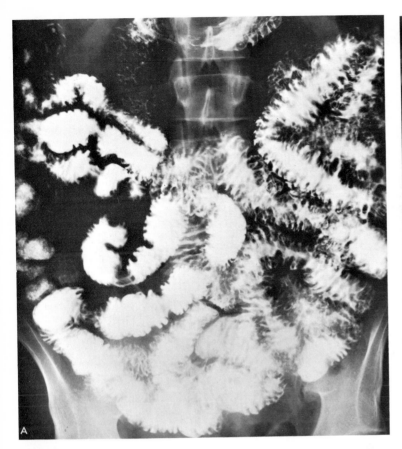

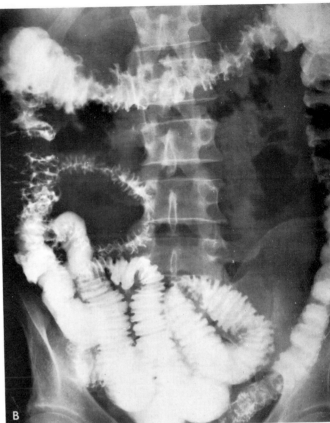

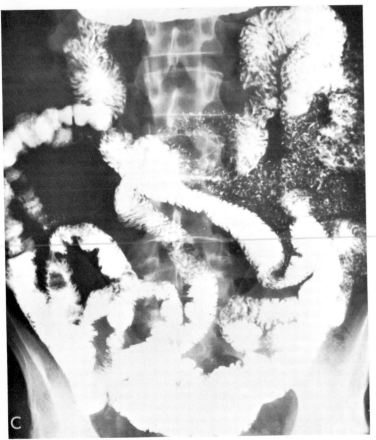

Figure 7-21   *A*, A 36 year old male presented with ascites and edema. Serum albumin was 1.0 grams per cent. Small bowel biopsy showed intestinal lymphangiectasis and clubbing and tufting of the villi with a heavy cellular infiltrate. The films demonstrate marked intestinal edema.

B, Edema of right side of colon of the same patient. He responded initially to a gluten-free diet, but his condition subsequently worsened.

C, Reexamination of the small bowel six months later demonstrates several intraluminal nodules and contour defects. The intestinal edema has disappeared. Autopsy shortly thereafter revealed lymphosarcoma of the entire gastrointestinal tract. The initial manifestation of lymphosarcoma may have been masked by the massive intestinal edema.

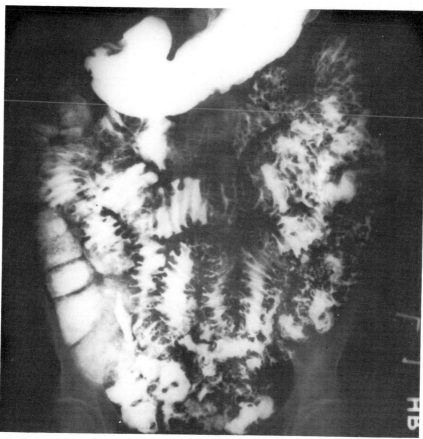

Figure 7-22 *Eosinophilic enteritis.* There is moderate thickening of the folds of the jejunum and most of the ileum, associated with spasm, irritability and a moderate amount of increased secretions. The roentgen changes in this case of eosinophilic enteritis are probably secondary to marked eosinophilic infiltration and edema of the bowel wall. (Courtesy of Dr. Barry Epstein.)

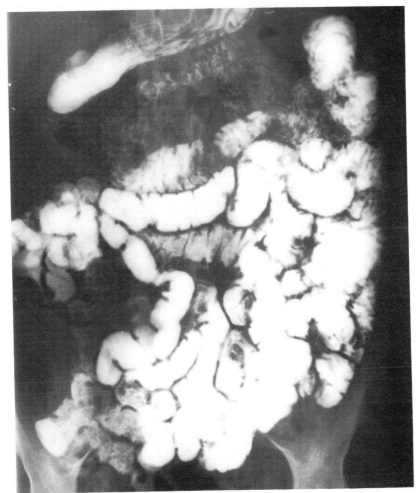

Figure 7-23 Eosinophilic enteritis. Same patient as in Figure 7-22, six months after start of prednisone therapy. The small bowel now appears normal.

and irregular. The mucosal folds appear thickened, somewhat indistinct, and distorted, but there is no ulceration or nodularity. It is also possible that ischemia of the colon is an associated condition in some of these cases and is responsible for part of the changes.

How great a role the changes of intestinal edema play in causing the characteristic roentgen appearance of such hypoproteinemic intestinal disorders as sprue, Whipple's disease, intestinal lymphangiectasia, or lymphosarcoma and eosinophilic enteritis is not known (Figs. 7-21, 7-22, 7-23). Certainly in intestinal lymphangiectasia the marked thickening of the folds is closely correlated with the degree of protein loss.

References

1. Waldmann, T. A., Steinfeld, J. L., Dutcher, T. F., Davidson, J. D., and Gordon, R. S.: The role of the gastrointestinal system in "idiopathic hypoproteinemia." *Gastroenterology,* 41:197-207, 1961.
2. Shimkin, P. M., Waldmann, T. A., and Krugman, R. L.: Intestinal lymphangiectasia. *Amer. J. Roentgen.*, 110:827-841, 1970.

3. Dobbins, W. B.: Electron microscopic study of the intestinal mucosa in intestinal lymphangiectasia. *Gastroenterology*, 51:1004-1017, 1966.
4. Pomerantz, M., and Waldmann, T. A.: Systemic lymphatic abnormalities associated with gastrointestinal protein loss secondary to intestinal lymphangiectasia. *Gastroenterology*, 45:703-711, 1963.
5. Strober, W., Wochner, R. D., Carbone, P. P., and Waldmann, T. A.: Intestinal lymphangiectasia: a protein-losing enteropathy with hypogammaglobulinemia, lymphocytopenia and impaired homograft rejection. *J. Clin. Invest.* 46:1643-1656, 1967.
6. Jeffries, G. H., Chapman, A., and Sleisenger, M. H.: Low-fat diet in intestinal lymphangiectasia. *New Eng. J. Med.*, 270:761-766, 1964.
7. Marshak, R. H., Khilnani, M., Eliasoph, J., and Wolf, B. S.: Intestinal edema. *Amer. J. Roentgen.*, 101:379-387, 1967.
8. Steinfeld, J. L., Davidson, J. D., Gordon, R. S., Jr., and Greene, F. E.: Mechanism of hypoproteinemia in patients with regional enteritis and ulcerative colitis. *Amer. J. Med.*, 29:405-415, 1960.
9. Marshak, R. H., Wolf, B. S., Cohen, N., and Janowitz, H. D.: Protein-losing disorders of the gastrointestinal tract: roentgen features. *Radiology*, 77:893-906, 1961.
10. Peterson, V. P. and Hastings, J. Protein-losing enteropathy in constrictive pericarditis. *Acta Med. Scand.*, 173:401-410, 1963.
11. Khilnani, M. T., Marshak, R. H., Eliasoph, J., and Wolf, B. S.: Intramural intestinal hemorrhage. *Amer. J. Roentgen.*, 92:1061-1071, 1964.

8

The Zollinger-Ellison Syndrome

The Zollinger-Ellison syndrome was first described in 1955[1] and was found to consist of a triad of clinical features:

1. A fulminating peptic ulcer diathesis with marked hypersecretion of hydrochloric acid by the stomach;

2. Persistent and recurrent ulceration despite medical and surgical treatment;

3. The presence of a non-beta islet cell tumor of the pancreas.

Since the time of the initial report, diarrhea has been recognized as a common feature of the syndrome, occurring in perhaps half the patients.

A recent review[2] notes that the reported cases may represent only the more flagrant forms of the disease. Many patients probably remain undiagnosed because their symptoms do not distinguish them from patients with ordinary duodenal ulcer disease.

Etiology

The possibility that the pancreatic tumor might elaborate a potent stimulant of gastric acid secretion was suggested early in the clinical history of the Zollinger-Ellison syndrome. Indeed, the presence of a gastric secretagogue had been demonstrated in the blood and urine of patients with the syndrome by means of a bioassay using the rat stomach.[3] Although it had been suspected for some years that the secretagogue derived from the pancreatic tumor might be gastrin, the hormone of the gastric antrum, proof of that identity has only recently been achieved.

One of the most remarkable advances in gastrointestinal physiology has been the coming of age of gastrin, a hormone which was discovered and named at the turn of the century but which had to wait some 60 years for confirmation and vindication.[4]

In a paper that he read before the Royal Society of London in 1905, John Edkins showed that crude extracts of mucosa from the antral region of the stomach stimulated gastric secretion in anesthetized cats, but extracts from the fundal region did not. Only a few years earlier Bayliss and Starling had dis covered the first hormone, secretin. Edkins called his active principle "gastrin," which, it is said, is a contraction for "gastric secretin."

Unfortunately for Edkins, and for gastrin, in the ensuing years investigators who attempted to confirm his work found that although a gastric secretory stimulant could be extracted from antral mucosa, an apparently identical stimulant could be extracted similarly from many other tissues. With the discovery of histamine in 1910 it seemed clear that Edkins' stimulant was nothing more than histamine. Little further attention was paid to the gastrin concept until the late 1930's when Komarov presented evidence that the antral mucosa contains a gastric stimulant in addition to histamine.[5] Komarov's nonhistamine extracts were not always active, however, and it was not until the work of Grossman, Robertson and Ivy in 1948[6] that physiologic proof of the existence of an antral hormone mechanism for gastric secretion was established.

The reliable extraction of that antral hormone had to wait until 1961, when Gregory and Tracy[7] reported the isolation of gastrin from hog antrums. Subsequently this group of investigators purified the material, established that there are two gastrins, characterized them as polypeptides, determined their amino acid sequence, and synthesized them.

The first of the gastrins, Gastrin I, is a 17-amino-acid polypeptide. Gastrin II differs from Gastrin I only by the presence of a sulfate group on the tyrosine molecule occupying position number 12 in the sequence. The two hormones exhibit identical physiologic properties.

The gastrins of a number of species—hog, dog, sheep, and man—have similar structures, and all have at the carboxyl end of the molecule an identical tetrapeptide, consisting of tyrosine, methionine, aspartic acid and phenylalanine. This tetrapeptide possesses all the physiologic properties of the complete gastrin molecule, and lengthening the amino acid sequence toward the complete molecule affects these properties only quantitatively.

A number of the physiological actions of gastrin have been identified and studied. Most important, of course, is its effect on gastric secretion of hydrochloric acid. Gastrin is approximately 500 times more potent a stimulant of acid secretion than histamine, on a molar basis. In addition, gastrin stimulates—although weakly—the secretion of pepsinogen by the gastric chief cells, increases gastric and—to a lesser degree—small bowel motility, relaxes the lower esophageal sphincter, stimulates the pancreas to secrete a fluid high in enzyme content but low in bicarbonate output, stimulates the liver to increase the output of water and bicarbonate in bile, and weakly contracts the gallbladder.

In 1960, Gregory,[8] using the same technique he employed in extracting gastrin from hog antrums, was able to extract a substance with biologic characteristics of gastrin from the tumor of a patient with the Zollinger-Ellison syndrome. In 1967 Gregory[9] reported isolating from two ulcerogenic pancreatic tumors a material which stimulated gastric secretion, was free of histamine, and had an amino acid composition identical to that of gastrin. Subsequently McGuigan and others have identified gastrin immunochemically in extracts derived from pancreatic islet cell tumors.

There seems no doubt, therefore, that the islet cell tumor of patients with the Zollinger-Ellison syndrome elaborates gastrin and that this hormone is responsible for hypersecretion of gastric acid and most of the clinical manifestations of the syndrome.

McGuigan[10] and Berson and Yalow[11] have described a radioimmunoassay method for determining serum gastrin levels. Normal subjects and patients with duodenal ulcer have fasting serum gastrin concentrations between 20 and 150 picograms per ml. Patients with the Zollinger-Ellison syndrome usually have clearly elevated fasting serum gastrin levels, with values from 150 pg. per ml. to 1000 pg. per ml. or more. Interestingly, these high serum values are also found in patients with pernicious anemia, whose antral mucosa releases gastrin unopposed by inhibitory effects of gastric hydrochloric acid. Such hypergastrinemia, of course, is without effect on production of HCl in the absence of parietal cells, and pernicious anemia causes no clinical diagnostic confusion with the Zollinger-Ellison syndrome.

Unfortunately some patients with documented Zollinger-Ellison syndrome have had fasting serum gastrin levels within the normal or borderline range. A number of stimulation tests have been devised in an effort to distinguish the patient with ordinary duodenal ulcer from the one with Zollinger-Ellison syndrome.[2] One test simply requires measurement of the serum gastrin levels after a meal; the autonomous gastrin-secreting Zollinger-Ellison tumor is not affected by feeding, while the antral mucosa of patients with hypergastrinemia of antral origin is stimulated by the meal and the serum gastrin level rises. Another test measures the effect of calcium infusion; serum gastrin levels of the patient with Zollinger-Ellison syndrome increase markedly, but normal subjects and patients with duodenal ulcer respond with only modest elevations. The third test measures response to an infusion of secretin; this hormone causes an increase in the serum gastrin level of some patients with Zollinger-Ellison syndrome but a decrease in the serum gastrin of normal subjects and patients with duodenal ulcer.

Patients with the Zollinger-Ellison syndrome have markedly elevated outputs of gastric acid. Typical patients demonstrate a 1-hour basal secretion of greater than 15 mEq. of acid or a 12-hour overnight secretion of greater than 100 mEq. Unfortunately, measurement of gastric acid alone will not provide a secure diagnosis of the Zollinger-Ellison syndrome because as many as one-third of patients do not achieve these characteristic values, and a few patients with ordinary duodenal ulcer will do so. A high ratio of basal to peak histamine-stimulated secretion is usually found in patients with the Zollinger-Ellison syndrome, a response of parietal cells to chronic basal stimulation by the gastrin-producing tumor.

Zollinger has estimated that the fulminating ulcer diathesis is present in 90 per cent of cases, and approximately half of these are associated with severe diarrhea and sometimes steatorrhea. In these patients the extraordinary acid secretion is believed to be responsible for the diarrhea, probably by lowering the pH in the duodenum and inhibiting pancreatic enzymes, by increasing motility of the intestine, and by inducing morphologic and functional changes in the small bowel epithelial cells.

Of great interest are patients with non-beta islet cell tumors who have hypokalemia and diarrhea so profound that it has been called "pancreatic cholera."[2] Yet they have low gastric acidity or even achlorhydria. Peptic ulcer disease is not a feature of this syndrome. Serum gastrin levels are not increased and the tumors do not contain gastrin. The hormone or hormones responsible have not yet been identified, but suggested candidates include secretin, glucagon, and gastric inhibitory polypeptide.[12, 13, 14]

Pathology

The pancreatic tumor of the Zollinger-Ellison syndrome is composed of non-beta islet cells; the specific gastrin-producing cell has otherwise not yet been identified. The tumor, sometimes an adenoma but more commonly a carcinoma, may occur anywhere in the pancreas but especially in the body and tail; aberrant adenomas also occur. There may be multiple tumors within the pancreas, rather than a single adenoma, or diffuse hyperplasia of islet cells may occur throughout the gland. In approximately two-thirds of patients the tumor is malignant. The degree of malignancy is low, and in terms of growth the tumor is not aggressive.

The pancreatic tumor of the Zollinger-Ellison syndrome may be part of the syndrome of multiple endocrine adenomatosis (Wermer's syndrome), a familial condition characterized by the presence of coexisting multiple tumors of hyperplasias of the parathyroid, pituitary, adrenal, or thyroid gland, and the pancreatic islets.

Gastric mucosal folds are large. The folds in the proximal small bowel are thickened. Ulcers may occur in the esophagus and stomach but are uncommon. Approximately two-thirds of all ulcers occur in the first portion of the duodenum and one-fourth in the jejunum distal to the ligament of Treitz. Multiple ulcers are common.

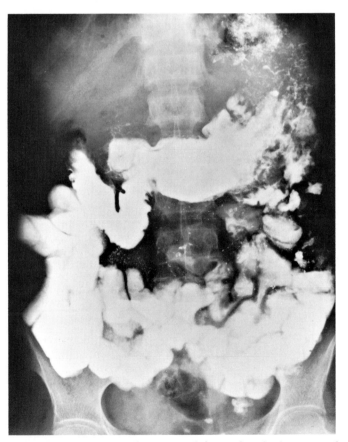

Figure 8-1   Zollinger-Ellison Syndrome. One hour study. The barium in the stomach and proximal small bowel has a granular appearance. The folds in the second and third portions of the duodenum are slightly coarsened. Increased fluid, pseudosegmentation and fragmentation are identified in the proximal jejunum.

Clinical Features

The clinical features of the Zollinger-Ellison syndrome are those of severe peptic ulcer disease and, in approximately half the patients, severe diarrhea, sometimes with evidence of malabsorption syndrome. Hypoglycemia is not a feature of the disease.

Marked hypersecretion of gastric acid characterizes approximately 90 per cent of patients, and the measured output of acid may be enormous. Typically, gastric analysis shows basal secretion of hydrochloric acid greater than 15 mEq/hour (normal less than 5 mEq/hour) and values greater than 60 mEq/hour following maximal doses of histamine (normal less than 20 mEq/hour).

A few patients with islet cell tumors have profound diarrhea and hypokalemia without gastric hypersecretion. This is the group of patients with so-called "pancreatic cholera." The clinical presentation is therefore without upper gastrointestinal manifestations, and the association with the Zollinger-Ellison syndrome is usually developed only as diagnostic studies progress.

Most patients with the Zollinger-Ellison syndrome are first thought to have ordinary peptic ulcer disease. The ulcer diathesis proves resistant to medical treatment, however, and the patients ultimately require surgical intervention. With greater awareness of the syndrome, diagnosis can now usually be made, or at least suggested, preoperatively. Clinical clues to the diagnosis of this entity include laboratory and roentgen evidence of marked gastric hypersecretion, ulcers in atypical locations, and the presence of severe diarrhea. A preoperative search for an islet cell tumor may be made with pancreatic scan and with celiac and superior mesenteric arteriography. Careful exploration of the pancreas is mandatory in all operations for duodenal ulcer to avoid overlooking a previously undiagnosed islet cell tumor.

If a tumor is unrecognized at laparotomy and conventional surgery for duodenal ulcer is performed, recurrent ulceration will invariably occur, and subsequent resections short of total gastrectomy will not prevent still further ulcer recurrence. In the presence of the gastrin-secreting islet tissue, ulceration recurs as long as acid-producing gastric tissue remains.

If the pancreatic tumor is benign and can be resected, conventional surgery may be adequate and curative. Unfortunately, over half the tumors are malignant and the majority have metastasized to liver or regional lymph nodes at the time of laparotomy. Since both the primary tumor and the metastases secrete gastrin, total gastrectomy has been advocated as the only successful palliative treatment. Most deaths have been associated with multiple resections and complications of ulcer, including hemorrhage and perforation. Because the islet cell tumor is slow-growing, few deaths have been attributed to the malignancy itself.

Roentgen Manifestations

The following roentgen features[15, 16] are associated with the Zollinger-Ellison syndrome:
1. Gastric hypersecretion.
2. Large gastric folds (hyperrugosity).
3. Single or multiple peptic ulcers.
4. Dilatation of the second portion of the duodenum, with coarsening of the folds.
5. Edema and inflammatory changes of the proximal small bowel.

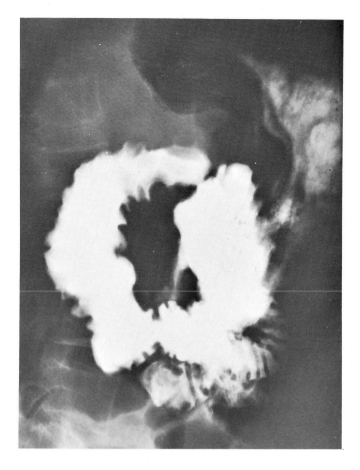

Figure 8-2   Zollinger-Ellison Syndrome. The stomach is moderately enlarged, associated with prominence of the rugal folds. Moderate dilatation of the second portion of the duodenum is identified, as well as coarsened, thickened mucosal folds. There is no discrete ulceration.

6. Early recurrent marginal ulceration following subtotal gastric resection.
7. Marked increase in intraluminal small bowel fluid.
8. Hypermotility.

Gastric hypersection is readily recognized during barium meal examination. Fluid is present despite overnight fasting and lack of pyloric obstruction. The barium appears less dense than normal and is granular in appearance (Fig. 8-1). The dilution of barium is frequently best seen in the small bowel where it produces a moulage effect, obliterating the fold pattern. Increased intraluminal fluid may also produce pseudo-segmentation and sacculation of the barium column (Fig. 8-1).

Hypertrophy of the rugal folds has been attributed in part to a thickened mucosa containing increased numbers of parietal cells. Intramural edema is another important factor, and an appearance resembling Menetrier's disease may be found. Indeed, on pathologic examination of a resected stomach it may be difficult to distinguish the two entities without knowledge of the clinical features (Figs. 8-2 and 8-3).

Esophageal ulcer is rare but has been reported after subtotal gastric resection. Gastric ulcer is also not common, occurring in approximately 10 per cent of cases. Although the duodenal bulb is the usual location of ulcer, the presence of ulcers distal to the bulb should always arouse the suspicion of Zollinger-Ellison syndrome. This has been a frequent finding in many of the reported cases. Small superficial ulcers are not rare throughout the duodenum and proximal small bowel. On occasion they are large and easily recognized on roentgen examination (Figs. 8-4 to 8-9).

(*Text continued on page 100.*)

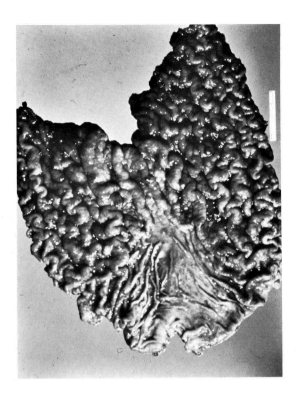

Figure 8-3 Zollinger-Ellison Syndrome. Same case as in Figure 8-2. Specimen of stomach revealing the tremendous enlargement of the rugal folds. This appearance resembles that of Menetrier's disease on gross examination.

Figure 8-4 Zollinger-Ellison Syndrome. There is a large ulcer crater at the apex of the duodenal bulb with an area of narrowing proximally and distally. The distal half of the second portion of the duodenum is considerably dilated and the folds are thickened and coarsened. Coarsening of the folds with segmentation is identified in the proximal jejunum.

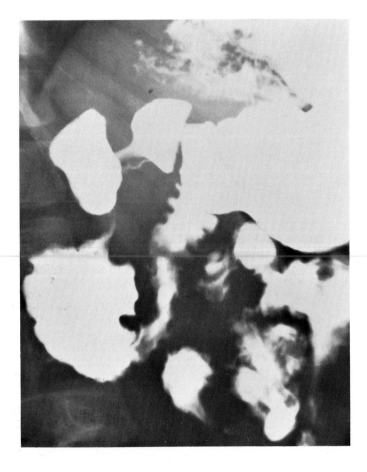

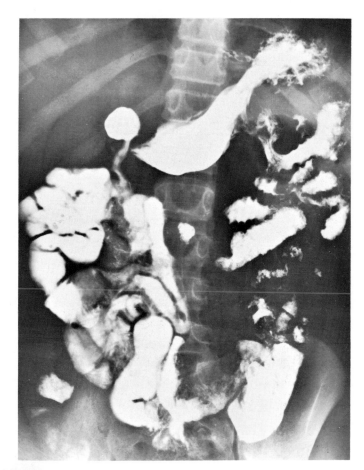

Figure 8-5 Zollinger-Ellison Syndrome. The same patient as in Figure 8-4, following gastroenterostomy. The ulcer crater has been left in situ. The proximal small bowel reveals segmentation, increased fluid and coarsening of the folds.

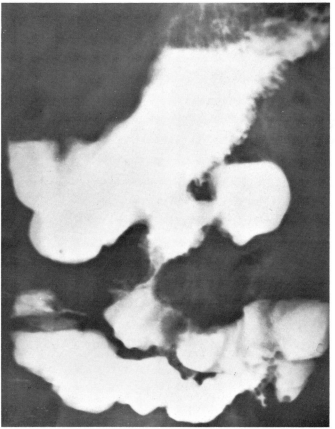

Figure 8-6 Zollinger-Ellison Syndrome. The same case, six weeks later. There are now two large marginal ulcerations, one pointing toward the left lobe of the liver, the other at the stoma. The folds and the proximal loops of small bowel are thickened and edematous.

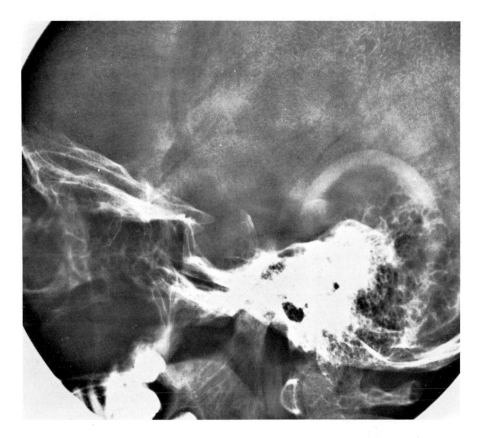

Figure 8-7 Zollinger-Ellison Syndrome. Same case as in Figure 8-6. There is a large sella turcica with thinning of the anterior and posterior clinoids, due to a chromophobe adenoma. This is an example of multiple endocrine adenomas in association with Zollinger-Ellison syndrome. A total gastrectomy was ultimately performed.

Figure 8-8 Zollinger-Ellison Syndrome. The stomach is slightly enlarged and the rugal folds are prominent. The second portion of the duodenum is dilated, associated with coarsened folds. An ulcer crater is seen in the midpart of the second portion of the duodenum.

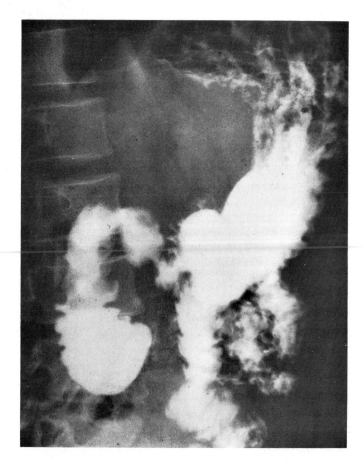

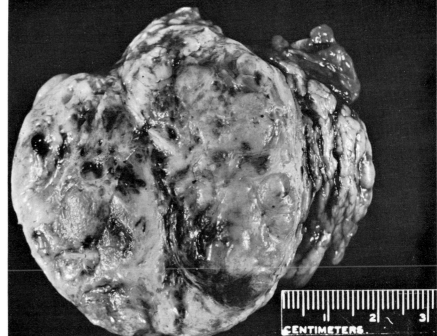

Figure 8-9 *Zollinger-Ellison Syndrome.* Same case as in Figure 8-8. Resected specimen of pancreatic tumor. At surgery, the tumor was thought to be a benign adenoma, but histologic examination demonstrated an islet cell carcinoma invading the capsule.

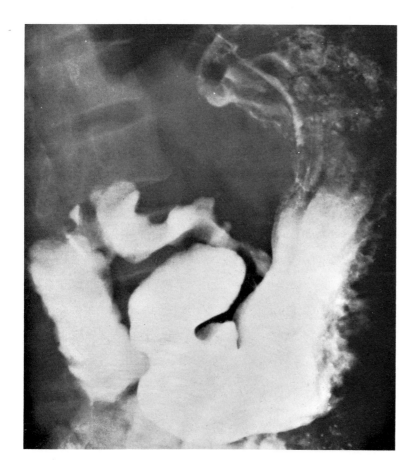

Figure 8-10 *Zollinger-Ellison Syndrome.* This patient has Wermer's syndrome and hyperparathyroidism. The folds in the stomach are enlarged. The duodenal bulb is markedly deformed. No definite crater is identified. The second portion of the duodenum is dilated and the folds are coarsened. This patient died of heart block. Autopsy revealed multiple endocrine tumors, including a pancreatic adenoma, and a scarred, healed duodenal bulb.

One of the striking manifestations of this syndrome is a dilated second portion of the duodenum with coarsened, thickened folds (Figs. 8-4 and 8-8 to 8-10). This radiologic finding is frequently present and should immediately suggest the possibility of Zollinger-Ellison syndrome. Earlier, before dilatation occurs, marked spasm and irritability are often present, and unless sufficient barium is employed a string sign may be seen, simulating the findings in regional enteritis. The cause of the dilatation of the duodenum is unknown. It is probably related to extensive edema of the mucosal folds over a prolonged period of time. The coarsening and edema of the folds frequently extend throughout the proximal small bowel and are undoubtedly related to the high concentration of hydrochloric acid in this region. The roentgen findings diminish in the distal portion of the small intestine, where the striking alteration is the marked accumulation of fluid in the small bowel.

Many times the correct diagnosis of the Zollinger-Ellison syndrome is not made and a subtotal gastric resection is performed. In these circumstances stomal ulcers, multiple jejunal ulcers, or both are found in the majority of patients. Some of these ulcers appear only a few weeks following partial gastric resection and are characteristically large (Fig. 8-6).

References

1. Zollinger, R. M., and Ellison, R. H.: Primary peptic ulcerations of the jejunum associated with islet cell tumor of pancreas. *Ann. Surg.*, 142:709-722, 1955.
2. Isenberg, J. I., Walsh, J. H., and Grossman, M. I.: Zollinger-Ellison syndrome. *Gastroenterology*, 65:140-165, 1973.
3. Lai, K. S.: Studies on gastrin. *Gut*, 5:327-341, 1964.
4. Walsh, J. H., and Grossman, M. I.: Gastrin. *New Eng. J. Med.*, 292:1324-1334 and 1377-1384, 1975.
5. Komarov, S. A.: Gastrin. *Proc. Soc. Exp. Med.* 38:514-516, 1938.
6. Grossman, M. I., Robertson, C. R., and Ivy, A. C.: Proof of hormonal mechanism for gastric secretion: humoral transmission of distention stimulus. *Amer. J. Physiol.*, 153:1-9, 1948.
7. Gregory, R. A., and Tracy, H. J.: Preparation and properties of gastrin. *J. Physiol.*, 156:523-543, 1961.
8. Gregory, R. A., et al: Extraction of a gastrin-like substance from a pancreatic tumor in a case of Zollinger-Ellison syndrome. *Lancet*, 1:1045-1048, 1960.
9. Gregory, R. A., Grossman, M. I., Tracy, H. J., and Bentley, P. H.: Nature of gastric secretagogue in Zollinger-Ellison tumors. *Lancet* 2:543-544, 1967.
10. McGuigan, J. E., and Trudea, W. L.: Immunochemical measurement of elevated levels of gastrin in the serum of patients with pancreatic tumors of the Zollinger-Ellison variety. *New Eng. J. Med.*, 278:1308-1313, 1968.
11. Berson, S. A., and Yalow, R. S.: Radioimmunoassay in gastroenterology. *Gastroenterology*, 62:1061-1084, 1972.
12. Barbezat, G. O., and Grossman, M. I.: Intestinal secretion: Stimulation by peptides. *Science*, 174:422-424, 1971.
13. Elias, E., Bloom, S. R., Welbourn, R. B., et al.: Pancreatic cholera due to production of gastric inhibitory polypeptide. *Lancet*, 2:791-793, 1972.
14. Verner, J. V., and Morrison, A. B.: Endocrine pancreatic islet disease with diarrhea. *Arch. Int. Med.*, 133:492-500, 1974.
15. Christoforidis, A. J., and Nelson, S. W.: Radiologic manifestations of ulcerogenic tumors of the pancreas. *J.A.M.A.*, 198:511-516, 1966.
16. Zboralske, F. F., and Amberg, J. R.: Detection of the Zollinger-Ellison syndrome: The radiologist's responsibility. *Amer. J. Roentgenol.*, 104:529-543, 1968.

9

Parasitic Infection of the Small Bowel

Several of the parasitic infections of man may be associated with roentgen findings on small bowel examination. Parasites that may cause radiologically demonstrable alterations in the small bowel include Giardia lamblia, Necator (hookworm), Strongyloides stercoralis, tapeworm, and Ascaris lumbricoides.

GIARDIASIS

Giardia lamblia is a flagellated protozoan. Trophozoites, which tend to inhabit the duodenum and proximal jejunum of the host, are believed to attach themselves to the mucosa by their sucking discs, and they are not usually found in the stool. Reproduction of the organisms is accomplished by formation of cysts, which are passed in the stool. Following ingestion by a host, the cysts reach the duodenum where excystation and infection occur.

Giardia lamblia has long been known to be a common parasite of the human proximal small bowel. The reported incidence of infection in institutional populations has varied from 2 to 50 per cent.[1] In the past the organism was believed to be a harmless commensal of no clinical significance. Recently, however, a number of studies have demonstrated diarrheal disease and malabsorption in association with giardiasis.[2, 3, 3a] These clinical findings are reversible following treatment with quinacrine (Atabrine) or metronidazole (Flagyl) and elimination of the parasites. Several epidemics have been reported of an acute diarrheal illness due to drinking water contaminated with Giardia lamblia.

The response of a given patient to infection with Giardia lamblia appears to be variable, depending on the infecting dose and on such host-related factors as age, previous surgery, presence or absence of bacterial infection in the intestine, nutrition, and the status of the body's immune mechanisms.[4]

Some authors have found significant mucosal alterations on small bowel biopsy in patient with giardiasis.[2, 4] Reported changes include acute and chronic inflammation, abnormal villous configuration, damage to epithelial cells, and increased epithelial mitoses. Of interest is the observation that some patients with giardiasis have hypogammaglobulinemia, and reduced susceptibility to infection may be responsible for the giardia infection.[5] (See Chapter 10, The Small Bowel in Immunoglobulin Deficiency Syndromes.) Some investigators have demonstrated tissue invasion by the parasite.[6] There seems to be no consistent correlation between the severity of the mucosal changes and the occurrence of malabsorption, for malabsorption has been reported in patients with no significant mucosal alterations.[3] The mechanism of malabsorption in giardiasis remains uncertain.

Roentgen Findings

The radiologic findings in Giardia infection have rarely been discussed and have often been confused with the sprue pattern. The roentgen appearance of giardiasis, however, is that of an inflammatory process.

In an early report Welch[7] described duodenal cap irritability with coarsening of the duodenal mucosal pattern in three-fourths of 29 reported cases of giardia infestation. Peterson[1] described prolonged transit time, marked segmentation, and a moderate degree of dilatation of loops and coarsening of the mucosal folds in the loops of mid-small bowel. He ascribed these findings to the "deficiency pattern," a term which has been used to describe the features of sprue.

More recent publications have commented upon the radiologic findings in certain conditions which are *associated* with giardiasis. Giardia infection has been noted to be frequent in cases of hypogammaglobulinemia with nodular lymphoid hyperplasia of the small intestine.[8, 9] In addition to the nodular filling defects, coarsening of the mucosal folds and clumping of barium were also observed by these authors, but they did not attribute the latter changes to giardiasis.

Our observation has been that the roentgen findings in giardiasis are inflammatory in character.[10] The roentgen alterations are usually limited to the duodenum and jejunum. Mucosal folds appear thickened, blunted, and, in many areas, distorted and fragmented (Figs. 9-1 and 9-2). Associated with the mucosal changes is a marked degree of spasm and irritability, which produces a rapid change in the direction and configuration of the valvulae conniventes (Fig. 9-3). The lumen of the bowel is frequently narrowed because of spasm. Dilatation, when present, is minimal. Increased secretions are frequent and cause blurring and indistinctness in the appearance of the folds, and sometimes there is fragmentation and slight segmentation. Motility through the jejunum may be so rapid that multiple filming with considerable amounts of barium is necessary to study the roentgen features. The ileum appears normal. In several cases we have observed complete return to normal of the fold pattern following treatment (Fig. 9-4).

The radiologic abnormalities we have described appear to correlate with the degree of inflammatory response to giardia infection. In the case reported by Morecki and Parker[3] the parasite was seen intraluminally and within some mucosal cells, but there was no increase in leukocytes in the mucosa or submucosa; the roentgen appearance of the small bowel was described as normal. On the other hand, in the first of the patients described by Hoskins,[2] the jejunal biopsy showed marked infiltration of the lamina propria and crypt epithelium. In this patient the small bowel series showed thickened mucosal folds, most marked in the proximal jejunum, and both the jejunal biopsy and the roentgen abnormalities returned to normal following quinacrine therapy.

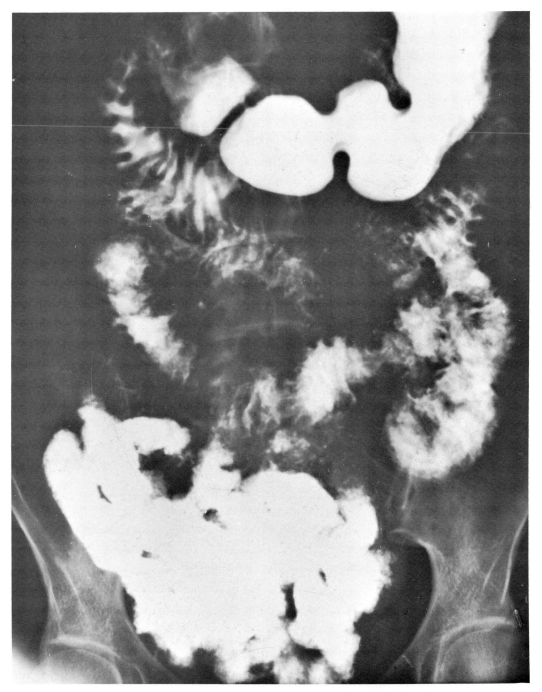

Figure 9-1 Giardiasis. There is marked spasm and irritability of the jejunum, associated with narrowing of the lumen. Thickening of the folds is associated with increased secretions, secondary to the inflammatory edema.

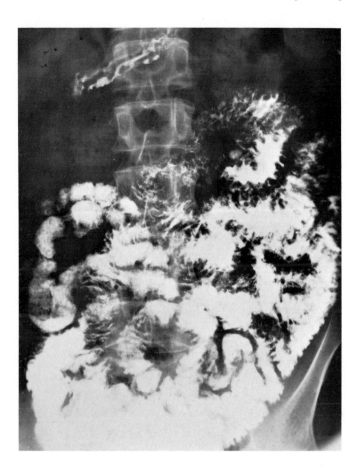

Figure 9-2 Giardiasis. Marked spasm and irritability of the jejunum with slight narrowing of the bowel lumen is noted. The valvulae conniventes are distorted, thickened, and fragmented. The findings in giardiasis are usually limited to the duodenum and jejunum.

When giardiasis complicates a hypogammaglobulinemic enteropathy, the above roentgen changes may be associated with the multiple tiny filling defects of nodular lymphoid hyperplasia (Fig. 9-5) or, less commonly, with the sprue (malabsorption) pattern. Elimination of the parasite results in disappearance of

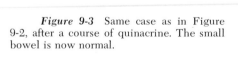

Figure 9-3 Same case as in Figure 9-2, after a course of quinacrine. The small bowel is now normal.

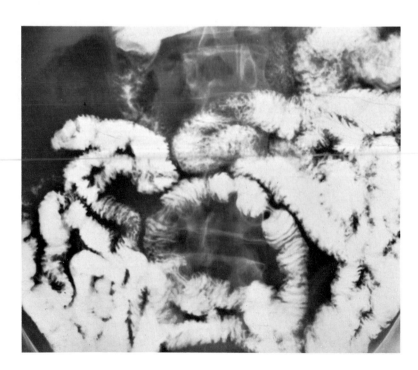

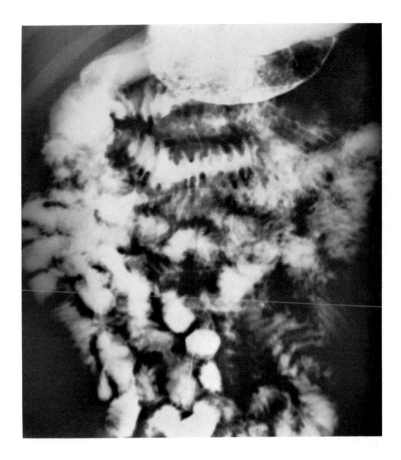

Figure 9-4 *Giardiasis.* Thickening of the valvulae conniventes throughout the visualized portions of the small bowel is identified. The alterations are more prominent in the jejunum.

the inflammatory changes. The number and size of the nodular follicles are not affected, however, by treatment of the Giardia infection.

HOOKWORM

The hookworms infecting man include Necator americanus, which is the common genus in the United States but is also found in Africa and the Far East; Ancylostoma braziliense in Central and South America and in Africa; and Ancylostoma duodenale in the Far East and along the Mediterranean shore.

Hookworms, which have a lifespan of several years, tend to inhabit the proximal small bowel of the infected host. Fertilization occurs in the human small intestine. Ova are passed in the feces and hatch in the soil. Under favorable conditions the larvae grow and penetrate the skin of the host. The larvae enter the blood, reach the lungs, ascend to the pharynx, are swallowed, and reach the intestine where they mature.

Adult worms attach to the mucosa of the small bowel by their buccal capsules, sucking blood and tearing off bits of mucosa, thus, it has been presumed, causing chronic inflammation and anemia. Actual invasion of the intestinal wall by the parasite appears to be uncommon.

Reports in the literature have been in conflict concerning the intestinal reaction in patients with hookworm infection. Reports such as that of Sheehy et al.[11] indicate that symptomatic patients with hookworm disease can be shown to

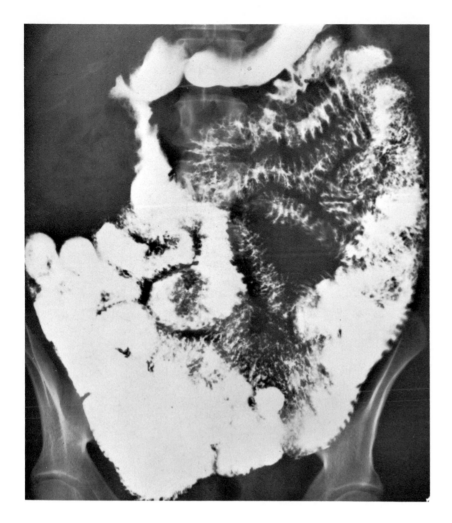

Figure 9-5 *Giardiasis and hypo-gammaglobulinemia.* There is moderate thickening of the valvulae conniventes in the jejunum, associated with slight rigidity and narrowing of the lumen. These changes are secondary to giardiasis. Numerous tiny filling defects, due to lymphoid hyperplasia, are also seen within the lumen of the jejunum; these changes are presumed to be secondary to the hypogammaglobulinemia. Giardiasis is a common finding in patients with hypogammaglobulinemia.

have morphologic inflammatory changes on small bowel biopsy and also biochemical evidence of malabsorption; both the mucosal changes and the malabsorption disappear after treatment and eradication of the parasite. On the other hand, a number of more recent studies[10, 11] demonstrate, on small bowel biopsy, inflammatory changes which vary from being merely mild to moderately severe; these do not change significantly after treatment and clinical improvement, and fail to correlate with malabsorption. The interpretation of small bowel biopsy changes is difficult in tropical populations in which malnutrition and other enteric infections are also common. For the time being, however, it would appear that one must be cautious in attributing inflammatory changes in the small bowel and malabsorption syndrome to hookworm infection.

The symptoms of acute intestinal hookworm infection include abdominal tenderness and discomfort, anorexia, nausea and vomiting, diarrhea, and flatulence. When the infection becomes chronic, long-standing diarrhea and anemia occur. Tetrachlorethylene is the treatment of choice and is effective in approximately 90 per cent of cases.

The roentgen findings on small bowel examination resemble those of giardiasis, with thickening and distortion of the folds in the proximal intestine and increased secretions. (Fig. 9-6). The radiologic features suggest a mild

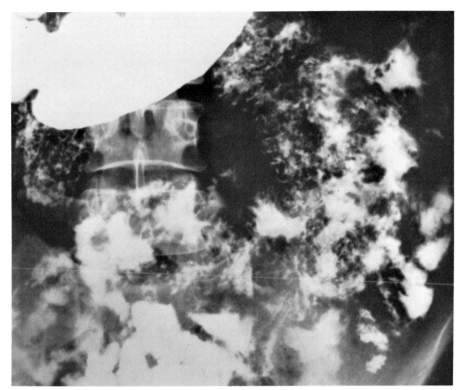

***Figure 9-6** Hookworm infection.* There is thickening of the jejunal folds with spasm, irritability, and increased secretions. Slight segmentation and fragmentation are also noted. These changes resemble the findings in giardiasis and are probably inflammatory.

inflammatory reaction. In view of the difficulties in evaluating pathologic changes in the small bowel in hookworm infestation, the roentgen findings require further study and correlation with clinical and pathologic manifestations.

STRONGYLOIDES STERCORALIS

Strongyloides ova and larvae resemble those of hookworm. The adult worms inhabit the mucosal crypts of the proximal small bowel. Although hookworms are only attached to the mucosa, Strongyloides larvae and adults invade the mucosa, causing inflammation, fibrosis, and sometimes granuloma formation. Autoinfection is a phenomenon of Strongyloides infestation, for larvae may develop within the bowel and penetrate the intestinal mucosa or the perianal skin, producing a developmental cycle within the host.

The patient with Strongyloides infection may be asymptomatic or may have abdominal symptoms of pain, diarrhea, nausea and vomiting, flatulence, and malabsorption.[14] Autoinfection may lead to hepatitis, pneumonia, severe diarrhea, and fever. Effective treatment of strongyloides infestation is provided by a course of thiabendazole.

Roentgen findings in Strongyloides infection are those of inflammatory

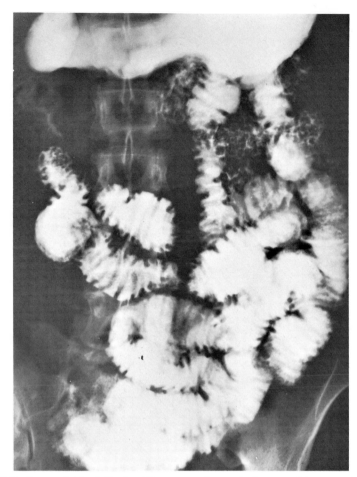

Figure 9-7 Strongyloides infection. There is moderate thickening of the jejunal folds.

disease in the proximal small bowel, with edema, ulceration, and in advanced cases stenosis. The ileum and colon are usually normal radiologically (Fig. 9-7).

TAPEWORM

Tapeworms inhabit the small bowel of man, and although the patient usually remains asymptomatic, the worms may be responsible for abdominal pain and distention, flatulence, and nausea. Treatment with quinacrine (Atabrine) is effective.

Occasionally the adult tapeworm may be visualized radiologically. Characteristically it appears in the lower jejunum or ileum as a long, gradually tapering radiolucent line within the barium column (Figs. 9-8 and 9-9). The worm may become folded upon itself because of its great length. The tapeworm has no alimentary canal.

The tapeworm can be distinguished from Ascaris because of its greater length and because of the absence of the thread of barium often found within the alimentary tract of Ascaris.

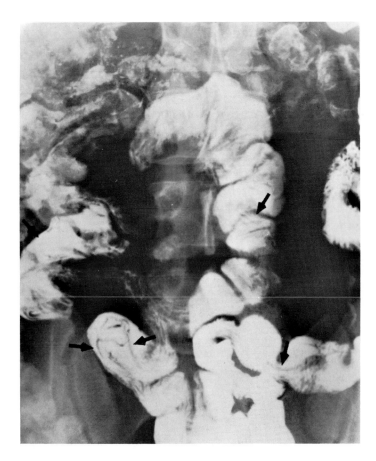

Figure 9-8 Tapeworm infection. Several radiolucent stripes are seen in various segments of the small bowel.

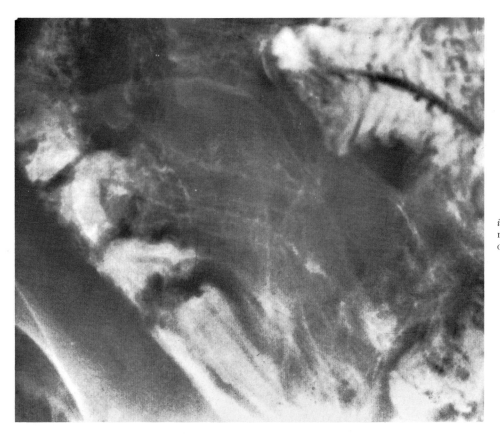

Figure 9-9 Tapeworm infection. There are numerous radiolucent stripes in the lumen of the bowel.

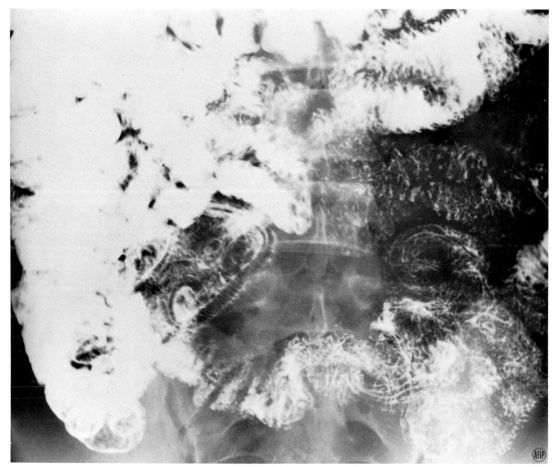

Figure 9-10 *Ascaris infection.* Multiple ascarides are outlined by barium in the small bowel. The alimentary tracts of several worms contain ingested barium. (Courtesy of Dr. Maurice Reeder, Armed Forces Institute of Pathology.)

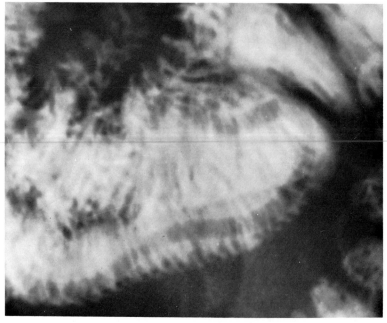

Figure 9-11 *Ascaris in a loop of jejunum.*

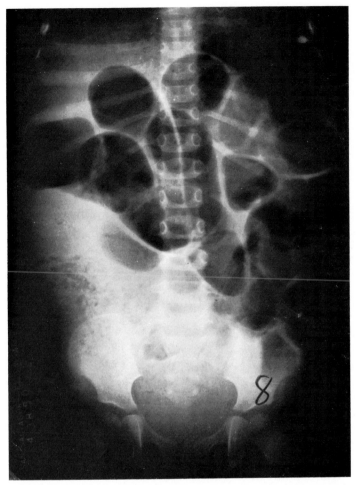

Figure 9–12   Ascaris infection. The ascarides produce multiple defects in the terminal ileum and cecum. (Courtesy of Dr. Maurice Reeder, Armed Forces Institute of Pathology.)

Larval forms of tapeworm, which sometimes develop in soft tissues, may calcify, becoming visible on plain abdominal films.

ASCARIS LUMBRICOIDES

Ascaris lumbricoides, the largest intestinal roundworm that infects man, inhabits the small bowel. In mild infections the worm causes no symptoms, but presence of larger numbers may cause abdominal pain and masses of worms may produce intestinal obstruction, volvulus, or intussusception. Treatment with piperazine is effective.

On small bowel examination the outlines of the worms stand out clearly as radiolucent filling defects within the barium column. They are long, smooth, cylindrical, and sometimes coiled in outline (Figs. 9-10 and 9-11). If the patient has been fasting before the examination the Ascaris may ingest barium, and its alimentary tract will then be seen as a thread-like string along the length of the worm's body. Masses of Ascaris worms can occasionally be visualized without the use of contrast media. So many worms may be present that the abdomen is distended, and numerous positive shadows may be seen against the gas in the bowel (Fig. 9-12).

References

1. Peterson, G. M.: Intestinal changes in giardia lamblia infestation. *Amer. J. Roentgen.*, 77:670-677, 1957.
2. Hoskins, L. C., Winawer, S. J., Broitman, S. A., Gottlieb, L. S., and Zamcheck, N.: Clinical giardiasis and intestinal malabsorption. *Gastroenterology*, 53:265-279, 1967.
3. Morecki, R., and Parker, J. G.: Ultrastructural studies of the human Giardia lamblia and subjacent jejunal mucosa in a subject with steatorrhea. *Gastroenterology*, 52:151-164, 1967.
3a. Petersen, H.: Giardiasis (Lambliasis). *Scand. J. Gastroenterol.* 7: Supplement 14, 1–44, 1972.
4. Yardley, J. H., and Bayless, T. M.: Giardiasis. *Gastroenterology*, 52:301-304, 1967.
5. Marshak, R. H., Hazzi, C., Lindner, A. E., and Maklansky, D.: Small bowel in immunoglobulin deficiency syndromes. *Amer. J. Roentgen.*, 122:227-240, 1974.
6. Brandborg, L. L., Tankersley, C. B., Gottlieb, S., Barancik, M., and Sartor, V. E.: Histological demonstration of mucosal invasion by Giardia lamblia in man. *Gastroenterology*, 52:143-150, 1967.
7. Welch, P. B. Giardiasis with unusual findings. *Gastroenterology*, 3:98-102, 1944.
8. Hermans, P. E., Huizenga, K. A., Hoffman, H. N., II, Brown, A. L., Jr., and Markowitz, H.: Dysgammaglobulinemia associated with nodular lymphoid hyperplasia of the small intestine. *Amer. J. Med.*, 40:78-89, 1966.
9. Hodgson, J. R., Hoffman, H. N., II, and Huizenga, K. A.: Roentgenologic features of lymphoid hyperplasia of the small intestine associated with dysgammaglobulinemia. *Radiology*, 88:883-888, 1967.
10. Marshak, R. H., Ruoff, M., and Lindner, A. E.: Roentgen manifestations of giardiasis. *Amer. J. Roentgen.*, 104:557-560, 1968.
11. Sheehy, T. W., Meroney, W. H., Cox, R. S., Jr., and Soler, J. E.: Hookworm disease and malabsorption. *Gastroenterology*, 42:148-156, 1962.
12. Cuttani, H. K., Puri, S. K., and Misra, R. C. Small intestine in hookworm disease. *Gastroenterology*, 53:381-388, 1967.
13. Aziz, M. A., and Siddqui, A. R.: Morphological and absorption studies of small intestine in hookworm disease (ancylostomiasis) in West Pakistan. *Gastroenterology*, 55:242-250, 1968.
14. Milner, P. F., Irvine, R. A., Barton, C. J., Bras, G., and Richards, R.: Intestinal malabsorption in Strongyloides stercoralis infestation. *Gut*, 6:574-581, 1965.

10

The Small Bowel in Immunoglobulin Deficiency Syndromes

Congenital agammaglobulinemia was first described by Bruton[1] in 1952. Not long after, it became apparent that various degrees of *acquired hypo*gammaglobulinemia are much more frequent and that gastrointestinal disturbances are common findings in the immunoglobulin deficiency syndromes. In fact, diarrhea and steatorrhea were features of the first reported case of idiopathic acquired (late onset) hypogammaglobulinemia in 1954.[2] A few years later hypogammaglobulinemia was found in association with occasional cases of sprue syndrome[3] and with pernicious anemia and atrophic gastritis.[4,5] In the mid-1960s a unique group of patients with hypogammaglobulinemia was identified,[6] characterized by nodular lymphoid hyperplasia of the small bowel mucosa and submucosa, diarrhea, and an unusual susceptibility to infection with Giardia lamblia. This infection has also been detected with remarkable frequency in other immunodeficiency syndromes.[7]

The purpose of this chapter is to review the clinical and radiological features of small bowel involvement in the various immunodeficiency (hypogammaglobulinemic) syndromes.

Immunological Background

Recent advances in clinical immunology have contributed greatly to our understanding of the pathogenesis of disease related to immune mechanisms. The body's immunologic defenses fall into two broad groups: (1) humoral immunity, vested in a protein component of the serum called the immunoglobulins, or antibodies; and (2) cellular or delayed immunity which resides in the lymphocytes.

The immunoglobulins are gamma globulins when measured by serum protein electrophoresis. They are classified according to antigenic specificity as IgG, IgA, IgM, IgD, and IgE. These globulins are synthesized by different

113

classes of plasma cells. IgG comprises approximately 80 per cent of normal serum gamma globulin. Most of the acquired antibodies are in this group. IgA, making up approximately 15 per cent of normal serum gamma globulin, exhibits a variety of antimicrobial activities. IgA is the principal type of antibody present in external secretions—that is, in saliva and in bronchial and intestinal secretions. In the small bowel, IgA is formed in plasma cells in the intestinal mucosa and enters the intestinal epithelial cells where conjugation to another protein ("secretory piece") takes place and the larger molecule is secreted as "secretory IgA" into the intestinal lumen. IgM, comprising perhaps 5 per cent of total serum gamma globulins, are large molecules that include such familiar antibodies as the hemagglutinins and some of the heterophile antibodies. IgD, constituting only a tiny fraction of serum gamma globulin, is of unknown significance, and IgE antibodies appear to be responsible for immediate hypersensitivity reactions such as atopic dermatitis and allergic asthma.

Structurally the immunoglobulins are symmetrical molecules made up of two pairs of polypeptide chains termed L (light) and H (heavy) chains. The light chains are common to all immunoglobulins; the heavy chains differ in the five principal immunoglobulin families and give them their distinctive characteristics. Bence-Jones proteins are closely related to light chains and are possibly identical to them.

A diffuse increase in serum immunoglobulin is a nonspecific response to many chronic diseases. Neoplastic processes involving plasma cells and lymphocytes (which are the precursors of plasma cells) may cause elevated serum levels of specific immunoglobulins or of their structural units. These appear as "spikes" on the electrophoretic pattern. Such diseases include multiple myeloma, Waldenström's macroglobulinemia, and the heavy chain diseases in which the plasma cells elaborate the H chain of an immunoglobulin (e.g., IgG heavy chain disease and IgA heavy chain disease, which is also termed alpha chain disease). These neoplastic overproductions of specific immunoglobulins may be associated with decreased levels of the other normal immunoglobulins.

Immunologic deficiency states are usually characterized by increased susceptibility to infection. Sex-linked agammaglobulinemia (Bruton) involves an almost complete absence of plasma cells and exceedingly low levels of all the immunoglobulins. The more frequent "common variable," late onset forms of hypogammaglobulinemia include a variety of disorders with low serum levels of one or more of the immunoglobulin classes, but not as low as in Bruton's disease.

The second form of the body's immunologic defenses is cellular or delayed immunity. This mechanism does not involve the immunoglobulins but is dependent upon lymphocytes that have been conditioned or processed by passage through the thymus gland. Because of their thymic origin, these thymus-dependent lymphocytes have been called T-lymphocytes. The T-lymphocytes are not antibody-forming cells in themselves nor do they evolve into antibody-producing cells.

Cells that produce antibodies (immunoglobulins) derive from a distinctive population of lymphocytes. Like the T-cells, they originate in the bone marrow, but they do not require processing in the thymus gland. Such lymphocytes are called B-cells, in recognition of their relationship to the bone marrow. It is the B-cells that are the precursors of the plasma cells.

B-cells and T-cells may share functions and influence each other. In some patients there is evidence that hypogammaglobulinemia may be caused or perpetuated by an abnormality of regulatory T-cells, which act to suppress B-cell maturation and antibody production.[8]

CLASSIFICATION

The enteropathic immunoglobulin deficiencies are predominantly of the acquired, adult-onset type, since the infantile forms are rarely associated with gastrointestinal symptoms.[9] They may be either primary (idiopathic) or secondary to some other disease involving the gastrointestinal tract, such as the exudative enteropathies and various lymphoreticular malignancies.

For the purposes of this chapter, it is useful to classify the various immunoglobulin disorders associated with gastrointestinal manifestations into the following main groups (Table 10–1):

I. Primary Immunoglobulin Disorders with Gastrointestinal Manifestations

    A. Variable Immunoglobulin Deficiency
        1. Hypogammaglobulinemic sprue.[3,10] Uniform depression of all immunoglobulin levels, with malabsorption and villous atrophy, but with absence of plasma cells in the lamina propria and no response to gluten exclusion.
        2. Hypogammaglobulinemia with pernicious anemia[5] and atrophic gastritis, but with absence of antibodies to parietal cells and intrinsic factor, frequent lack of response of the B_{12} malabsorption to exogenous intrinsic factor, and lack of the expected elevation of the fasting serum gastrin level.[11] There is villous atrophy and lack of plasma cells in the small bowel.
        3. Nodular lymphoid hyperplasia of the small bowel.[6] The immunoglobulin defect is incomplete and affects especially IgA and IgM in most cases. There is malabsorption and a high incidence of intestinal

Table 10–1.   *Immunoglobulin Disorders with Gastrointestinal Manifestations: Clinical Classification*

I. PRIMARY
    A. *Variable Immunoglobulin Deficiency*
        1. Hypogammaglobulinemic sprue
        2. Hypogammaglobulinemia with pernicious anemia and atrophic gastritis
        3. Nodular lymphoid hyperplasia of the small bowel and giardiasis
    B. *Selective IgA Deficiency*
        1. IgA deficient sprue
        2. Nodular lymphoid hyperplasia of the small bowel (uncommon)
II. SECONDARY
    A. Decreased immunoglobulin synthesis or increased synthesis of abnormal immunoglobulins (e.g., plasma cell dyscrasias, including Waldenström's macroglobulinemia and alpha-chain disease, lymphosarcoma, chronic lymphatic leukemia)
    B. Increased immunoglobulin breakdown and loss (e.g., exudative gastroenteropathies, intestinal lymphangiectasia)
    C. Amyloidosis

infection with Giardia lamblia, Strongyloides, Monilia, bacteria, and possibly viruses. Respiratory infections are frequent. The villi appear normal on small bowel biopsy, but there are few or no plasma cells found; lymphoid aggregates are seen.

B. Selective IgA Deficiency

    1. IgA deficient sprue.[12, 13] Isolated IgA deficiency with gluten enteropathy, villous atrophy and presence of ample plasma cells in the lamina propria, although these are abnormal in that they contain IgM and no IgA. There is no unusual susceptibility to infection.

    2. Isolated IgA deficiency with nodular lymphoid hyperplasia also occurs.[14]

It must be noted that in some instances a single patient will show a combination of features, such as nodular lymphoid hyperplasia and Giardiasis together with sprue-like villus atrophy,[15] rendering his disease difficult to classify according to the above scheme. There is an increased incidence of gastric[16] and colonic[17] carcinoma as well as lymphoma of the bowel[18] in all these enteropathic types of immunoglobulin deficiency.

One or more of the following factors may contribute to the etiology of the malabsorption that is so frequent in primary hypogammaglobulinemia: intramural intestinal infection, intraluminal bacterial overgrowth, Giardia lamblia, gastric achlorhydria, pancreatic insufficiency, and gluten sensitivity. The intestinal mucosal alterations may be secondary to infection by bacteria or parasites and often improve after their eradication.[7, 9]

II. Secondary Immunoglobulin Disorders with Gastrointestinal Manifestations

A. Decreased immunoglobulin synthesis and/or increased synthesis of abnormal immunoglobulin fragments. This disorder is found in Waldenström's macroglobulinemia, alpha-chain disease and other plasma cell dyscrasias. It has also been found in well-differentiated lymphosarcoma (lymphocytic lymphoma) and chronic lymphatic leukemia. It is of interest that whereas these latter two represent disorders of humoral immunity, Hodgkin's disease reflects a derangement of T-cell function and cell-mediated immunity.[19]

    Alpha-chain disease ("Mediterranean lymphoma") is a condition characterized by a diffuse plasma cell proliferation affecting the IgA secretory system and synthesizing an abnormal immunoglobulin fragment which is part of the heavy chain of IgA (alpha-chain).[20, 21] In nearly all cases the plasma cell infiltrate has involved the whole length of the small intestine and mesenteric lymph nodes, although a respiratory form of the disease has also been reported. The clinical picture is usually that of a severe malabsorption syndrome affecting males or females, generally in their second or third decades. The serum contains a free alpha-chain with reduced levels of IgG, IgM, and albumin. The pathologic counterpart is an abdominal lymphoma, originally termed "Mediterranean lymphoma" because of the peculiar ethnographic distribution of most of the earlier reported cases. Whether alpha-chain disease starts as a benign hyperplastic process or is malignant from its onset has not been determined.

B. Increased immunoglobulin breakdown and loss secondary to exudative gastroenteropathies, including intestinal lymphangiectasia.[22] The effect is similar to the losses that occur with the nephrotic syndrome and exfoliative dermatitides. The major fall here is in IgG associated with loss of albumin, together with lymphopenia when secondary to intestinal lymphangiectasia.

C. Amyloidosis.[23] Nonspecific immunoglobulin abnormalities, such as elevated or depressed serum levels of IgA, IgG, and IgM, are frequently encountered in all types of amyloidosis, while M-components are found in the serum or urine of most patients with amyloidosis associated with lymphoproliferative disorders.

ROENTGEN FEATURES

With this clinical classification in mind, we have organized the roentgenographic manifestations of the enteropathic immunoglobulin deficiency syndromes into the following groups:

1. *Sprue (malabsorption) pattern,* as seen in hypogammaglobulinemic sprue and in IgA deficient sprue.

2. *Multiple nodular defects,* as seen in variable immunoglobulin deficiency and in lymphoma.

3. *Inflammatory changes* secondary to giardiasis.

4. *Thickening of small intestinal folds,* as in amyloidosis, lymphoma, macroglobulinemia, plasma cell dyscrasias, and intestinal lymphangiectasia.

The roentgen alterations are not necessarily confined to just one of the above findings and a patient may exhibit more than one of these features either simultaneously or on successive examinations.

Sprue (Malabsorption) Pattern

The roentgen findings in hypogammaglobulinemic sprue and in IgA deficient sprue are indistinguishable from those seen in celiac sprue, with dilatation of the small bowel, segmentation, fragmentation and scattering of the barium column, and with hypersecretion causing dilution of barium distally (Fig. 10–1). Transient nonobstructive intussusceptions may be observed.

Rarely a sprue pattern is seen in diffuse intestinal lymphosarcoma. In such patients the distinctive roentgen features of lymphosarcoma are also present, such as nodularity, ulceration, and irregular thickening of the folds.

Multiple Nodular Defects

Multiple nodular defects are most commonly seen in association with immunoglobulin variable disease, selective IgA deficiency, and lymphosarcoma.

Nodular lymphoid hyperplasia associated with hypogammaglobulinemia predominantly affects the small intestine. Less frequently the colon and rectum are involved. The characteristic roentgen feature is a uniform distribution throughout the involved segment of intestine of innumerable tiny, smooth, nodular filling defects measuring 1 to 3 mm. in diameter.[16] The nodules are

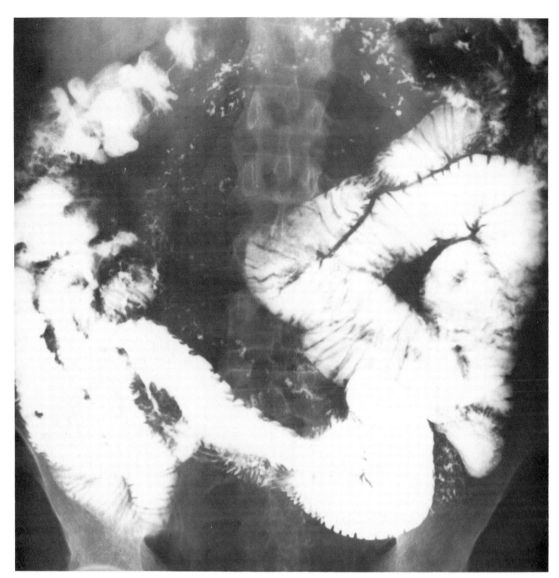

Figure 10-1 *Hypogammaglobulinemic sprue.* The roentgen alterations are indistinguishable from celiac sprue. They include dilatation, especially of the jejunum, associated with thinning of the folds, fragmentation, segmentation, and increased secretions. Hypogammaglobulinemic sprue is rare and a diagnosis by roentgen examination alone cannot be made.

round and regular in outline and are not associated with other mucosal alterations. The small bowel is not dilated and the valvulae conniventes are not thickened or blunted. Microscopic examination of a peroral small bowel biopsy specimen reveals the characteristic enlarged lymphoid follicles within the lamina propria causing effacement of the villus pattern of the overlying mucosa and imparting a nodular or polypoid appearance[6] (Fig. 2–9).

Although it is true that nodular lymphoid hyperplasia is usually associated with immunoglobulin abnormalities, it can be seen in the absence of such serum alterations. Normal serum values are more common when it is the colon that is involved. In children and young adults the terminal ileum alone may

(Text continued on page 123.)

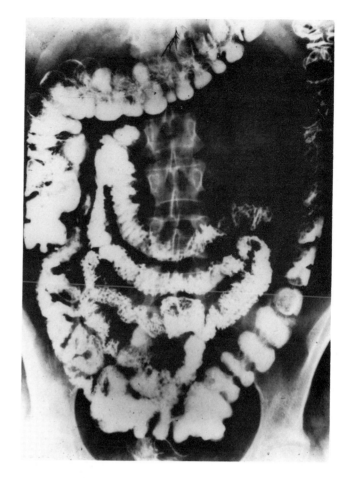

Figure 10-2 Variable immunoglobulin deficiency. This patient was investigated because of diarrhea. Her IgA levels were markedly reduced, with borderline IgG and IgM. There are numerous small, symmetrical 2–4 mm. nodules throughout the jejunum and ileum without evidence of ulceration. It is of interest that despite the administration of 20 fluid ounces of barium, the nodules were easily demonstrated. The colon is normal.

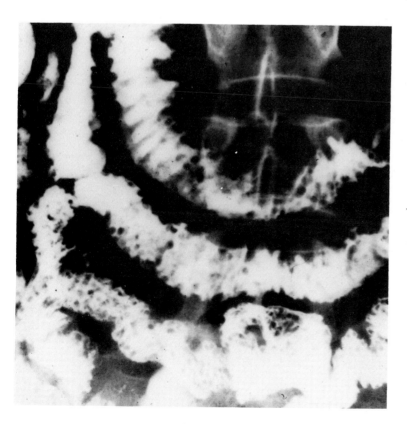

Figure 10-3 Variable immunoglobulin deficiency. (Magnified view of Figure 10-2.) Symmetrical small nodules are identified. This is an excellent example of the typical nodules of nodular lymphoid hyperplasia.

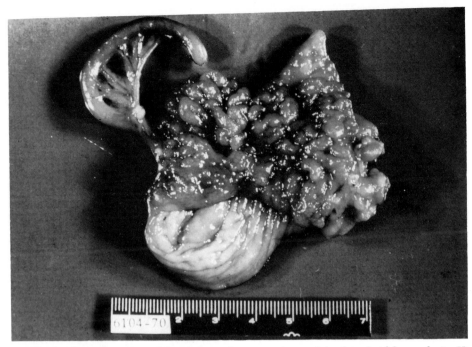

Figure 10–4 *Specimen of distal ileum demonstrating nodular lymphoid hyperplasia.* Histologic section revealed marked lymphoid hyperplasia. The appendix is visualized and is normal.

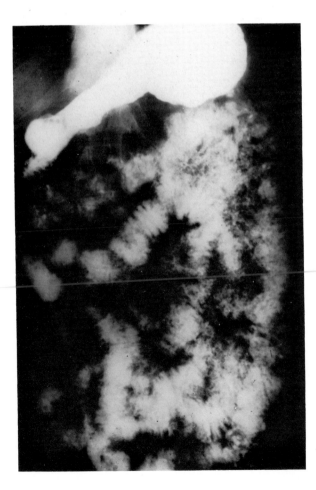

Figure 10–5 *Variable immunoglobulin deficiency with reduced IgA, IgG and IgM.* Numerous small nodules are seen distributed throughout the small bowel.

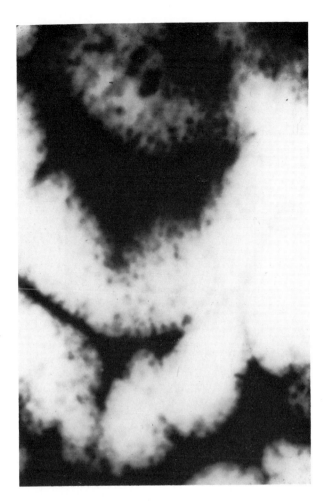

Figure 10–6 *(Same patient as Figure 10–5. Magnified view.)* The nodules are well demonstrated. They are characteristically small, round, regular, symmetrical, and demonstrate no evidence of ulceration.

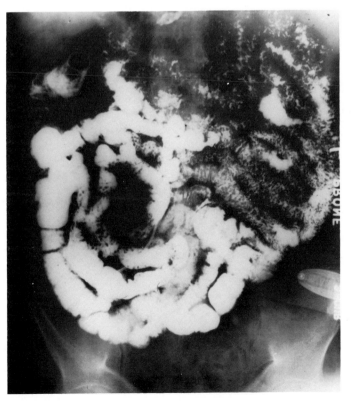

Figure 10–7 *Selective immunoglobulin A deficiency.* There are numerous tiny nodules distributed throughout the entire small bowel, best visualized in the distal jejunum and proximal ileum. There is no evidence of increased secretions or ulcerations. This patient had vague abdominal complaints with diarrhea. Follow-up studies revealed no change after a period of three years. Small bowel biopsy confirmed the diagnosis of nodular lymphoid hyperplasia.

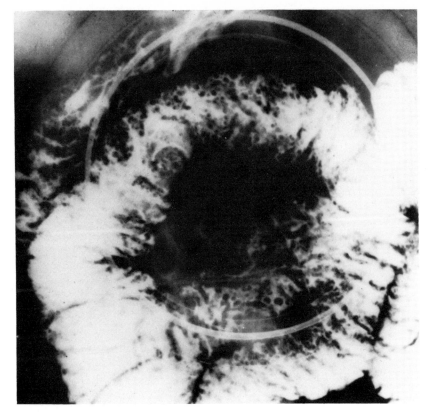

Figure 10-8 *(Same patient as Figure 10-7)*. Close-up of distal duodenum and jejunum, exquisitely delineating the tiny nodules typical of nodular lymphoid hyperplasia.

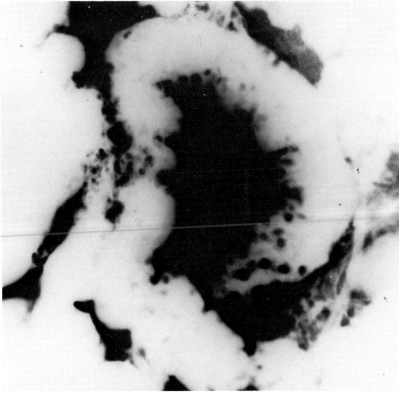

Figure 10-9 *(Same patient as Figures 10-7 and 10-8)*. Magnified view of ileum. The multiple small nodules described above are again seen throughout the ileum.

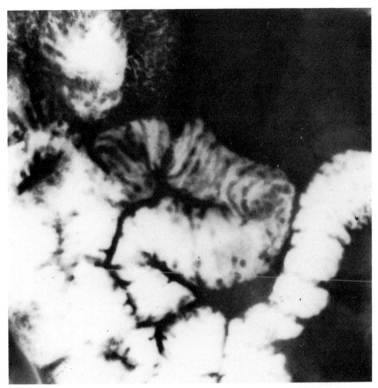

Figure 10–10 *Lymphosarcoma.* This case demonstrates the occasional difficulty in differentiating nodular lymphoid hyperplasia from lymphosarcoma. There are multiple small nodules, varying in size from 3 to 6 mm. in diameter. Some are irregular and others appear submucosal. There is no evidence of ulceration. Because the nodules varied in size, lymphosarcoma could not be excluded and follow-up study was advised.

demonstrate multiple small symmetrical nodules as a normal finding (see Fig. 13–72).

Diffuse lymphosarcoma of the small intestine may also result in multiple nodules visualized on the roentgen study. These are usually larger and may produce irregular scalloping of the bowel contour or a cobblestone appearance. Ulcerations can frequently be demonstrated within the nodules. Rarely it can be very difficult to distinguish nodular lymphoid hyperplasia from lymphosarcoma, and in these patients follow-up roentgen studies and small bowel biopsy may be required for differentiation (Figs. 10–10, 10–11).

Inflammatory Changes Secondary to Giardiasis

The roentgen findings in Giardia lamblia infection are inflammatory in character and are usually limited to the duodenum and jejunum.[24] There is spasm and irritability, slight narrowing of the lumen with thickening, and distortion of the folds. Increased intestinal secretions frequently cause blurring of the folds and sometimes fragmentation and slight segmentation of the barium column. Transit through the jejunum may be rapid. The ileum usually appears normal (Fig. 10–12. See also Fig. 9–1 and Fig. 9–2).

When giardiasis complicates a hypogammaglobulinemia enteropathy, the above roentgen changes may be associated with the multiple tiny filling defects

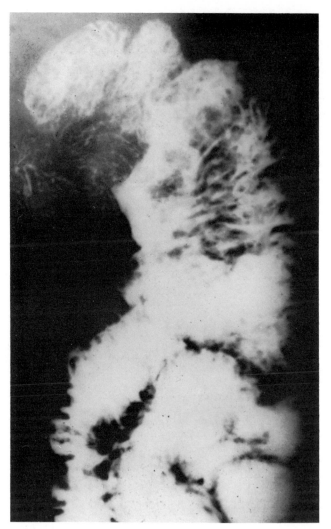

Figure 10–11 Lymphosarcoma. Same patient as Figure 10–10 four months later. There is a segment in midjejunum measuring three inches in length in which the mucosa is ulcerated, with a nodular configuration along the contours. There is no obstruction. Some of the tiny defects previously described are seen in adjacent loops of bowel. At surgery, almost the entire small bowel was involved with lymphosarcoma. (Courtesy of Dr. Roger Blahut.)

of nodular lymphoid hyperplasia (see Fig. 9–5), or, less commonly, with the sprue (malabsorption) pattern. Eradication of the parasite results in return of the fold pattern to normal as well as improvement of the villus structure in hypogammaglobulinemic sprue,[7] regression of diarrhea, steatorrhea and malabsorption, and of lactose intolerance and abnormal intestinal protein loss.[9] The number and size of the nodular follicles are not affected, however, by treatment of the Giardia infection.

It is important to note that the presence of Giardia lamblia in the stool does not necessarily mean that the small bowel roentgen study will be abnormal; indeed, small bowel changes are not seen in most patients with giardiasis. In epidemics of the infection and in patients with hypogammaglobulinemia the roentgen studies are more likely to be abnormal. Conversely, Giardia lamblia may be absent from the stool yet be present on duodenal aspirate or small bowel biopsy.

Thickening of the Small Intestine Folds

Thickening of the small bowel folds is not characteristic of the primary enteropathic immunodeficiencies, as classified earlier in this text, except for superimposed Giardia lamblia infection. It is, however, a feature of the secondary immunoglobulin disorders.

Amyloidosis, by infiltration of the bowel wall, produces conspicuous thickening of the folds and this process tends to be uniform throughout the entire small bowel on roentgen study.[25] Enlargement of the folds in the ileum gives an appearance resembling the normal feathery pattern of the jejunum, a configuration that has been termed "jejunization of the ileum." There is no significant dilatation or increase in secretions, and nodules are not present (see Fig. 6–1).

When amyloidosis involves the colon, it produces roentgen alterations that are similar to those of chronic ulcerative colitis, with absent haustral markings but no significant shortening (Figs. 10–13, 10–14). Ascites is often present and can be recognized by separation of the loops of small bowel. In the stomach

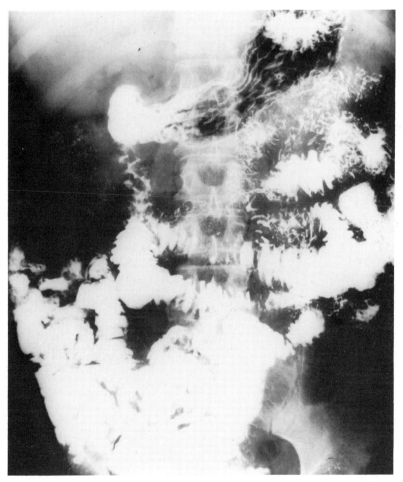

Figure 10–12 *Giardiasis.* There is moderate thickening of the duodenal and jejunal folds, associated with slight spasm.

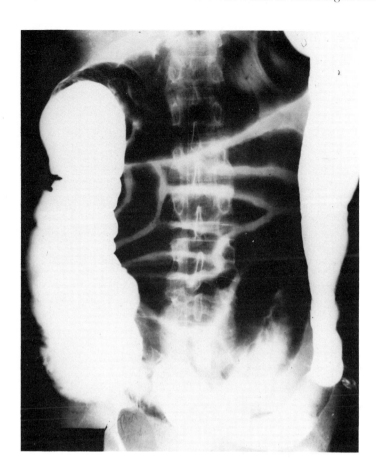

Figure 10–13 Amyloidosis. There is a complete absence of the haustral markings throughout the colon, and the configuration resembles ulcerative colitis. The air-filled loops of small bowel are separated by the presence of fluid in the abdomen.

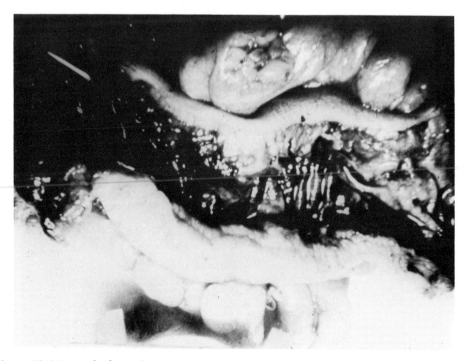

Figure 10–14 Amyloidosis. Gross specimen reveals marked thickening of the wall. This thickening is responsible for the roentgen findings described above.

amyloid infiltration produces a polypoid tumor or features similar to those of scirrhous carcinoma.

Lymphosarcoma may also appear as a smooth, diffuse thickening of the intestinal folds throughout the small bowel, without hypersecretion. The thickened folds are more commonly irregularly nodular, and coarse marginal scalloping of the bowel contour may be seen (see Fig. 20–1).

The roentgenographic features of *alpha-chain disease* are variable. The small intestinal folds may be thickened in an irregular fashion (Fig. 10–15). Multiple nodular defects may be demonstrated having the same characteristics as in lymphosarcoma and involving the whole length of the small bowel. A sprue-like pattern may also be seen with dilatation, which may be quite marked, involving both jejunum and ileum, increased secretions, and flocculation and segmentation of the barium. Masses of enlarged mesenteric lymph nodes may produce extrinsic compression or dislocation of the small bowel.

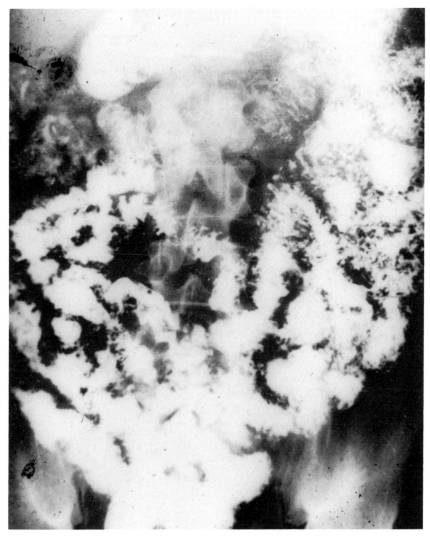

Figure 10–15 Alpha-chain disease. There are numerous small nodules of varying size distributed throughout the small bowel. The roentgen features are indistinguishable from those of diffuse lymphosarcoma, in the cases we have seen.

A group of patients has been described with marked plasma cell and lymphocyte infiltration of the small bowel in whom the process, over a follow-up of years, has not become lymphoma. Such patients have a variety of serum immunoglobulin defects ranging from deficiency to excessive levels. This group probably represents a heterogeneous collection of abnormalities that await classification.[26] They have in common, however, roentgen alterations of thickening of the folds and at times submucosal or intraluminal nodules. Patients with these findings frequently present clinically with diarrhea and malabsorption[5] (Fig. 10–16).

Uniform thickening of the folds of the small bowel is also found in some cases of *Waldenström's macroglobulinemia.*[27] The wall of the intestine is thickened, as evidenced by separation of the loops on small bowel series, and the lumen may be moderately dilated. The mucosal surface itself may have a fine granular appearance, perhaps caused by club-like dilatation and distention of the tips of the villi (see Fig. 22–27). The roentgen characteristics of sprue are not present. It must be said, however, that only a few cases of Waldenström's macro-

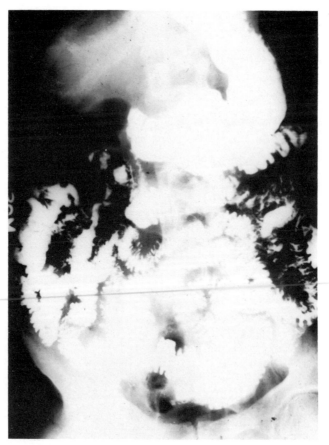

Figure 10–16 *Plasma cell infiltration of the small bowel.* There is moderate thickening of the valvulae conniventes, especially in the jejunum. Increased secretions are present. The relationship of these cases to alpha-chain disease has not been established.

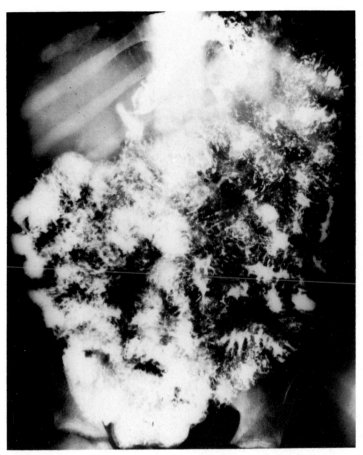

Figure 10–17 Intestinal lymphangiectasia. The entire small bowel is involved. There is minimal segmentation and fragmentation, associated with diffuse thickening of the valvulae conniventes and moderate secretions. There is no dilatation. The serum albumin in this patient was one gram per cent. The alterations described above are probably due to intestinal edema secondary to hypoalbuminemia.

globulinemia involving the intestinal tract have been studied thus far and these observations must be considered provisional.

Intestinal lymphangiectasia is an exudative, protein-losing enteropathy with gross dilatation of the lymphatics of the lamina propria of the small bowel reflecting a generalized disorder of the development of lymphatic channels.[22] Hypogammaglobulinemia, mainly affecting IgG, is associated with a fall in serum albumin and, to a lesser degree, other proteins, as well as with the loss of lymphocytes into the bowel lumen. Enlargement of folds on roentgen examination usually affects both the jejunum and the ileum. The pattern of fold enlargement is uniform, orderly, and symmetrical in a single loop. A stacked-coin appearance is not uncommon and the folds may have a regular biconvex appearance (Figs. 10–17, 10–18). Large folds in the ileum may result in its "jejunization" as described in some cases of amyloidosis. Excessive intestinal secretions result in dilution of the barium column distally in most cases and are an important distinguishing feature. Dilatation is minimal or absent. The thickening of the folds noted radiologically in intestinal lymphangiectasia represents mucosal and submucosal edema secondary to hypoproteinemia.

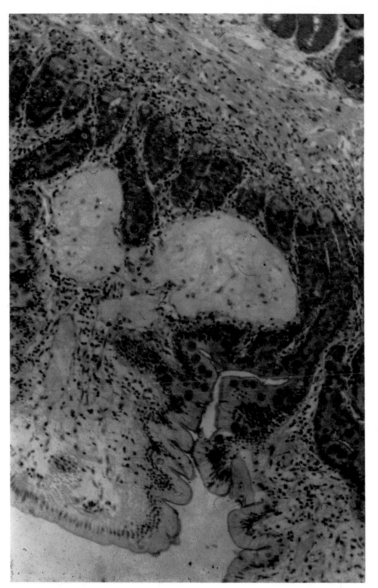

Figure 10–18   *Intestinal lymphangiectasia.* Histologic sections demonstrate marked dilatation of the lymphatics as well as edema of the mucosa.

SUMMARY

Recent advances in immunology have permitted recognition of a group of patients who have gastrointestinal manifestations as part of an immunoglobulin deficiency syndrome. Such immunoglobulin deficiency may be primary or may be secondary to a variety of diseases. We have classified and described the small bowel roentgen features associated with the various immunoglobulin deficiency syndromes as follows: (1) the sprue pattern, as seen in hypogammaglobulinemic sprue and in IgA deficient sprue; (2) multiple nodular defects; (3) inflammatory changes secondary to Giardiasis, associated with immune deficiency diseases; (4) thickening of the small intestinal folds, as seen in the plasma cell dyscrasias, lymphoma, intestinal lymphangiectasia, and amyloidosis.

References

1. Bruton, O. C.: Agammaglobulinemia. *Pediatrics*, 9:722–728, 1952.
2. Sanford, J. P., Favour, C. B., and Tribeman, M. S.: Absence of serum gamma globulins in an adult. *New Eng. J. Med.*, 250:1027–1029, 1954.
3. Cohen, N., Paley, D., and Janowitz, H. D.: Acquired hypogammaglobulinemia and sprue: Report of a case and review of the literature. *J. Mount Sinai Hosp.* N.Y., 28:421–427, 1962.
4. Lewis, E. C. II, and Brown, H. E. Jr.: Agammaglobulinemia associated with pernicious anemia and diabetes mellitus. *Arch. Intern. Med.*, 100:296–299, 1957.
5. Twomey, J. J., Jordan, P. H., Jarrold, T., et al.: The syndrome of immunoglobulin deficiency and pernicious anemia. *Amer. J. Med.*, 47:340–350, 1969.
6. Hermans, P. E., Huizenga, K. A., Hoffman, H. N. II, et al.: Dysgammaglobulinemia associated with nodular lymphoid hyperplasia of the small intestine. *Amer. J. Med.*, 40:78–89, 1966.
7. Ament, M. E., and Rubin, C. E.: Relation of Giardiasis to abnormal intestinal structure and function in gastrointestinal immunodeficiency syndromes. *Gastroenterology*, 62:216–226, 1972.
8. Waldman, T. A., Broder, S., Blaese, R. M., et al.: Role of suppressor T cells in pathogenesis of common variable hypogammaglobulinemia. *Lancet*, 2:609–613, 1974.
9. Ament, M. E., Ochs, H. D., and Davis, S. D.: Structure and function of the gastrointestinal tract in primary immunodeficiency syndromes: a study of 39 patients. *Medicine*, (Balt.) 52:227–248, 1973.
10. Eidelman, S., Davis, S. D., and Rubin, C. E.: Immunologic studies in "hypogammaglobulinemic sprue." *Clin. Res.*, 16:117, 1968.
11. Hughes, W. S., Brooks, P. E., and Conn, H. O.: Serum gastrin levels in primary hypogammaglobulinemia and pernicious anemia: Studies in adults. *Ann. Intern. Med.*, 77:746–750, 1972.
12. Crabbe, P. A., and Hermans, J. F.: Lack of gamma-A-immunoglobulin in serum of patients with steatorrhea. *Gut*, 7:119–127, 1966.
13. Mawhinney, H., and Tomkin, G. H.: Gluten enteropathy associated with selective IgA deficiency. *Lancet*, 2:121–124, 1971.
14. Gryboski, J. D., Self, T. W., Clemett, A., et al.: Selective immunoglobulin A deficiency and intestinal nodular lymphoid hyperplasia: Correction of diarrhea with antibiotics and plasma. *Pediatrics*, 42:833–837, 1968.
15. Hughes, W. S., Cerda, J. J., Holtzapple, P., et al.: Primary hypogammaglobulinemia and malabsorption. *Ann. Intern. Med.*, 74:903–910, 1971.
16. Hermans, P. E., and Huizenga, K. A.: Association of gastric carcinoma with idiopathic late-onset immunoglobulin deficiency. *Ann. Intern. Med.*, 76:605–609, 1972.
17. Hodgson, J. R., Hoffman, H. N. II, and Huizenga, K. A.: Roentgenologic features of lymphoid hyperplasia of the small intestine associated with dysgammaglobulinemia. *Radiology*, 88:883–888, 1967.
18. Peterson, R. D. A., Cooper, M. D., and Good, R. A.: The pathogenesis of immunologic deficiency diseases. *Amer. J. Med.*, 38:579–604, 1965.
19. Aisenberg, A. C.: Malignant lymphoma. *New Eng. J. Med.*, 288:883–890, 1973.
20. Rambaud, J. C., and Matuchansky, C.: Alpha-chain disease: Pathogenesis and relation to Mediterranean lymphoma. *Lancet*, 1:1430–1432, 1973.
21. Bonoma, L., Dammacco, F., Marano, R., et al.: Abdominal lymphoma and alpha chain disease. *Amer. J. Med.*, 52:73–86, 1972.
22. Shimkin, P. M., Waldmann, T. A., and Krugman, R. L.: Intestinal lymphangiectasia. *Amer. J. Roentgen.*, 110:827–841, 1970.
23. Glenner, G. G., Ein, D., and Terry, W. D.: The immunoglobulin origin of amyloid. *Amer. J. Med.*, 52:141–147, 1972.
24. Marshak, R. H., Ruoff, M., and Lindner, A. E.: Roentgen manifestations of Giardiasis. *Amer. J. Roentgen.*, 104:557–560, 1968.
25. Korelitz, B. I., and Spindell, L. N.: Gastrointestinal amyloidosis: Report of a case and review of the clinical and radiologic aspects. *J. Mount Sinai Hosp.*, 23:683–696, 1956.
26. Ruoff, M., Lindner, A. E., and Marshak, R. H.: Malabsorption syndrome with plasma cell infiltration of the small bowel. *Amer. J. Gastroenterol.*, 55:602–608, 1971.
27. Khilnani, M. T., Keller, R. J., and Cuttner, J.: Macroglobulinemia and steatorrhea: Roentgen and pathologic findings in the intestinal tract. *Radiol. Clin. N. Amer.*, 7:43–55, 1969.

11

Vascular Disease: Ischemic Ileitis, Jejunitis, and Colitis

Disturbances of the arterial or venous blood supply to the small bowel or colon may be responsible for a variety of clinical manifestations[1] and roentgenographic findings.[2]

The clinical features of vascular occlusion of the bowel are sudden onset of abdominal pain, sometimes associated with vomiting and fever, and passage of blood from the rectum. The episode may vary in severity from a catastrophe of extensive infarction to an incident so mild that the patient does not consult a physician and the event is recalled only in retrospect, perhaps after roentgen examination discloses a lesion.

The consequences of vascular occlusion depend upon the rapidity of onset, the length of gut involved, and the efficiency of the collateral circulation.[1-3] Rapid occlusion of the major vessels supplying the gut results in massive tissue necrosis and death from peritonitis and shock. Such catastrophic events usually allow little opportunity for roentgenographic study and are not reviewed in this chapter. When, however, the insult involves segmental rather than trunk vessels, or when closure is slow enough for collateral flow to provide an adequate blood supply, total infarction of intestine may not occur. In this circumstance complete healing may subsequently take place.

Of great radiologic interest is an intermediate situation in which blood flow is sufficient to prevent death of the intestine yet not adequate for complete recovery of the damaged bowel wall. Such partial recovery may be associated with a variety of pathologic changes, including muscle atrophy or hypertrophy, fibrosis, and stricture formation. These changes may produce roentgenographic features which must be distinguished from inflammatory bowel disease and from tumor.

The layers of a segment of bowel are not equally sensitive to impairment of their blood supply. The mucosa appears to be most dependent on intact blood flow, and the initial change in vascular occlusion is superficial ulceration, often circumferential. The ulcer may subsequently heal or perforate, or, with ensuing fibrosis, produce a stricture. The muscular layers are next involved, but the connective tissue layers of the submucosa and the subserosa may retain viability for considerable periods. Submucosal hemorrhage and edema cause localized nodularity or diffuse thickening of the mucosal folds. Ileus develops, either local or diffuse, and fluid accumulates within the lumen of the damaged gut. After the vascular injury, recovery may be complete, since the intramural blood and edema fluid are resorbed and the ulcerations heal without scars. On the other hand, fibrosis may result from the healing process, causing permanent stricture and proximal dilatation.

Clinically significant impairment of blood supply can occur even in the absence of gross changes in the bowel wall. When blood flow is sufficient to maintain function of the bowel at rest but inadequate to support the work of absorption and transit of a meal, the syndrome of intestinal angina may occur.[4] Characteristic clinical features are anorexia, weight loss, and postprandial abdominal pain. At times intestinal angina may be associated with a biochemically demonstrable malabsorption syndrome.

MESENTERIC THROMBOSES AND EMBOLI

Mesenteric arterial thrombosis is a complication of atherosclerosis. Gradual thrombosis, even if complete, may cause no changes in the gut be-

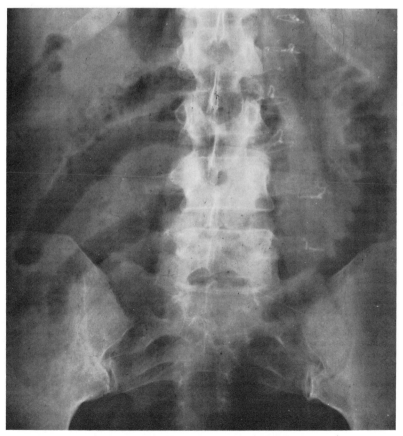

Figure 11–1 Infarction of the small bowel. Two loops of jejunum in the right upper quadrant are moderately narrowed, rigid, and separated. The separation is the result of thickening of the walls, secondary to the venous congestion. The valvulae conniventes are absent. An additional loop of jejunum on the left side is involved to a lesser extent.

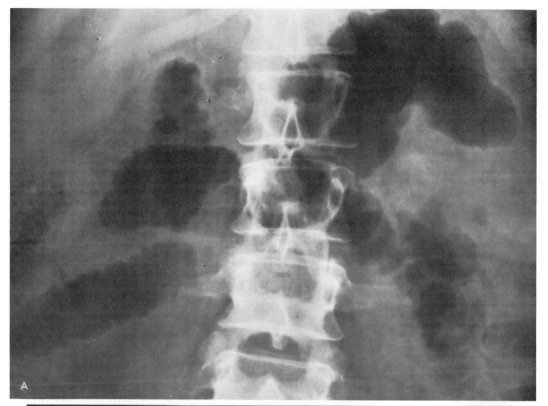

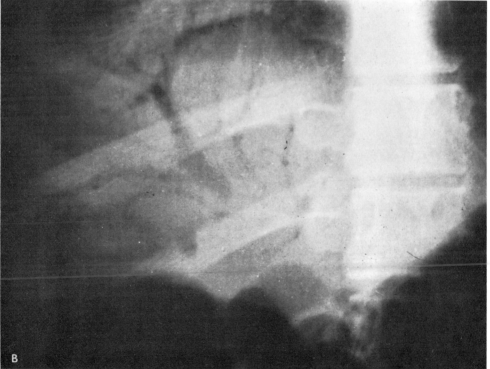

Figure 11-2 A, *Ischemia of the small bowel and colon.* Several gas-filled loops of small bowel and transverse colon are affected. The valvulae conniventes and haustral markings are absent or altered. The bowel wall is thickened and rigid. These changes were due to mesenteric venous thrombosis.

B, *Infarction of small bowel and colon.* Gas in the portal venous system is seen only in severe cases and has not been observed in segmental infarctions.

cause collateral flow is adequate. Sudden occlusion, however, or gradual closure in the absence of collaterals, leads to infarction of the bowel.

Venous thrombosis is less common than arterial thrombosis and tends to occur in diseases characterized by venous impairment, such as thromboangiitis obliterans or thrombophlebitis. It has been reported in association with intra-abdominal infection, polycythemia, pancreatitis, portal hypertension, polyarteritis nodosa, systemic lupus erythematosis, and, recently, with oral contraceptive medications.[2a]

Arterial emboli usually originate as mural thrombi in the heart after a myocardial infarction or as thrombi in a fibrillating atrium. These emboli tend to lodge in the branches of the superior mesenteric artery. It is generally considered that all varieties of vascular accidents involve the branches of the superior mesenteric vessels more commonly than the inferior mesenteric vessels. It has become apparent, however, that segmental vascular occlusion of the colon may be clinically mild, reversible, and difficult to diagnose,[3,5] and is more common than had been thought.

Nonocclusive Mesenteric Ischemia

With the development of angiographic studies and early surgery in the management of acute mesenteric vascular disease, a surprising finding became apparent: in a large proportion of patients with mesenteric infarction, neither thrombosis nor embolism can be demonstrated. This entity, which appears to

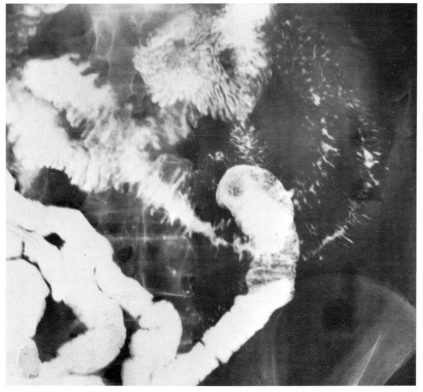

Figure 11–3 Segmental infarction of the small bowel. There is marked spasm and irritability of several jejunal loops as well as separation and uncoiling.

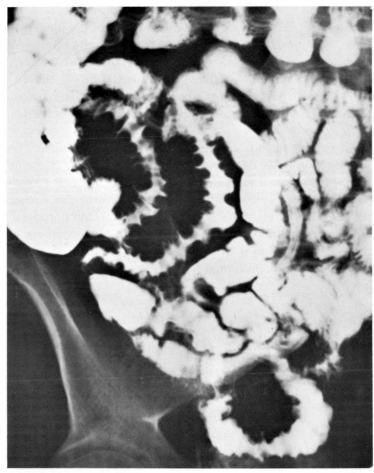

Figure 11–4 Segmental infarction. Moderate narrowing and rigidity of the distal loops of ileum, associated with thickening and blunting of the folds, are shown. The involved loops of bowel are moderately separated. These findings are similar to those of regional enteritis.

be common, has been termed "nonocclusive mesenteric ischemia." Although the mechanisms remain to be clarified, it probably represents a perfusion defect within the wall of the bowel.

SEGMENTAL ISCHEMIC DISEASE

The term "ischemic colitis" has been used to designate the changes that occur in the colon after vascular occlusion.[3] The terms "ischemic ileitis" and "ischemic jejunitis" might be applied to similar processes in the small bowel. The roentgenologic findings in segmental ischemic disease in small bowel and colon are remarkably similar, except for differences in location. Any segment of the small bowel may be involved. In the colon the most common locations appear to be the distal transverse colon, the splenic flexure, and the cecum. Any segment of the colon, however, including the rectum,[6] may be implicated. Right-sided ulcerative colitis is rare. Many such reported cases are probably examples of ischemic disease of the right colon.

A preliminary film of the abdomen is sometimes diagnostic. In the initial stages, no significant alterations may be identified. As the process continues, however, paralytic ileus occurs with edema of the valvulae or haustral markings and thickening of the wall. Fibrinous deposits on the serosa may cause fixation of the loops of bowel (Fig. 11-1). As edema increases, the valvulae or haustra disappear. Segmental dilatation of the colon can be distinct (Fig. 11-2). Localized perforations may be identified; these occur more frequently in the colon, where they appear as pneumatosis coli. The presence of intramural gas and gas in the portal vein are diagnostic signs of infarction.

Barium studies in the early stages reveal a marked degree of spasm associated with separation and uncoiling of the loops (Fig. 11-3). The involved segment may be difficult to fill because of spasm and irritability. The indi-

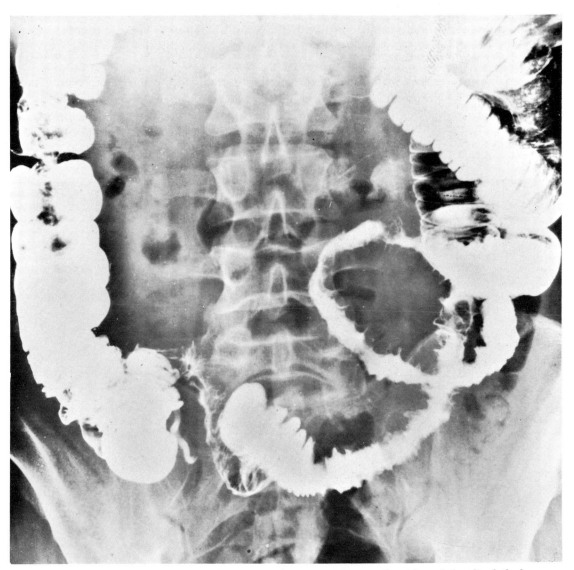

Figure 11-5 Segmental infarction. Moderate narrowing and rigidity of the distal ileal loops is shown. The narrowing is most pronounced in the terminal ileum. The proximal loops are dilated. The mucosal folds are thickened and blurred, and there is increased secretion.

vidual loops of bowel are separated from one another as if by thickening of the mesentery. The bowel lumen is narrowed, but there is no significant proximal dilatation at this stage. The folds are thickened and blunted, and in some segments a rigid picket fence, as seen in regional enteritis, is identified (Fig. 11-4). Multiple indentures, which have been described as "scalloping" or "thumb-printing," are seen along the contours of the bowel (Fig. 11-4). When seen face-on they appear as multiple polypoid filling defects. As edema progresses the folds become more thickened and hazy (Fig. 11-5). Although ulcerations are frequently seen in resected specimens of bowel with ischemic ileitis and colitis, the ulcerations are rarely deep enough to be recognized as individual ulcers on roentgenographic studies. With diffuse ulceration the entire mucosa may be completely effaced, and the barium column presents a smooth, homogeneous configuration.

As healing and fibrosis progress, flattening and rigidity of one border may ensue. The antimesenteric border then becomes pleated or plicated, forming multiple sacculations or pseudodiverticula (Fig. 11-6). As fibrosis continues, a long tubular segment with smooth contours and a concentric lumen is identified, and finally a stricture with proximal dilatation is seen (Figs. 11-7 and 11-8). The strictures may be short, but more commonly they are three or four inches long.

The sequence of findings just described is rapid. In a period of several weeks the lesion progresses from the initial stage of spasm and edema to stricture formation (Figs. 11-9 to 11-12). In the stages before fibrosis develops,

(Text continued on page 142.)

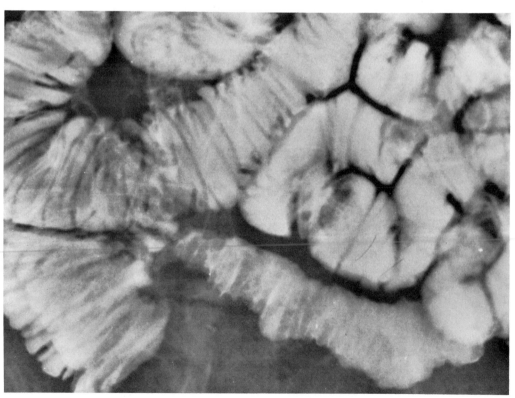

Figure 11–6 Segmental infarction. In a view during the healing stage, a loop of proximal ileum reveals slight narrowing, slight thickening of the folds, and rigidity. The inferior aspect of the loop is irregular as a result of pseudodiverticula or sacculations.

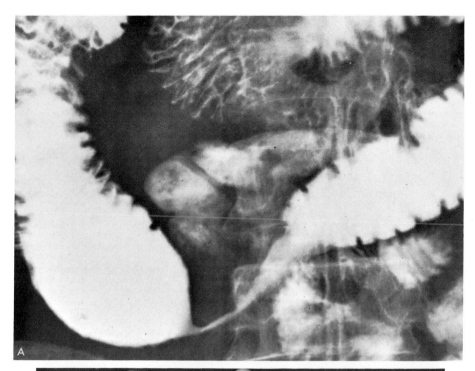

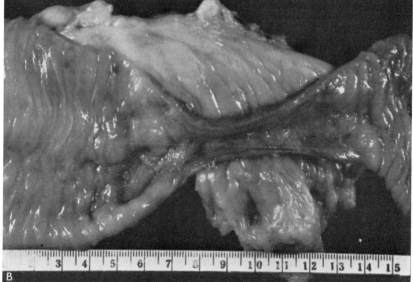

Figure 11-7 *Segmental infarction.* A, In the same patient as in Figure 11–3, four weeks later there is a strictured segment of bowel with smooth contours. The stricture is concentric and joins the proximal and distal bowels in a fusiform tapering fashion. The proximal and distal bowels are dilated.

B, Gross specimen of incomplete infarction in the same patient. A tubular fibrotic segment 7 cm. long with a conical transition to the adjacent bowel is shown. Microscopic examination revealed partial necrosis of all the walls of the bowel associated with the fibrosis.

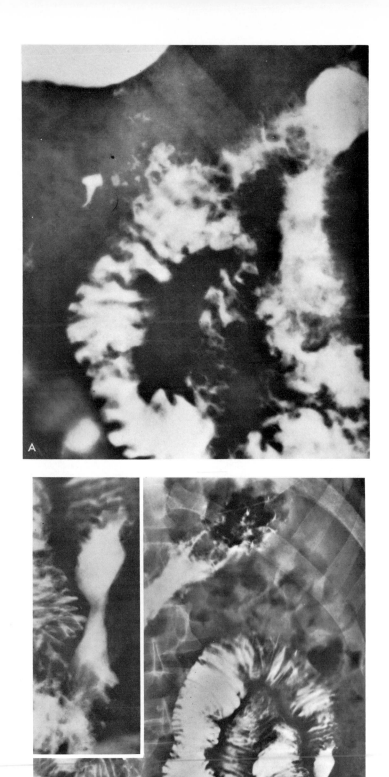

Figure 11–8 Segmental infarction. A, There is thickening and blurring of the folds with increased secretions, in a short segment of proximal jejunum.

B, In the same patient the short segment now has a castlike configuration owing to mucosal ulceration. There is more narrowing and rigidity.

140

(Illustration continued on opposite page.)

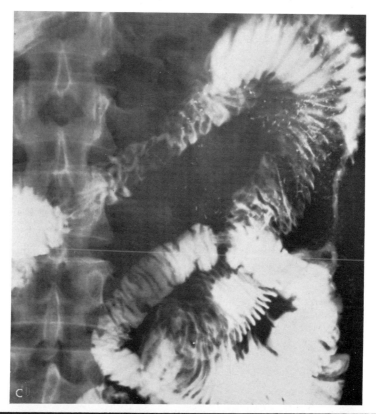

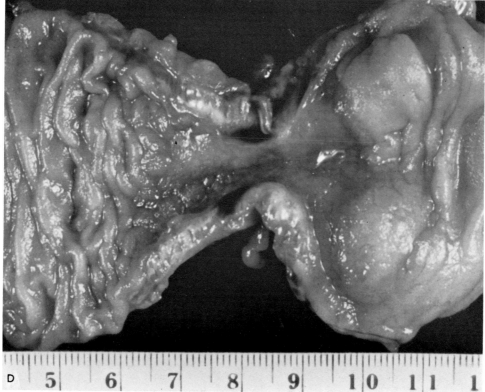

Figure 11–8 *Continued* C, One month later a stricture is identified in this region. *D,* Resected specimen.

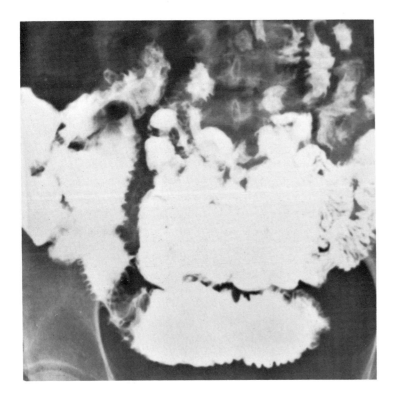

Figure 11–9 Incomplete infarction. In a 22 year old female patient one month following an uncomplicated pregnancy and delivery, the distal ileum is slightly spastic and irritable, with slight thickening of the folds.

partial or complete reversibility may occur (Figs. 11-13 and 11-14). The process may stop at any one of the stages described above, and the patient may be first seen at any stage. In some cases not only is the bowel dilated proximal to the stricture, but poststenotic dilatation is also seen. The fact that the stricture is

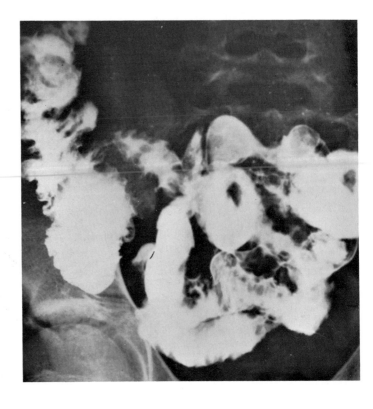

Figure 11–10 Incomplete infarction. Same patient as in Figure 11–9. Three weeks later there is more narrowing and rigidity of the ileum. The folds are more thickened and polypoid defects are identified.

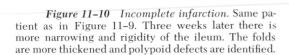

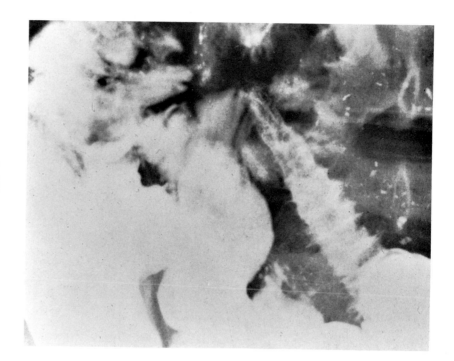

Figure 11-11 Segmental infarction. Same case as in Figure 11-10. Two weeks later there is further narrowing of the involved segment.

usually shorter than the initial area of involvement suggests that at the onset there was probably more widespread impairment of the blood supply. Since ulcerations are rarely deep, sinus tracts and fistulas are unusual.

In the colon a similar sequence of roentgenographic findings is iden-

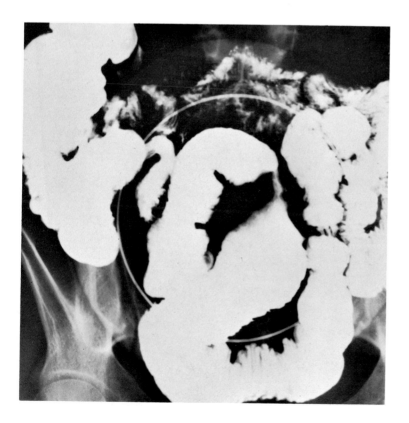

Figure 11-12 Segmental infarction. Same case as in Figure 11-11, one month later. A stricture is now seen with pre- and post-stenotic dilatation. The terminal ileum is moderately narrowed. The stricture is considerably smaller than the initial area of involvement.

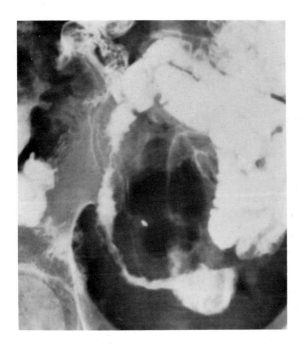

Figure 11–13   *Incomplete infarction.* Considerable narrowing and moderate rigidity of the distal ileum are demonstrated. The proximal bowel is not dilated, indicating that some of the narrowing is secondary to spasm.

tified, but pleating and sacculations are common (Figs. 11-15 to 11-31). The entire colon, including the rectum, may be infarcted. Radiologically the appearance simulates ulcerative colitis. On pathologic examination the intense necrosis, multiple thrombi, and lack of leukocytic infiltration help to distinguish ischemic disease from ulcerative colitis. A toxic megacolon resembling that occurring in ulcerative colitis has been reported.[7] In these cases marked colonic

(*Text continued on page 154.*)

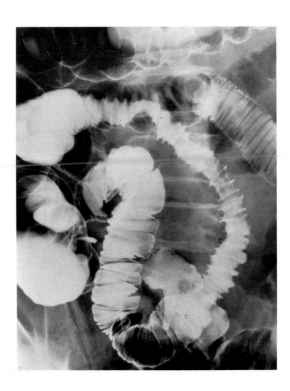

Figure 11–14   In the patient of Figure 11–13, reexamination three weeks later reveals only minimal narrowing and rigidity of the distal ileum, with slight blunting of the folds. The terminal ileum itself is normal except for slight dilatation. The patient was a 72 year old man who experienced severe right lower quadrant pain associated with the passage of dark red stools. He made an uneventful recovery.

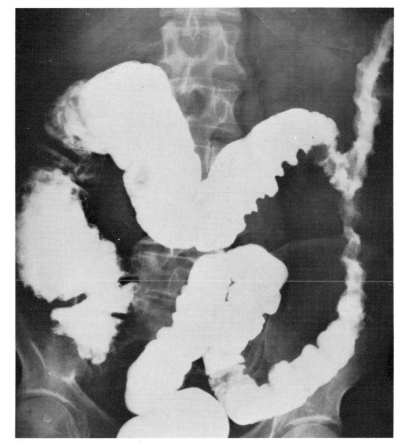

Figure 11–15 *Segmental infarction of the colon.* This 67 year old man had a coronary occlusion four years previously. There is a moderate degree of spasm and rigidity of the distal transverse and descending colon. The folds are thickened, in association with scalloping of the contours. No discrete ulcerations are identified. The segmental infarction was confirmed at autopsy.

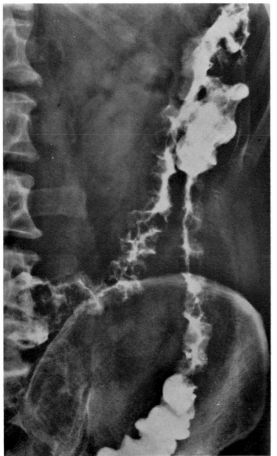

Figure 11–16 *Segmental infarction of the colon.* An evacuation film demonstrates the findings shown in Figure 11–15.

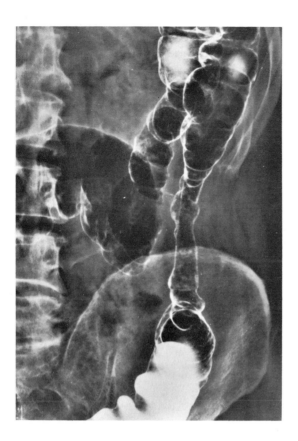

Figure 11–17 Segmental infarction in the patient of Figures 11–15 and 11–16, one month after the original examination. In the mid descending colon there is a narrowed segment of bowel approximately 5 in. long with smooth contours.

Figure 11–18 In the patient of Figure 11–15, two months after the original episode, moderate reversibility of the lesion is demonstrated. At this time there is slight flattening of the inferior wall of the distal transverse colon. The descending colon reveals sacculation and a moderate number of pseudodiverticula.

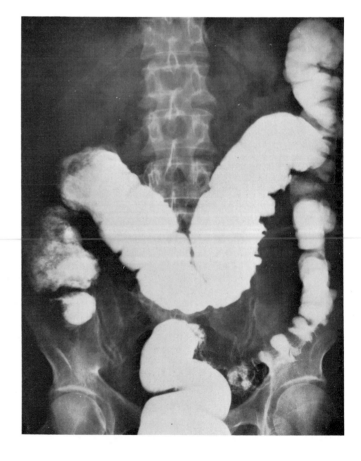

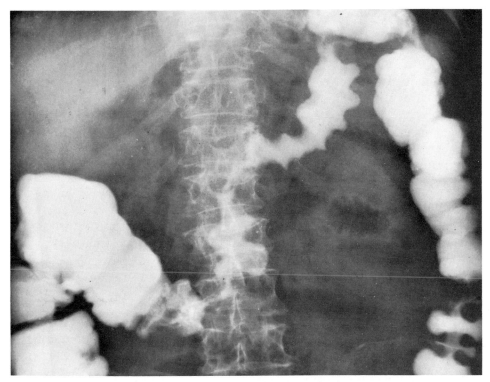

Figure 11–19 Incomplete segmental infarction of the colon in a 70 year old woman, with acute onset of abdominal pain and subsequent passage of bright red blood in the stool. Considerable spasm and irritability of the transverse colon is noted, associated with thickening of the folds. A moderate degree of scalloping of the contours is present.

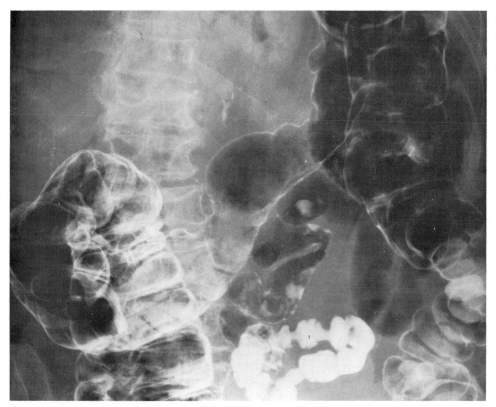

Figure 11–20 In the patient of Figure 11–19, one month later, the transverse colon reveals slight narrowing and rigidity with irregularity of the superior contour. These alterations persisted for one year after the onset of infarction.

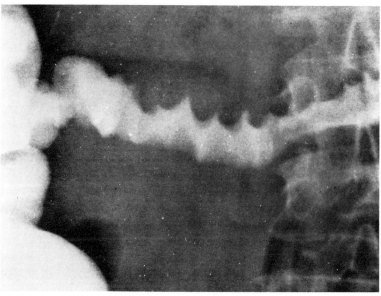

Figure 11–21 *Incomplete segmental infarction.* A spot film of the transverse colon reveals narrowing, rigidity, and a moderate degree of scalloping. The patient is a 70 year old woman who presented with severe abdominal pain and rectal bleeding. This examination was performed two days after the acute episode. The barium enema was normal one month later.

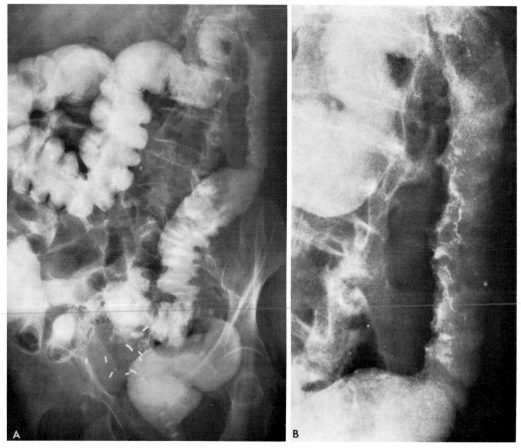

Figure 11–22 *Early stage of segmental infarction.* A, The barium enema was performed two days after an episode of acute abdominal pain followed by bright red bleeding. The proximal descending colon is moderately narrowed and rigid and shows thickened and edematous folds with scalloping of the contours. *B*, Closeup of *A*. It is frequently difficult to obtain adequate films in these cases because of the marked edema and increased fluid content.

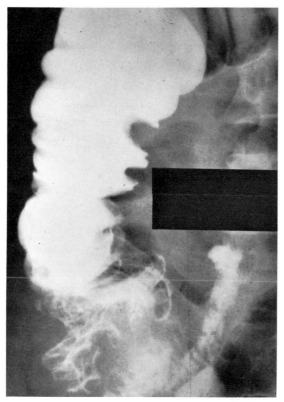

Figure 11–23 *Segmental incomplete infarction* with reversibility in a 60 year old woman. The cecum and ascending colon are slightly narrowed and rigid. There is a moderate degree of scalloping on the medial aspect of the colon. This is the type of case that has been mistakenly called "right-sided ulcerative colitis."

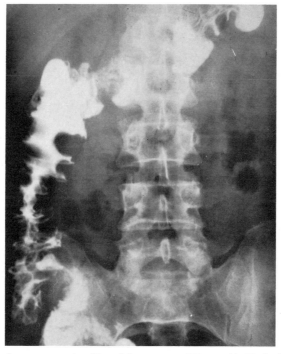

Figure 11–24 In an evacuation film of the patient of Figure 11–23, thickening of the folds is shown.

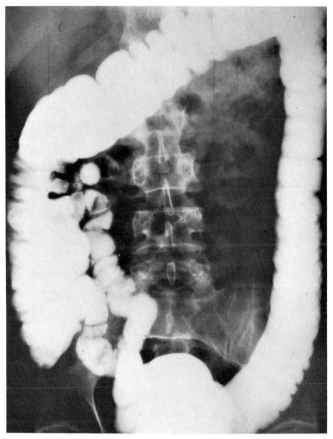

Figure 11–25 Barium enema examination of the patient of Figures 11–23 and 11–24 shows complete reversibility of the previous findings.

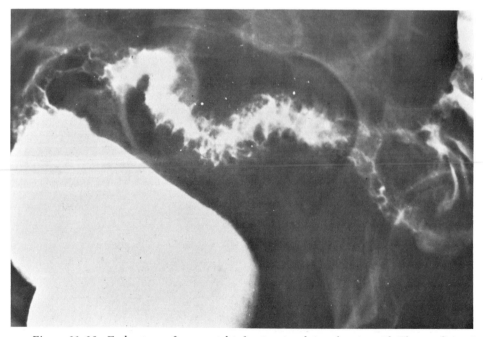

Figure 11–26 Early stage of segmental infarction involving the sigmoid. The condition is characterized by a moderate degree of narrowing, rigidity, and thickening of the folds.

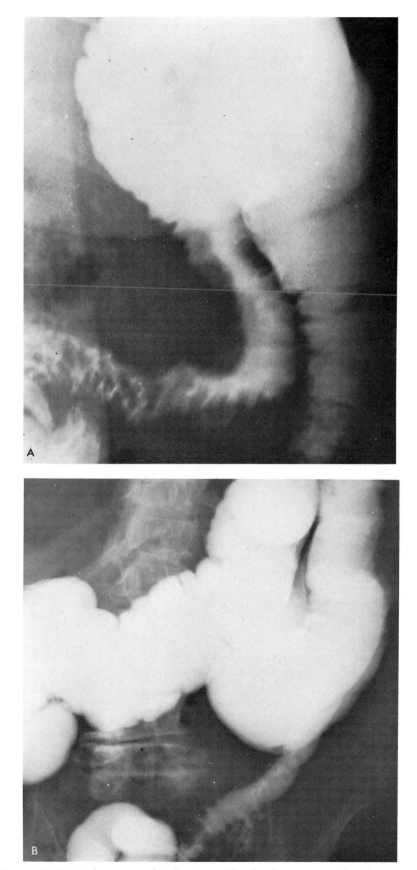

Figure 11–27 *Early segmental ischemia.* A, The distal transverse colon shows narrowing, moderate rigidity, and thumb-printing along its superior contour. This could easily be mistaken for a tumor. B, One month later there has been complete resolution.

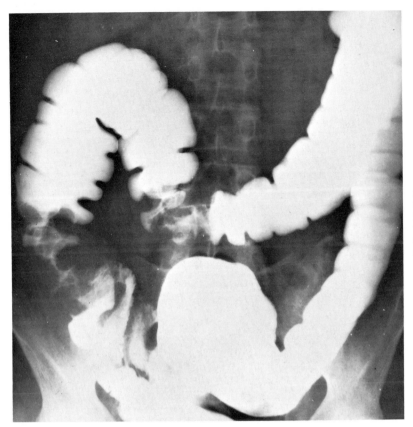

Figure 11-28 Segmental infarction of the right colon with two skip lesions. Skip lesions are unusual, and the roentgen findings cannot be distinguished from amebic or granulomatous colitis. The history, however, was characteristic of infarction, and one month later a barium enema was normal.

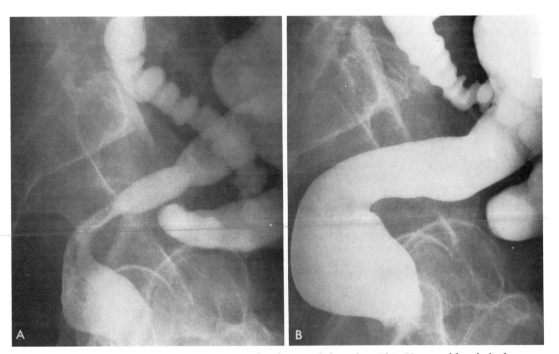

Figure 11-29 Regression in segmental ischemia of the colon. This 68 year old male had a sudden attack of abdominal pain and rectal bleeding two weeks prior to this examination. *A,* There is considerable narrowing and rigidity of the rectum and lower sigmoid. The contours are smooth. The presacral space is increased. *B,* One month later there is only minimal lack of distensibility and rigidity. In several other cases involving the rectum and sigmoid we have seen discrete ulcerations, but this has been an unusual finding in our patients.

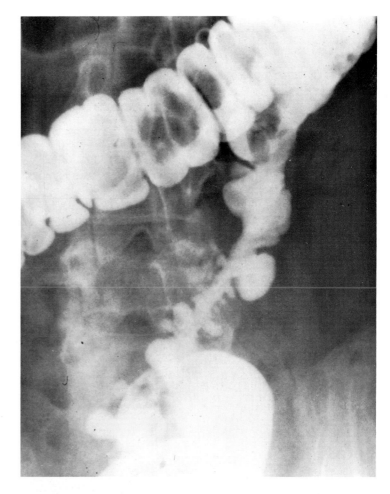

Figure 11–30 Late stage of segmental incomplete infarction of the colon. Narrowing and rigidity of the colon are revealed, as well as multiple sacculations or pseudodiverticula of the descending colon.

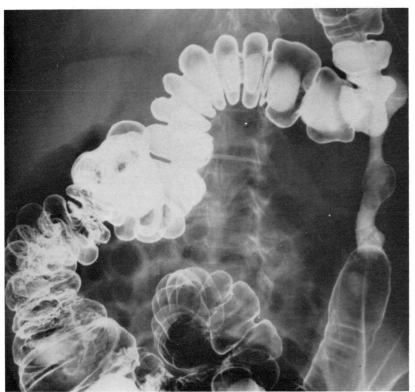

Figure 11–31 Stricture. Localized segment of narrowing in the proximal descending colon with smooth contours and a single sacculation. This type of stricture probably represents the end stage in some cases of ischemia of the colon.

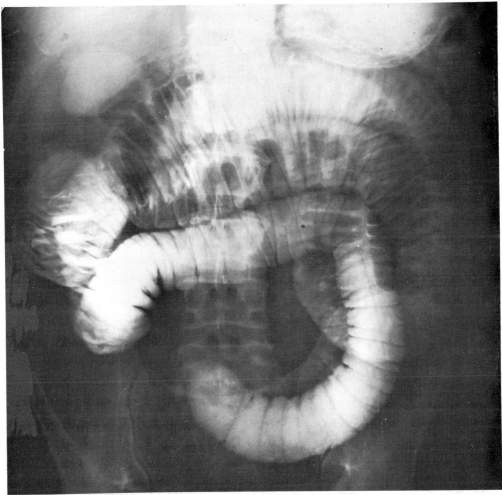

Figure 11-32 Unusual case of segmental infarction of the small bowel producing complete obstruction in the distal jejunum. This film was taken two weeks after the onset of abdominal pain.

distention occurred in association with large penetrating ulcers and pseudo-polypoid changes.

Ischemic colitis may develop proximal to a colonic carcinoma. It is therefore important to rule out a neoplasm by appropriate clinical and roentgenologic studies in all patients with vascular disease of the colon. The mechanisms of development of colitis in association with colonic carcinoma are unclear, but experimental studies[8] suggest that large bowel obstruction may be responsible for interference with the intramural blood supply proximal to the lesion.

In summary, the characteristic roentgenographic features of ischemic ileitis and colitis are thumb-printing, picket fence thickening of the folds, sacculation, tubular narrowing and stricture. The differential diagnosis includes carcinoma and granulomatous inflammatory disease. The stricture in infarction is smooth and tapering, with a concentric lumen and without overhanging margins or discrete ulcerations. Sacculations are common, especially in the colon. Skip lesions are unusual. In contrast to these findings, longitudinal ulcerations, fissuring, and skip lesions are frequent findings in granulomatous disease. Carcinoma is easily excluded by the lack of overhanging margins and the absence of an eccentric lumen.

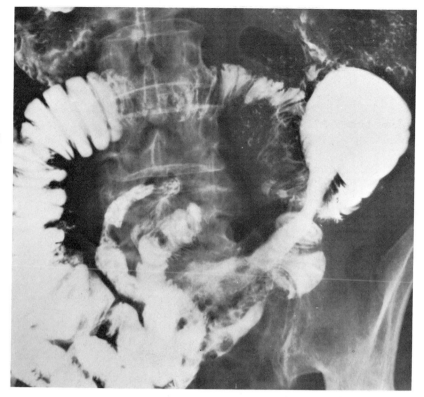

Figure 11–33 Reduced strangulated hernia. In a 54 year old woman with a right femoral hernia containing a loop of ileum, a segment of ileum about 6 in. long shows tubular stenosis with effacement of the mucosal pattern and conical transition to the proximal dilated bowel. The surgeon thought the loop of bowel was viable, despite the fact that it appeared discolored. The ileal loop was returned to the abdomen and the wound closed. Three weeks after operation symptoms of intestinal obstruction occurred.

SEGMENTAL VASCULAR COMPROMISE

Segmental vascular compromise may occur from incarceration of bowel in a hernial sac (Figs. 11-33 and 11-34), from bands of adhesions, and from volvulus or intussusception.[9] When infarction is incomplete but the bowel is not resected, stricture formation may occur, just as in segmental infarction of the bowel.

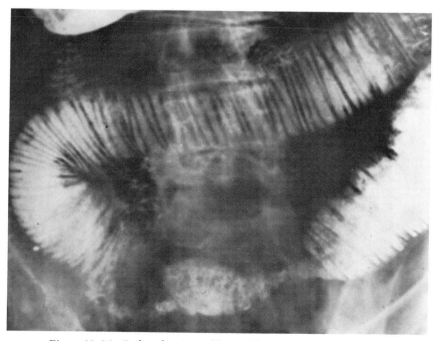

Figure 11–34 Reduced incisional hernia. Two strictures are identified.

References

1. Williams, L. F., Jr.: Vascular insufficiency of the intestines. *Gastroenterology,* 61:757-777, 1971.
2. Schwartz, S., Boley, S., Schultz, L., and Allen, A.: A survey of vascular diseases of the small intestine, *Seminars Radiol.,* 1:178-218, 1966.
2a. Ruoff, M., and Ranson, J. H. C.: Persistent hypercoagulability after venous mesenteric infarction and oral contraceptive. *N.Y. State J. Med.,* 73:791-793, 1973.
3. Marston, A., Pheils, M. T., Thomas, M. L., and Morson, B. C.: Ischemic colitis, *Gut,* 7:1-15, 1966.
4. Bircher, J., Bartholomew, L. G., Cain, J. C., and Adson, M. A.: Syndrome of intestinal arterial insufficiency ("abdominal angina"). *Arch. Intern. Med.,* 117:632-638, 1966.
5. Marshak, R. H., Maklansky, D., and Calem, S. H.: Segmental infarction of the colon, *Amer. J. Dig. Dis.,* 10:86-92, 1965.
6. Kilpatrick, Z. M., Forman, J., Yesner, R., et al.: Ischemic proctitis. *J.A.M.A.,* 205:74-80, 1968.
7. Miller, W. T., Scott, J., Rosato, E. F., et al.: Ischemic colitis with gangrene. *Radiology,* 94:291-297, 1970.
8. Glotzer, D. J., and Pehl, B. G.: Experimental obstructive colitis. *Arch. Surg.,* 92:1-8, 1966.
9. Wolf, B. S., and Marshak, R. H.: Segmental infarction of the small bowel. *Radiology,* 66:701-707, 1956.

12

Intramural Intestinal Bleeding

In the years since the first edition of this volume, we are seeing fewer cases of intramural intestinal bleeding. It appears that patients receiving anticoagulants are achieving better control and monitoring of their medications, and replacement of some of the blood clotting factors deficient in hemorrhagic hematologic diseases has become available.

Bleeding into the intestinal wall may occur in healthy persons following trauma to the abdomen. It may also develop spontaneously in patients who are receiving anticoagulant drugs or as a consequence of underlying diseases which are associated with coagulation defects. These diseases include hemophilia, leukemia, multiple myeloma, lymphoma, and metastatic carcinoma. Thrombocytopenia, hypofibrinogenemia, circulating anticoagulants, activation of the fibrinolytic system, and dysproteinemia have all been implicated at times in intramural intestinal bleeding.

Intramural hemorrhage as a result of trauma is most often seen in children, especially boys, who are frequently involved in abdominal injuries from play or athletics. Abdominal trauma in adults commonly occurs as a result of automobile accidents, and with the use of seat belts crushing injuries to the abdomen may cause contusion of the small bowel. Pain following blunt trauma to the abdomen may be persistent or may disappear and recur in the next hours or days in association with nausea and vomiting. On examination a mass may be felt, and the abdomen is tender. Intramural hemorrhage following trauma is suggested clinically by the presence of a mass and the finding of intestinal (especially duodenal) obstruction. This localization may occur because the bowel tends to fix the duodenum between its ligamentous supports and the spine.[1] In spontaneously occurring hematomas there tends to be a diffuse infiltration of the bowel wall rather than a localized intramural mass, and any portion of the bowel may be involved, without predilection for the duodenum.[2] With passage of time and correction of coagulation defects, if these are present, the intramural hematoma is resorbed and the bowel returns to its normal appearance.

Histologic examination of the bowel involved in intramural hemorrhage shows thickening of the intestinal wall with submucosal extravasation of blood.

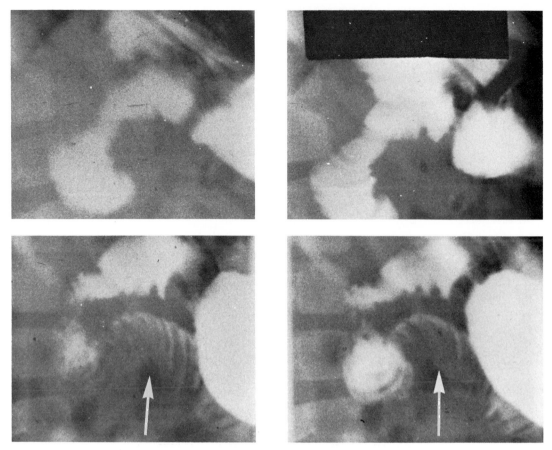

Figure 12-1   Intramural hematoma secondary to trauma of the third portion of the duodenum. The folds over the mass are stretched, producing a coiled-spring appearance.

Symptoms of intramural bleeding may range from mild abdominal discomfort to the clinical features of intestinal obstruction. Either gross or microscopic blood is often present in the stool, but it may be only a transitory finding, easy to overlook. Paralytic ileus commonly occurs, but if the lumen is narrowed the picture may be one of mechanical obstruction. Full clinical recovery following supportive medical treatment is the rule, and surgical intervention is rarely required if the diagnosis of intramural bleeding can be established from the clinical and roentgenologic features.

Roentgen Findings

The roentgen findings after trauma are usually localized in the region of the stomach and duodenum. A mass of varying size along the medial aspect of the duodenum, displacing the stomach, duodenum, or both,[3] may be seen on scout films. Psoas muscle outlines may be obliterated because of retroperitoneal bleeding. After the administration of barium the most common roentgen abnormality seen is a mass in the duodenum, associated with the coiled-spring appearance of intussusception. At times the mass is so large that it may narrow the lumen of the duodenum, which has an arcuate configuration. In such cases resolution may be slow and surgical evacuation of the clot may be required.

A preliminary roentgenogram of the abdomen in spontaneous bleeding may demonstrate significant findings. If there is a solitary hematoma of sufficient size, it may be recognized either by its increased density or by the displacement of loops of the small or large bowel. If the hemorrhage is confined to the bowel wall, varying degrees of paralytic ileus, narrowing of the bowel lumen, or localized filling defects producing marked scalloping of the bowel may be seen. Differentiation from infarction on the preliminary roentgenogram alone can be difficult.

With barium studies, the roentgenographic changes caused by intramural hemorrhage have many typical features.[4] The variation in the roentgenographic appearance seems to be a reflection of the difference in the extent of intramural hemorrhage and the presence of mucosal edema and intestinal secretions. Changes in the small intestine have been reported more frequently than changes in the large bowel, and involvement of the esophagus and stomach has not been documented.

The roentgenographic alterations are usually segmental but may be diffuse. The involved segments of small intestine reveal varying degrees of rigidity and uncoiling of the loops, depending on the amount and extent of bleeding into the bowel wall and mesentery. Marked rigidity and separation of the loops of bowel are rarely observed. As a rule, mechanical or clinical obstruction is not prominent, although some degree of narrowing of the bowel lumen is frequent. We have observed transient intussusception proximal to the lesion in one patient.

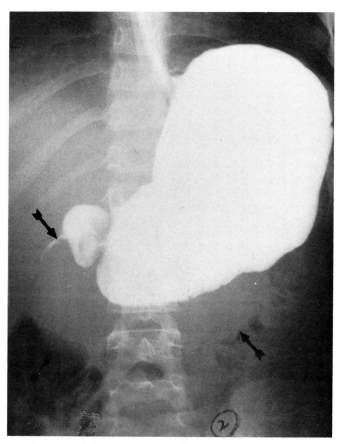

Figure 12–2 Intramural hematoma: secondary to trauma: Barium meal examination reveals a mass obstructing the duodenum from the apex of the bulb to the ligament of Treitz. The duodenal lumen is narrowed and beyond the apex of the bulb it is occluded. The mass also displaces the transverse colon.

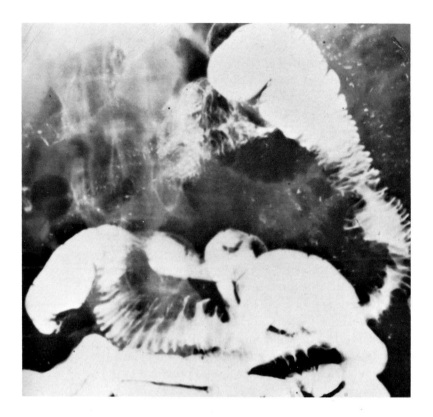

Figure 12–3 Intramural bleeding secondary to anticoagulant therapy. The distal jejunum is narrowed and shows some loss of flexibility. Marked alterations of the folds are present, characterized by sharp delineation, uniform thickening, a spike-like configuration, and symmetric, regular spacing simulating a stack of coins. There is no mucosal ulceration or nodularity suggestive of an inflammatory or neoplastic process. The bowel immediately proximal to this segment is slightly dilated.

Figure 12–4 In the patient of Figure 12–3 two days later, there has been considerable resolution of the degree and extent of involvement. The folds are less thickened and the bowel lumen has become wider. Autopsy nine months later showed no abnormality of the small bowel.

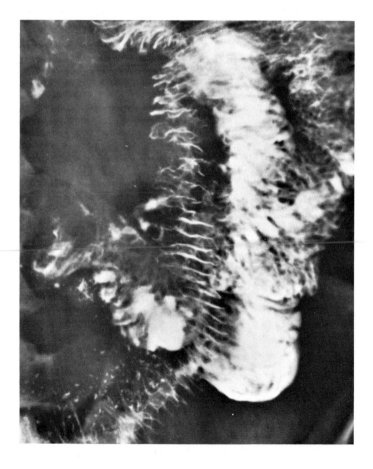

The small intestine fold pattern has a characteristic appearance. There is a uniform, regular thickening of the folds, sharp delineation of their margins, and a parallel arrangement, producing a symmetric, spikelike configuration which resembles a stack of coins. This stacked-coin appearance is the most prominent alteration and is more striking in the jejunum than the ileum because of the better developed jejunal folds (Figs. 12-3 and 12-4). There is a conspicuous lack of spasm or changeability of folds. Bleeding into the mesentery is an occasional finding, especially in patients receiving anticoagulants and in hemophiliac patients. Evidence of a mass, flattening of the folds on the mesenteric side of the bowel, and separation and uncoiling of the bowel loops is noted. If the mesenteric hemorrhage is large, a hammocklike configuration of the bowel segments may result (Fig. 12-5). Resolution of these findings in a short period of time is observed on follow-up examinations (Figs. 12-6 to 12-9).

The changes in the colon are similar to those seen in the small bowel, except that the scalloped areas may be large and are seen more frequently (Figs. 12-10 to 12-15).

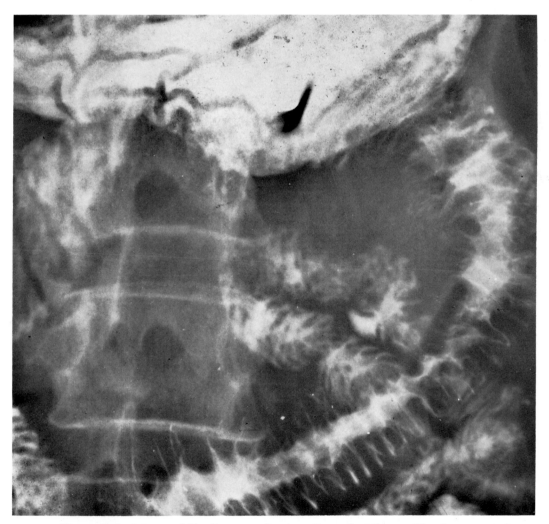

Figure 12–5 Intramural bleeding secondary to anticoagulant therapy. The changes noted in hemorrhage into the bowel wall are again seen. On the antimesenteric side the irregularly thickened folds have a uniform appearance. On the mesenteric side the folds are irregularly flattened, not only by the intramural hematoma but by blood in the mesentery as well.

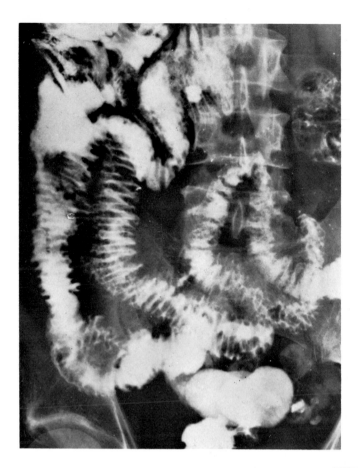

Figure 12-6 *Idiopathic thrombocytopenic purpura with hemorrhage into the small intestinal wall.* The folds in the distal ileum are thickened and have a stacked coin appearance. The appearance is similar to that noted in intramural bleeding secondary to anticoagulant therapy. The findings in this patient were confirmed at surgery during splenectomy.

Figure 12-7 In the patient of Figure 12-6, five weeks later, the abnormal findings have completely disappeared.

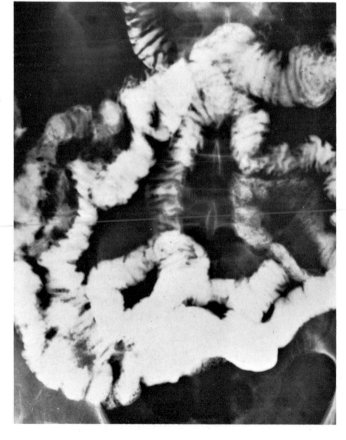

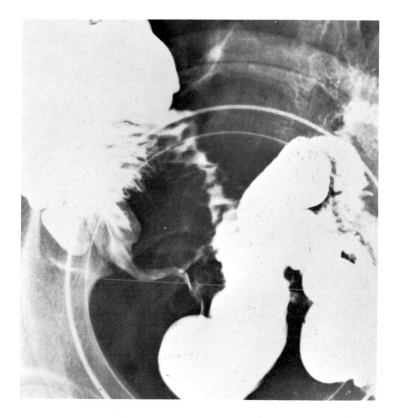

Figure 12-8 Intramural bleeding in a patient with hemophilia. The terminal ileum is moderately narrowed and rigid with irregularity of the contours. The folds are thickened. There was no evidence of spasm or irritability.

Differentiation of the roentgenographic changes of mesenteric vascular occlusion from those caused by intramural bleeding may be difficult. Indeed, a patient who is receiving anticoagulants may develop a mesenteric occlusion. In favor of anticoagulant-induced changes are the stacked-coin appearance, lack of

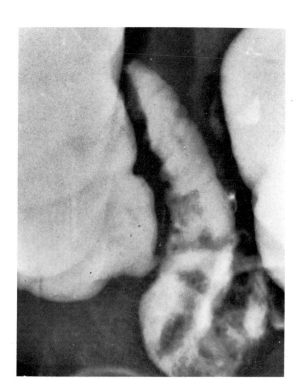

Figure 12-9 In the patient of Figure 12-8, two months later there is complete resolution of the changes.

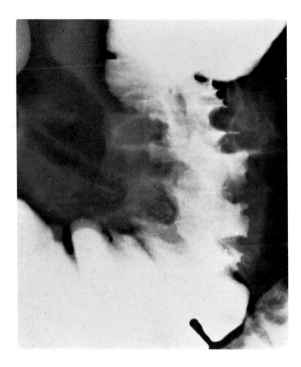

Figure 12-10 Intramural bleeding in hemophilia. A short segment of the transverse colon is slightly narrowed and the contours show scalloping or thumb-printing.

spasm or irritability, presence of a mesenteric mass, and complete resolution of the roentgenographic findings. In mesenteric vascular occlusion a localized mesenteric mass caused by bleeding is uncommon, and the folds exhibit varying degrees of edema, spasm, and irritability. The usual sequel of vascular occlusion is a stricture at the site of the maximally infarcted segment. In some cases, however, differential diagnosis is impossible since complete resolution of the roentgenographic changes has been noted in mesenteric vascular occlusion (Figs. 12-16 and 12-17).

(*Text continued on page 169.*)

Figure 12-11 Intramural bleeding in the colon. There is marked scalloping and thumb-printing of the distal transverse colon and proximal descending colon secondary to intramural hemorrhage following anticoagulant therapy.

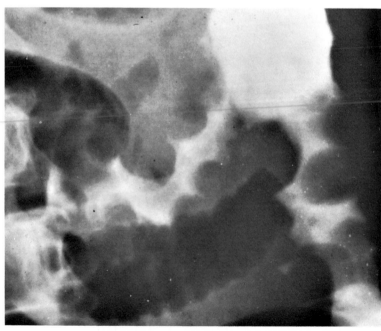

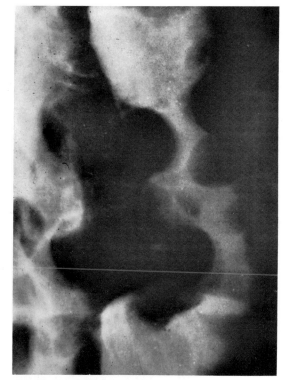

Figure 12-12 In the patient of Figure 12–11, a spot roentgenogram demonstrates the characteristic thumb-printing and scalloping in the colon. Except for the fact that the changes are more pronounced, the appearance is similar to that of infarction.

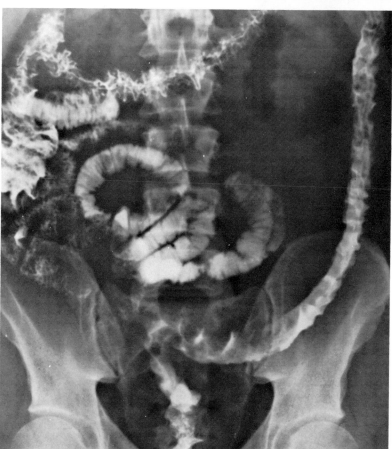

Figure 12-13 *Intramural bleeding in the colon simulating ulcerative colitis.* The patient had heart disease and was receiving anticoagulants. Sigmoidoscopy was normal. The findings returned to normal after anticoagulant therapy was discontinued.

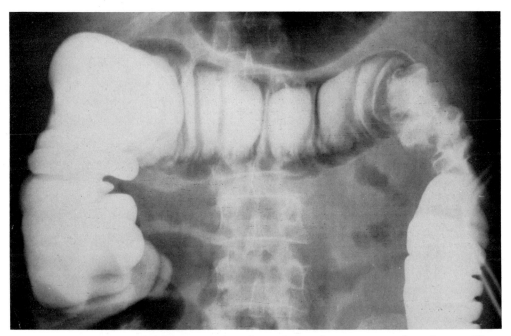

Figure 12-14 *Localized lesion in the splenic flexure due to anticoagulant therapy.* The lesion was resected because carcinoma was suspected. At laparotomy no tumor was found. The changes were secondary to intramural hemorrhage.

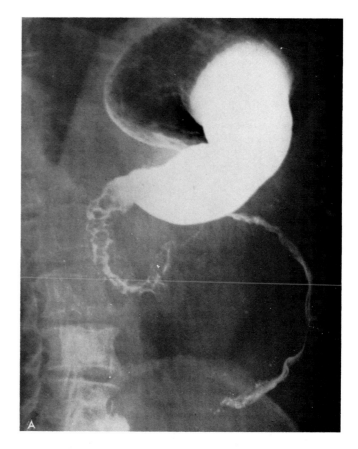

Figure 12-15A Massive hemorrhage in a patient with prostatic carcinoma. At three hours a barium study outlines only the duodenum and proximal jejunum. In the duodenum, the lumen is narrow and the folds are regularly thickened. The jejunum is markedly narrowed and the folds are obliterated. There is marked rigidity and C-shaped configuration secondary to intramural hemorrhage.

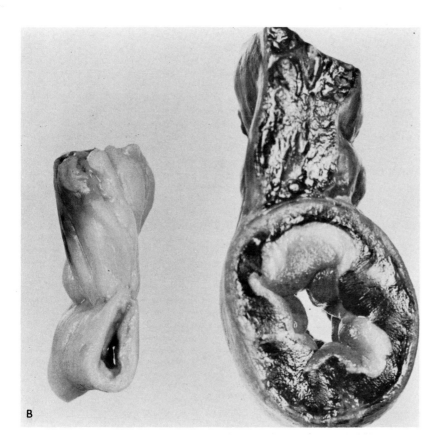

Figure 12–15B Cross section of the involved segment of the jejunum and mesentery revealing marked intramural bleeding with elevation of the mucosa and considerable narrowing of the lumen. Hemorrhage into the mesentery is also identified. (Courtesy of Dr. Isidore Katz, State University of New York.)

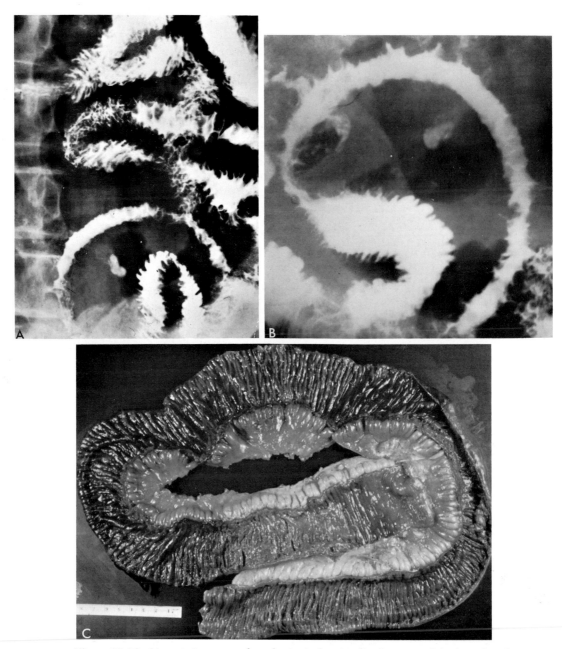

Figure 12–16 *Mesenteric venous thrombosis.* A, the visualized portion of the bowel in this film reveals a moderate degree of narrowing, rigidity, separation of the loops of bowel, and thickening and blunting of the folds. In the proximal bowel the alterations are highly suggestive of intramural hemorrhage. Distally the folds appear to be effaced. The patient was an 80 year old woman who died the day following the small bowel examination. Study of the small bowel at autopsy revealed an extensive mesenteric venous thrombosis. The mucosal changes were due to a combination of hemorrhage and edema.

B, Magnified view of the distal loops of Figure 12–16A, demonstrating narrowing, rigidity, edema, and ulceration of the mucosa.

C, Specimen illustrating an extensive mesenteric venous thrombosis, responsible for the roentgen changes shown in A.

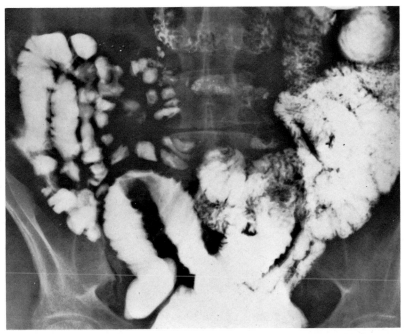

Figure 12–17 The film shows an abnormal loop of jejunum, characterized by thickening and flattening of the folds without ulceration or nodularity. Some abnormal motor activity is noted. The patient, a 58 year old woman receiving anticoagulant therapy following a myocardial infarction three months previously, developed midabdominal pain. Recovery was uneventful and follow-up examination of the small bowel was normal. It is impossible to determine whether these changes are due to anticoagulants or to mesenteric infarction.

Inflammatory lesions of the small bowel can readily be differentiated from intramural hemorrhage. In the early stages there is marked spasm and irritability; later, ulceration, inflammatory polyps, marked rigidity, and separation of the loops of bowel are evident. Neoplastic diseases of the small bowel, specifically lymphosarcoma, can be distinguished by ulceration, localized dilatation, tumor nodules, or multiple areas of involvement.

References

1. Wiot, J. F.: Intramural small intestinal hemorrhage—a differential diagnosis. *Seminars Radiol.*, 1:219-233, 1966.
2. Khilnani, M. T., Marshak, R. H., Eliasoph, J., and Wolf, B. S.: Intramural intestinal hemorrhage. *Amer. J. Roentgen.*, 92:1061-1071, 1964.
3. Felson, B., and Levin, E. J.: Intramural hematoma of duodenum; diagnostic roentgen sign. *Radiology*, 63:823-831, 1954.
4. Senturia, H. R., Susman, N., and Shyken, H.: Roentgen appearance of spontaneous intramural hemorrhage of small intestine associated with anticoagulant therapy. *Amer. J. Roentgen.*, 86:62-69, 1961.

13

Vasculitis

Vasculitis, which occurs in the connective tissue ("collagen") diseases, thromboangiitis obliterans (Buerger's disease), and Henoch-Schönlein syndrome may compromise the blood supply of segments of the small intestine and cause ischemic or hemorrhagic changes in the bowel wall. These alterations may be responsible for some of the obscure pain patterns in these diseases and also for mucosal ulceration and perforation.

CONNECTIVE TISSUE DISEASES

Gastrointestinal complications are not uncommon in the course of systemic connective tissue diseases and have been reported in rheumatoid arthritis[1] as well as in polyarteritis nodosa, systemic lupus erythematosus, and dermatomyositis.[2, 3] In these diseases, perforation, massive bleeding, and multiple infarctions may occur in the small bowel, and the underlying pathology in all appears to be a necrotizing vasculitis involving small arteries, arterioles, and veins.

The small intestinal manifestations of vasculitis must often be managed as surgical emergencies, but the prognosis depends largely upon the course of the underlying connective tissue disorder. Treatment is generally unsatisfactory. Although corticosteroids are usually employed their usefulness can be questioned, and in some patients an acceleration of the vasculitis by steroid therapy has been suggested.

The roentgenographic changes in vasculitis are remarkably similar to those in segmental infarction (Figs. 13-1 and 13-2). In the early stages there is narrowing of the lumen associated with a mild degree of rigidity. The folds are thickened, hazy, and blunted. Increased secretions are prominent because of the inflammatory process. Discrete ulcerations are usually not deep enough to be identified, but in more severe cases the ulcers are deep and at times the entire mucosa and submucosa may be sloughed. Skip lesions are not unusual. Perforations occur and sinus tracts and fistulas, with walled-off perforations,

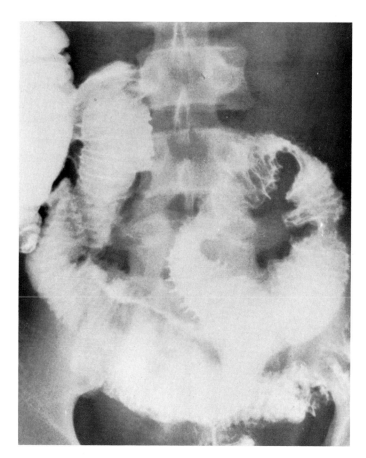

Figure 13–1A Polyarteritis nodosa. The distal loops of small bowel reveal edema of the folds, associated with moderate rigidity. (Courtesy of Dr. Sidney Nelson, Ohio State University.)

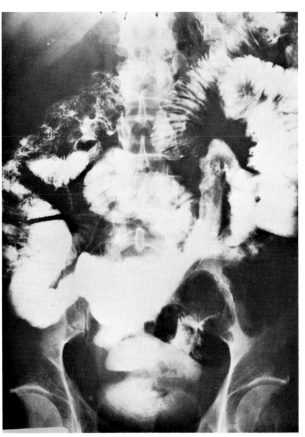

Figure 13–1B Polyarteritis nodosa producing infarction of the small bowel with perforation and abscess formation. (Courtesy of Dr. Alexander Margulis, University of California, San Francisco.)

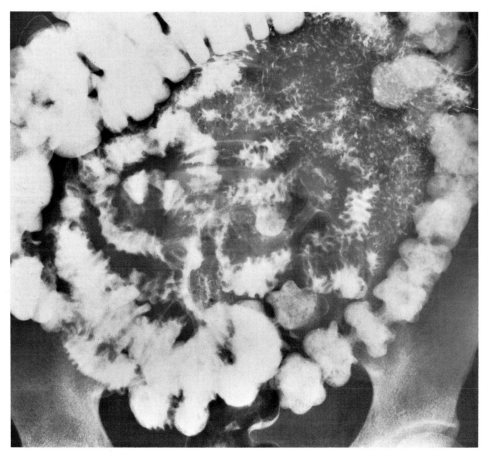

Figure 13–2 *Lupus erythematosus.* The distal jejunum and entire ileum reveal edema of the folds associated with some rigidity and narrowing of the lumen. Small bowel biopsy also demonstrated edema of the folds.

may be seen (Fig. 13-1*B*). Following resection, repeated infarctions may occur, in some cases culminating in massive small bowel infarctions.

THROMBOANGIITIS OBLITERANS

Although usually considered a peripheral vascular disease, thromboangiitis obliterans can also involve the mesenteric vessels and cause ischemic changes in the small bowel. The disease, which is of unknown etiology and is not always well distinguished from atherosclerosis, affects men more often than women and is reported to be more common in Jews than in other groups studied. In the extremities the clinical manifestations are coldness, pain, migratory phlebitis, cyanosis, and gangrene. Many patients are heavy cigarette smokers. Interdiction of tobacco, which causes vasoconstriction, is the mainstay of treatment. Bilateral sympathectomy may be of benefit.

The pathology of the disease is an inflammatory process involving both arteries and veins with formation of thrombi. The lesions tend to be segmental, with normal lengths of vessel between areas of disease. At varying intervals of time additional segments of vessel may be involved with acute inflammation.

In the small bowel, segmental infarction may occur. The roentgen findings (Fig. 13-3 and 13-4) resemble those of the connective tissue diseases.

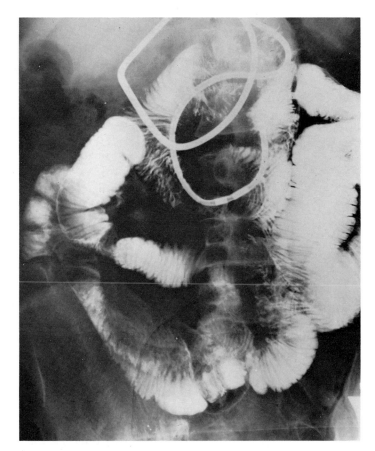

Figure 13–3 Thromboangiitis obliterans. There are two narrowed segments in the jejunum with effacement of the mucosa secondary to edema. There is probably diffuse superficial ulceration in both segments.

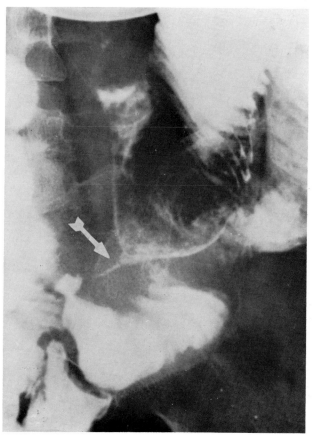

Figure 13–4 Thromboangiitis obliterans. Same patient as in Figure 13–3. Four weeks later a stenotic segment measuring 2 cm. in length is identified. This patient passed a cast of the small intestine prior to this examination. Pathologic examination of this material confirmed the fact that it represented necrotic small intestinal wall. At operation, two areas of stenosis and an obliterating endophlebitis of the mesenteric veins were revealed.

HENOCH-SCHÖNLEIN SYNDROME

Henoch-Schönlein syndrome is an acute arteritis characterized by purpura, nephritis, abdominal pain, and joint pain. The disease tends to be self-limited, often developing several weeks after a streptococcal infection. At times, however, it evolves into a syndrome that is indistinguishable from polyarteritis nodosa or glomerulonephritis. In the bowel, Henoch-Schönlein changes are marked by submucosal edema. All portions of the gastrointestinal tract except the esophagus have been reported to be involved.[4] Pain and tenderness in the abdomen are the principal clinical features, and when fever is present an acute abdomen may be found. Either diarrhea or constipation may occur. At exploratory laparotomy the involved bowel has been described as appearing reddened and edematous, but unlike the findings in infarction, the mesenteric vessels pulsate normally. Histologic section shows an arteritis with extensive edema of the mucosa and submucosa. The disease process is reversible, and healing is complete without fibrosis or stenosis.

In Henoch-Schönlein syndrome the most conspicuous roentgenographic alteration is the appearance of the fold pattern. The folds are thickened and blurred because of the marked edema and increased secretions (Figs. 13-5 to 13-8). The blurring and indistinctness of the folds may become so pronounced that complete effacement of the entire fold pattern may be seen (Fig. 13-9). As the edema and secretions increase, the barium column becomes segmented

(*Text continued on page 178.*)

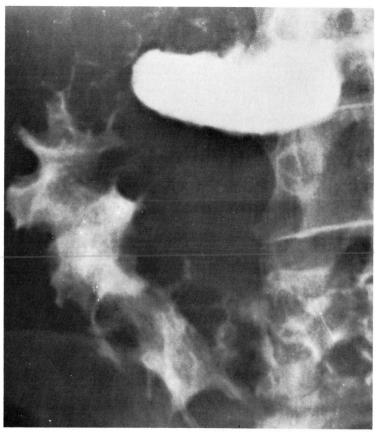

Figure 13–5 *Henoch's purpura.* The folds in the second portion of duodenum are markedly exaggerated and have a hazy, nodular appearance.

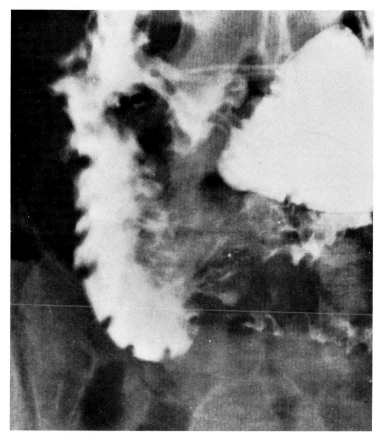

Figure 13-6 Henoch's purpura. In the patient of Figure 13–5, one month later, there is marked improvement in the appearance of the folds.

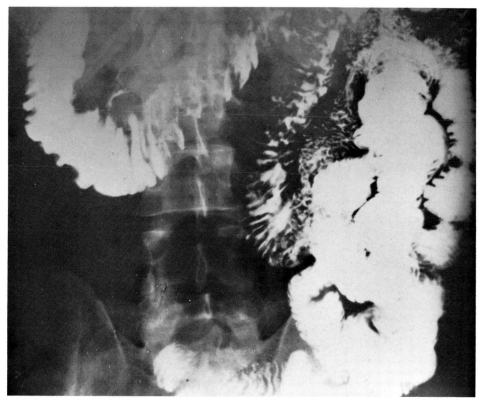

Figure 13-7 Henoch's purpura. Exaggerated thickened folds accompanied by spasm and irritability are seen in the fourth portion of the duodenum and in the proximal jejunum.

175

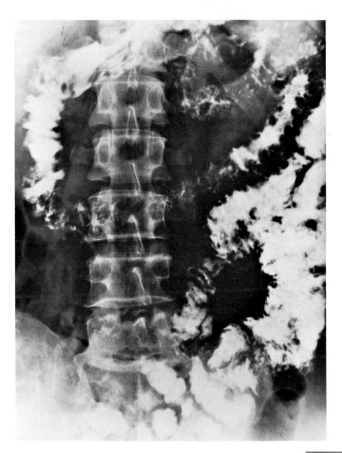

Figure 13-8 Henoch's purpura. Almost the entire small intestine is involved. The condition is characterized by an irregular thickening of the mucosal folds, increased secretions, and minimal segmentation. The bowel lumen is of normal caliber.

Figure 13-9 Henoch's purpura. The small intestine is slightly dilated. The mucosal pattern is completely effaced because of increased secretions and mucosal edema. This should not be confused with the diffuse ulceration seen in regional enteritis.

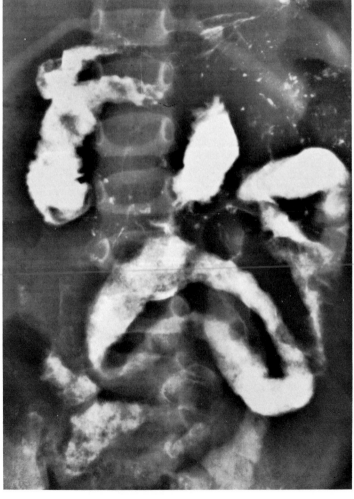

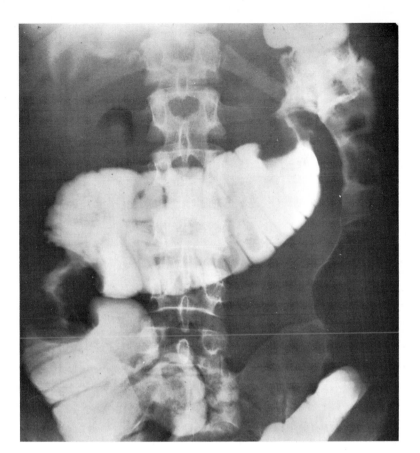

Figure 13–10 Henoch's purpura. Two segmental areas of narrowing in the colon are characterized by sharply defined margins, a concentric lumen which retains some degree of flexibility, and irregular thickening of the folds without mucosal ulceration. The appearance is consistent with a circumferential submucosal lesion.

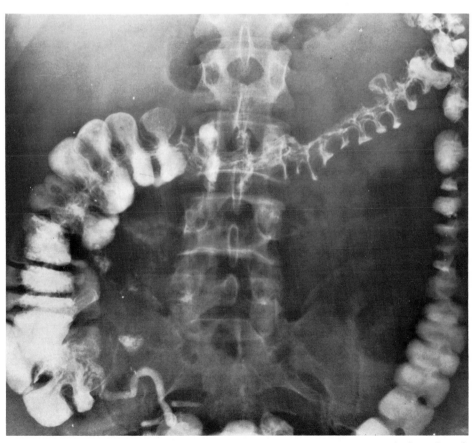

Figure 13–11 Henoch's purpura. In the patient of Figure 13–10, two weeks later the colon appears normal.

and fragmented. Occasionally, scalloping and marked thumb-printing resulting from excessive edema and hemorrhage may be identified. In the colon an appearance of carcinoma may be simulated (Figs. 13-10 and 13-11). Discrete ulcerations are not seen. Because of the increased secretions and the thickening of the folds, intestinal lymphangiectasia may be suggested in the differential diagnosis.

PRIMARY NONSPECIFIC ULCERATION OF THE SMALL BOWEL

Solitary ulcers of the small intestine are very rare, and although the cause is unknown a vascular etiology is suspected. The ulcers are more likely to appear in the ileum than in the jejunum; occasionally they are multiple. The lesions tend to be well-defined and free of surrounding inflammatory response, and they characteristically present with bleeding, perforation, or obstruction.

In some cases, enteric-coated potassium chloride tablets have been incriminated in the solitary small bowel ulcer. It is believed, with experimental support, that rapid release of potassium over a short segment of small bowel causes spasm of mural and mesenteric blood vessels with consequent infarction and ulceration, typically circumferential.[5]

References

1. Bienenstock, H., Minick, C. R., and Rogoff, B.: Mesenteric arteritis and intestinal infarction in rheumatoid disease. *Arch. Intern. Med.*, 119:359-364, 1967.
2. Couris, G. D., Block, M. A., and Rupe, C. E.: Gastrointestinal complications of collagen diseases. *Arch. Surg.*, 89:695-700, 1964.
3. Ettinger, A., and Perez-Tamayo, R.: Ulcerative jejunitis in polyarteritis. *Radiology*, 68:669-672, 1957.
4. Handel, J., and Schwartz, S.: Gastrointestinal manifestations of the Schönlein-Henoch syndrome. *Amer. J. Roentgen.*, 78:643-652, 1957.
5. Boley, S. S., Allan, A. C., Schultz, L. and Schwartz, S.: Potassium-induced lesions of the small bowel. *J.A.M.A.*, 193:997-1000, 1965.

14

Regional Enteritis

The chronic granulomatous inflammatory disease of the small bowel which is now termed regional enteritis, or Crohn's disease of the small intestine, was first described by Crohn, Ginzburg, and Oppenheimer[1] in 1932, under the name terminal ileitis or regional ileitis. Failure to recognize regional enteritis prior to 1932 can reasonably be attributed to diagnostic confusion with intestinal tuberculosis, and indeed the clinical, roentgenologic, and pathologic features of the two diseases have so much in common that even using the criteria of today the distinction may at times prove difficult.

Although the general recognition of granulomatous disease of the bowel can be dated quite precisely to 1932, it is interesting to speculate on when the disease first appeared in the literature. Wilks and Moxon,[2] in an 1875 collection of lectures in which they provide the first careful description of ulcerative colitis, also mention an acute ileitis with characteristics strongly suggestive of granulomatous disease:

> We have met several times with severe local acute ileitis in the shape of a thickening of the whole of the coats, including the valvulae conniventes which stood out stiffly, while the whole wall was thick with inflammatory lymph, the microscope showing a generalized charging of the whole tissue with pyroid corpuscles. This condition was found in . . . (circumscribed patches) . . . of from six inches to two or three feet.

Shapiro,[3] in an historical review, cites possible cases as early as 1806.

In 1923, Moschowitz and Wilensky,[4] of New York's Mount Sinai Hospital, reported in detail four patients with nonspecific granulomatous disease of the intestine. This paper is of notable interest, for the authors carefully described the clinical and pathologic features of the disease we now call granulomatous colitis (and ileocolitis) and were able to separate the entity from intestinal tuberculosis, carcinoma, lymphoma, syphilis, and diverticulitis. They recognized that similar cases had previously been reported and were even aware of remission after bypass procedures: "The most interesting and diagnosticable characteristic in connection with these granulomata is their disappearance after a simple side-tracking procedure."

A few years later, Leon Ginzburg and Gordon Oppenheimer at Mount Sinai Hospital continued with work begun by Moschowitz and Wilensky on nonspecific granulomas of the bowel. They utilized the extensive surgical material from the service of Dr. A. A. Berg, and in time they were able to identify among patients with nonspecific intestinal granulomas a dozen cases of a localized hypertrophic ulcerative stenosis of the terminal ileum. In 1930 Dr. Burrill Crohn had under his care two patients with a similar disease, and operation was performed by Dr. Berg. These workers now joined forces as the characteristics of the "new" disease evolved. In 1932 Crohn, Ginzburg, and Oppenheimer submitted their classic description of granulomatous inflammation of the small bowel. They reported 14 cases of the disease, which they called "terminal ileitis." The paper was presented at a meeting of the American Medical Association. Dr. J. A. Bargen, who was in the audience, protested that the name "terminal" suggested that this was a fatal illness, yet the reported patients had all survived. Dr. Crohn and his associates accepted his suggestion that the disease should be called "regional ileitis" and such was the name when the paper was published.

At the time of the original report, it was the concept of Crohn and his colleagues that this was a disease confined to the distal small bowel and that the process stopped abruptly at the ileocecal valve. Presumably the other nonspecific granulomas, such as those described in the colon by Moschowitz and Wilensky, were considered to be different diseases. In the years that have elapsed since the original paper, it has become apparent that although the disease which had been called "regional ileitis" commonly *does* involve the terminal ileum, it may be found in any part of the gastrointestinal tract. Rare cases of possible esophageal involvement have been reported, but there are a number of reports of cases involving the stomach, either alone or in association with disease in the intestine, and a few cases of duodenal involvement alone have been reported. In 1934, only two years after the description of regional ileitis, Colp[5] reported the first case of granulomatous colitis. The patient was a medical student who had involvement of the ileum and the cecum. Not much of the colon was involved, of course, but this case was sufficient to demonstrate that the ileocecal valve is no barrier to the development of granulomatous disease in the colon. Regional enteritis involving the colon alone or in conjunction with disease in the small bowel has been carefully studied and is the subject of a separate chapter in this book (*Granulomatous Colitis and Ileocolitis*).

British workers have used the term "Crohn's disease" for nonspecific granulomatous disease wherever it occurs in the gut. American writers, who generally avoid eponyms, have tended to vary the name with the area involved in the disease. Thus, in the stomach the process is termed granulomatous gastritis; in the small bowel, regional enteritis; in the colon, granulomatous colitis; and in the small bowel and colon, when both are involved, granulomatous ileocolitis. The pathological entity is the same at all levels of the intestinal tract.

Pathology

The bowel involved in regional enteritis is sharply delimited from contiguous gut and has a narrowed lumen, sometimes strictured. The intestinal wall is rigid and thick. The attached mesentery is thickened, and mesenteric lymph nodes are enlarged. The mucosa is red and swollen and has a cobblestone appearance as longitudinal and transverse ulcers intersect. Sinus tracts and fistulas may be present and may extend to adjacent viscera or to the body wall. Several areas of disease ("skip lesions") may be present in the bowel, separated by lengths of normal-appearing intestine. Mesenteric abscess may develop.

It is convenient to consider that there are four main gross pathologic features:

1. Stricturing and thickening of the bowel wall.
2. Discontinuous ulceration.
3. Cobblestoning of the mucosa.
4. Fistula formation.

Strictures are due to the combination of edema and more predominantly fibrosis which is so characteristic of this disease (Figs. 14-1 and 14-2). In fact, Crohn's disease in the intestine is a form of chronic elephantiasis with lymphatic blockade and the production of fibrous tissue, which gives it its characteristic appearance. The mesentery is also involved by edema and fibrosis, and excessive mesenteric fat overhangs the intestine. The strictures may be single or multiple and of varying length.

Discontinuous ulceration is one of the most typical features of Crohn's disease. The ulcers may be large and serpiginous or small and difficult to identify. The mucosa between the ulcerations may be normal, edematous, or reveal cobblestoning.

Cobblestoning is seen in approximately 25 to 35 per cent of the cases and is due to three principal causes. The first of these is edema of the mucosal and submucosal folds that are not closely attached to the underlying muscularis and bulge up to produce a cobblestone appearance.

The second mechanism is the presence of a network of longitudinal and transverse fissures that involve the mucosa and submucosa, leaving intervening intact portions of mucosa.

A third mechanism is seen in the stenotic phase of this disease. Marked fibrosis produces traction on the overlying mucosa in a compartmentalized fashion, which acts as as a pulley.

Fissures and *sinus tracts* in Crohn's disease extend to various depths of the bowel wall or into the mesentery. The fistulas may reach the skin or other surfaces, such as those of the bladder or vagina. If the disease involves primarily the small intestine, they may extend into either the large intestine, or rarely the stomach.

The histologic features of Crohn's disease are characteristic. The most typical single feature of established Crohn's disease is the presence of granulomas, which are found in about 90 per cent of the cases providing that adequate sections of the intestinal wall, mesentery, and regional lymph nodes are carefully examined. These granulomas are small, vaguely resembling tubercles or sarcoid granulomas. However, they lack caseous necrosis and are less tightly organized and uniform than is usual in sarcoidosis. They are located close to or sometimes within dilated lymphatics, which they apparently partly or completely obstruct. The granulomas are composed of epithelioid macrophages and may contain giant cells. These giant cells are of the Langhans type and frequently have peripheral lipid vacuoles. Granulomas may be found only in the regional lymph nodes and be absent from sections of the intestinal wall

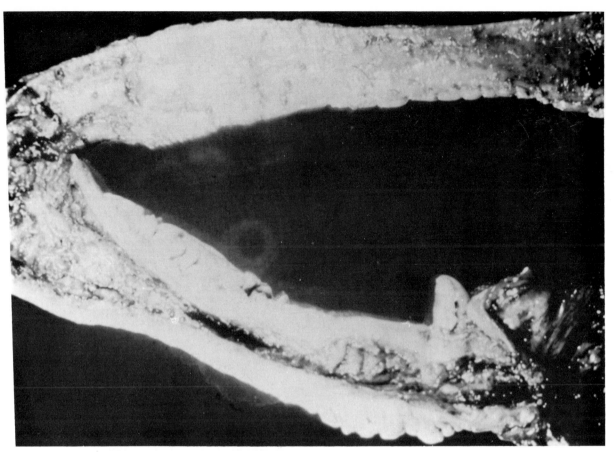

Figure 14-1 A longitudinal segment of bowel illustrates the marked thickening of the intestinal wall caused by a combination of edema and fibrosis. This results in a stenotic lumen with the characteristic "hose pipe" stricture of Crohn's disease.

and mesentery. Particularly since the advent of treatment with steroids, the incidence of granulomas in resected specimens seems to have decreased, and in steroid-treated patients probably they cannot be found in more than half.

The cause of granuloma formation in Crohn's disease is unknown, but as in other granulomatous diseases it appears to represent some inadequacy of the host response to an irritating agent which may be inorganic, organic, a virus, or other pathogenic organisms. Granulomas represent a stale-mated inflammation which does not heal rapidly, but eventually subsides with fibrous scarring.

A second characteristic finding in Crohn's disease is prominent lymph follicles in the mucosa and submucosa. These lymphoid follicles may or may not have germinal centers. The leukocytic infiltrate is that of nonspecific chronic inflammation with combinations of lymphocytes, macrophages, and plasma cells. Measurements of the plasma cells in Crohn's disease have shown them to be larger than the plasma cells found in other inflammatory diseases of the intestine, but the cause of this is unknown.

As we have mentioned in describing the gross pathology, a third very striking characteristic of Crohn's disease is persistent lymphangiectasis with lymphedema. Because of inflammation, granuloma formation, and fibrosis the lymphatics in the intestinal wall, mesentery, and mesenteric lymph nodes are obstructed at multiple points, and between the obstructions are very prominent dilated lymphatics with lymph stasis. This lymph stasis is essentially the same lesion as seen in elephantiasis, and it may in part be responsible for the productive fibrosis which once gave the name cicatrizing enteritis to Crohn's disease. The earliest lesions resulting in lymphatic blockade are produced by proliferation of the endothelium that lines the lymphatics. Endothelial cells form sheets which obstruct lymph drainage.

Another important histologic feature is the presence of knife-like clefts or a transverse fissure which sometimes branch and penetrate from the mucosa deep into the bowel wall, sometimes reaching the subserosal fat.

Crohn's disease characteristically involves all layers of the bowel wall, so that inflammation is seen in the mucosa, submucosa, intermuscular septa, and subserosa. It is thus a transmural inflammation, a term which has particular significance in the colon, where it is a feature used to differentiate Crohn's disease of the colon from ulcerative colitis.

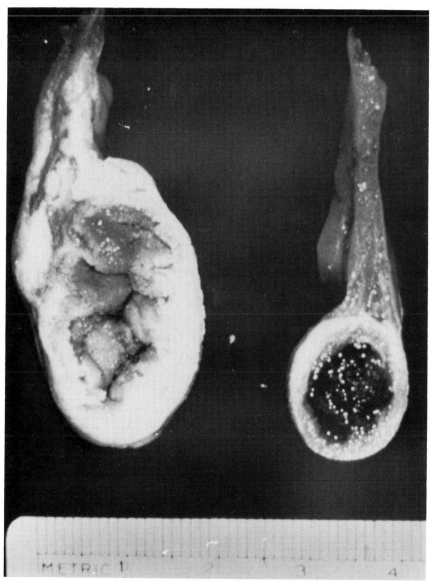

Figure 14-2 Cross sections of normal and diseased intestine. Marked thickening and encroachment on the lumen by fibrous tissue and edema is evident in Crohn's disease.

Etiology

The cause of regional enteritis remains unknown, despite years of extensive study and speculation. Families have now been reported in which regional enteritis occurred in a parent and one child, in a parent and several children, in two or more siblings, and in both monozygotic and dizygotic twins. Occurrence of the disease in members of the same family suggests a genetic predisposing factor, but studies so far do not permit conclusions concerning possible genetic mechanisms. In several studies the disease is statistically more common among Jews. Psychiatric factors have not been studied as extensively in regional enteritis as in ulcerative colitis, but thus far no specific emotional background or etiology is apparent. Many studies over the years have failed to demonstrate causative protozoa or tubercle bacilli, and bacteria appear to play only a secondary role. Virus isolation studies and measurements of antibody titers have failed to incriminate known agents.

The presence of granulomas early raised the question of whether regional enteritis might be a form of sarcoidosis, but the two diseases appear to affect quite different populations, and patients with sarcoidosis rarely have lesions in the intestinal tract. Variable results have been achieved with use of the Kveim test, some series showing positive tests in a proportion of patients with Crohn's disease, a finding not confirmed by other series. Further confusion about a possible relationship between Crohn's disease and sarcoidosis has been raised by uncertainty about the specificity of the Kveim test, which has been reported to be positive in a variety of diseases apparently having in common only the feature of lymphadenopathy.

Mitchell and Rees,[6a] in a series of studies, injected material from the bowel and regional lymph nodes of patients with Crohn's disease into the foot pads of mice, producing granulomatous lesions in a proportion of the animals. In some of these reacting mice it was possible to induce a positive Kveim reaction. It was the conclusion of these workers that they had demonstrated a transmissible agent in Crohn's disease and also had shown a relationship between sarcoidosis and Crohn's disease. These interesting findings need to be confirmed and interpreted.

None of the experimental methods attempted in animals has succeeded in producing lesions fully characteristic of regional enteritis. The possibility that autoimmune responses might be the cause of the disease is of current interest and has been reviewed in detail by Slaney.[7] He presents evidence that granulomatous lesions can be produced as part of a hypersensitivity response to foreign protein in a previously sensitized animal. However, circulating antibodies to intestinal cells have not been demonstrated in patients with regional enteritis, serum immunoglobulin levels are normal or slightly increased, and immunoglobulin cell populations in the bowel wall are normal.

Studies of immunologic reactivity have given confusing results: anergy is sometimes but not generally reported, with findings of decreased skin test and DNCB responsiveness and impairment of phytohemagglutinin-induced lymphocyte transformation.

On balance, at the present time, it is difficult to see immune mechanisms as the cause of Crohn's disease, but they may contribute to the pathologic process once underway.

Clinical Features

Although regional enteritis may occur at any age, most commonly the onset is in the late 'teens or the twenties. The clinical course usually begins with diarrhea, abdominal cramps, low-grade fever, anemia, anorexia, and weight loss. The onset is often insidious, and in the early stages there may be only a gradual increase in symptoms. At times the symptoms may be low-grade or so intermittent that the patient does not seek medical attention or appropriate diagnostic studies are not done for months or years; in these cases the true onset of disease is recognized only in retrospect. Occasionally the onset is acute, and the patient presents with what seems to be acute appendicitis. At surgical exploration on these occasions, however, the small bowel appears chronically inflamed, so it seems likely that what appeared to be "acute ileitis" is really an acute exacerbation of a previously quiescent chronic disease.

A characteristic finding on physical examination is the presence of a tender abdominal mass, usually in the right lower quadrant. The mass represents chronically inflamed bowel, thickened mesentery, enlarged lymph nodes, and sometimes an intra-abdominal abscess.

Partial small bowel obstruction and stricture formation are common in regional enteritis, but complete obstruction is unusual even in severe disease. For this reason obstruction may be a cause of disabling symptoms but it is rarely a cause of surgical emergency. Spasm and edema may cause obstruction which can be relieved by small bowel intubation and medical supportive measures.

Similarly, free perforation of the small bowel into the peritoneal cavity is extremely rare. On the other hand, small, sealed-off perforations of the bowel are not only common but are quite characteristic of the disease. These small perforations represent extensions of inflammatory disease through the bowel wall to the serosa and out into the mesentery. The leakage is slow, the perforation is small, and the leak becomes sealed off. Regional lymph nodes become enlarged and inflamed. Such small, sealed-off perforations are the basis of the fistulas which are so common in regional enteritis. Fistulas may extend from one loop of small bowel to another, from small bowel to colon, or from small bowel to vagina, bladder, or the abdominal wall. Perianal fistulas and abscesses are common features of the illness. It is especially interesting that perianal fistulas may be the first clinical finding in regional enteritis and may antedate the other clinical features by many months or even years. The source of the anorectal disease in regional enteritis is not clear. It has been considered to represent inflammation extending from the rectal crypts in association with diarrhea and poor anal hygiene, or spread of disease downward from loops of diseased small bowel lying on the pelvic floor. Recently Gray et al.[10] have presented evidence that anal granulomatous lesions may not be secondary to intestinal involvement at all, but rather a local manifestation of a granulomatous process that can involve any segment of a gastrointestinal tract—i.e., the anal disease represents, in effect, a skip lesion.

Microscopic bleeding is common in regional enteritis, and iron deficiency is one cause of the anemia that occurs in this disease. Stools are often guaiac positive. Gross blood in the stools is uncommon, however, and when it does occur it is usually only an occasional episode and not a regular feature of the course.

Extraintestinal findings, such as peripheral arthritis, ankylosing spondylitis, iritis, erythema nodosum, and pyoderma gangrenosum, all occur in patients with regional enteritis but are less common than in ulcerative colitis. In those patients with disease of the terminal ileum or with resection of this segment of bowel, cholesterol gallstones and oxalate renal calculi present with increased frequency.

Management

In most patients regional enteritis follows a chronic course with low-grade disability. About one-third of patients are managed medically throughout their course; two-thirds eventually require some sort of surgical intervention. Regional enteritis does not appear to spread anatomically, either proximally or distally, in the absence of surgery. As patients are followed with repeated small bowel roentgen examinations year after year on medical programs, the disease may worsen within a given area, and abscesses, strictures, or fistulas may develop, but the linear extent of disease throughout follow-up appears to be the same as on the initial examination. The failure of the disease to spread under medical treatment is remarkable, for the disease is notorious for its tendency to spread and to recur after surgery. Disease recurs in at least half the patients who are operated upon, usually within the first two years after operation but sometimes many years later. As a rule the disease recurs just proximal to the old diseased area, at the site of anastomosis, but sometimes the recurrence is quite distant and skip lesions may develop. A "cure" of regional enteritis either medically or surgically is unusual, but prolonged remissions of many years' duration may occur.

Medical Treatment

The goal of medical treatment in regional enteritis is to induce a remission and, failing this, to provide symptomatic and supportive treatment so that the patient can function in everyday life despite the activity of a chronic disease. Medical programs include dietary manipulation, rest and sedation, use of antidiarrheal agents, and correction of anemia. Antibiotics do not appear to affect the course of the disease and are reserved for treatment of complications such as abscess formation and management of fistulas. Adrenal corticosteroids reduce inflammation and may relieve both obstructive symptoms and the toxicity of fistulas and abscess formation. Steroids are thus useful in management of symptoms, although they are less likely to induce a remission than in ulcerative colitis. Although steroid therapy has been a major factor in making the life of the patient with regional enteritis more comfortable, there is no convincing evidence that it has influenced the incidence of surgery or altered the natural history of the disease. An immunosuppressive and anti-inflammatory agent, azathioprine (Imuran) has recently been employed in treating patients unresponsive to other medical measures. Anecdotal reports of clinical improvement, including closure of fistulas, have appeared,[9] but large controlled clinical trials, now underway, will be required to evaluate the effectiveness of the drug. Azulfidine, usually considered an effective drug only in ulcerative colitis, is sometimes of benefit in both regional enteritis and granulomatous colitis.

Surgical Treatment

Surgery is indicated for treatment of the complications of regional enteritis. These include obstruction, fistulas which are symptomatic or causing debility, abdominal masses and abscesses, and the very rare complications of perforation or hemorrhage. Usually intermittent partial obstruction or infection with abscess formation are the complications that require surgery. "Intractability" to a medical regimen, without development of complications, is a difficult surgical indication to define. It encompasses patients who, despite good medical management, simply don't do well; they have continuous disability with diarrhea, abdominal pain, and fever. In this group one must consider treating the diseased bowel surgically.

Because the risk of recurrent disease is high, many physicians prefer to treat even the severe case of regional enteritis medically as long as possible and reserve surgery for the time when complications occur or the clinical course is deteriorating.

The early operations for regional enteritis were bypass procedures in which the diseased loops of bowel were simply excluded from continuity with the fecal stream. More recent procedures emphasize resection of the diseased bowel and anastomosis of proximal normal small bowel to colon. The amount of bowel that is resected seems to have little to do with recurrence; the recurrence rate is about the same whether a minimal resection is done, taking out only obviously diseased bowel, or an extensive procedure, taking much apparently normal bowel, is performed. Moreover, the recurrence rate after resections appears to be no less than after bypass procedures. Nevertheless, most surgeons today prefer to remove diseased bowel, and the usual procedure is a resection of the diseased area with an end-to-end anastomosis. Bypass procedures today are generally reserved for cases in which the bowel is so matted down with fistulas and abscesses that it cannot be removed.

Roentgen Features

Several investigators have attempted to divide the roentgen findings in this disease into acute, subacute, and chronic stages. Since the classic form of regional enteritis is that of a low-grade inflammatory process with episodes of acute exacerbation, it is difficult to identify clear-cut patterns indicative of stages of the disease. It is possible that acute regional enteritis does occur, but the determination of the precise onset of the disease is almost impossible; what is described as acute regional enteritis may be a more active phase of the chronic illness.

Proximal and distal extension of the disease process, despite repeated roentgen examinations over a period of many years, is rarely seen. The maximum length of the involved area is determined by the initial roentgen studies. This is not true after exclusion operations or resections, when longitudinal spread is not infrequent.

One of the prominent features of this disease is the development of stenosis with obstruction. Roentgenologically, we have found that cases may be divided conveniently into stenotic and nonstenotic types. It is impossible to classify cases into early or late stages, since many may continue without stenosis for many years. Division into active and inactive phases seems inappropriate, since a patient with long segments of stenotic and probably fibrotic intestine may exhibit considerable evidence of clinical activity manifested by fever, abdominal pain, and leukocytosis.

Nonstenotic Phase

The roentgen findings closely parallel the pathologic features.[11] Early changes are blunting, flattening, thickening, distortion, or straightening of the valvulae conniventes. The folds may be markedly distorted or arranged in a fairly regular, symmetric, parallel fashion, appear rigid, and are perpendicular to the long axis of the intestine. The folds become thicker, irregular, indistinct, and partially fused (Figs. 14-3 to 14-6). The lumen and contour become irregular. Occasionally the irregularity of contour and of the valvulae conniventes is seen without distinct blunting or thickening of the folds (Figs. 14-7 and 14-8). These early changes are due to the inflammatory submucosal and mucosal thickening. When ulceration occurs, a more characteristic pattern is produced. Longitudinal streaks of barium recognizable as ulcers appear (Fig. 14-9) and are usually associated with transverse ulcerations, producing in some cases a cobblestone pattern (Figs. 14-10 to 14-12). This specific pattern is better seen in the jejunum, probably because the valvulae conniventes are more prominent in

(Text continued on page 192.)

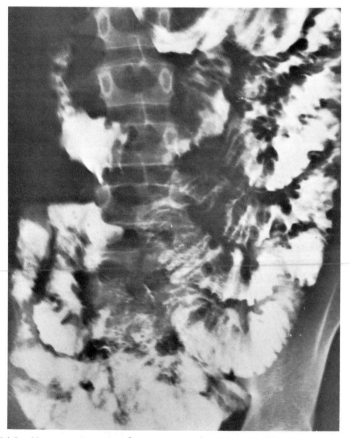

Figure 14-3 *Nonstenotic regional enteritis.* In this 10 year old girl there is thickening and blunting of the folds, with moderate irregularity of the contour of the bowel. Minimal rigidity and uncoiling of the loops of small bowel as well as increased secretions are noted.

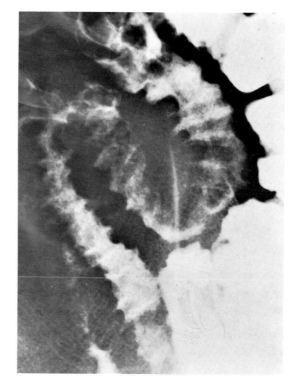

Figure 14-4 Nonstenotic regional enteritis. A young male with 10 days of fever and diarrhea. The folds in the distal ileum are hazy, thickened, and blunted, in association with slight narrowing, rigidity, and separation of the loops of bowel.

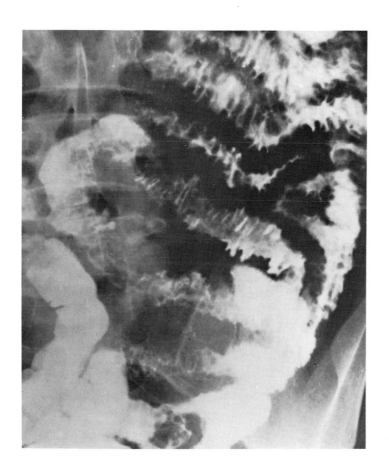

Figure 14-5 Nonstenotic regional enteritis. The mucosal folds are thickened, blunted, and in some areas fused. The contour of the bowel is irregular and associated with slight rigidity and separation of the loops of bowel, which also appear straightened and uncoiled.

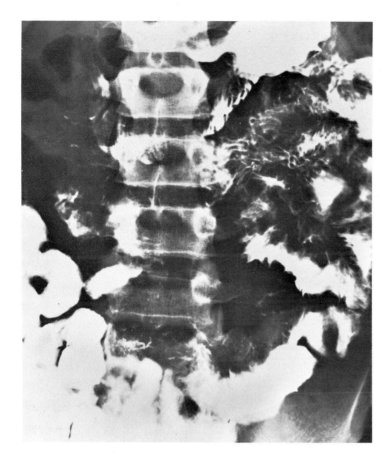

Figure 14-6   *Nonstenotic regional enteritis.* There is a moderate degree of spasm and irritability of the jejunum and proximal ileum, associated with slight narrowing of the lumen and slight rigidity. The folds are minimally thickened, and the contour is irregular.

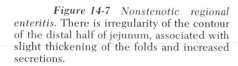

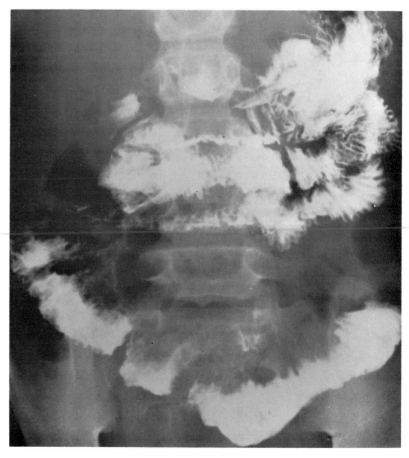

Figure 14-7   *Nonstenotic regional enteritis.* There is irregularity of the contour of the distal half of jejunum, associated with slight thickening of the folds and increased secretions.

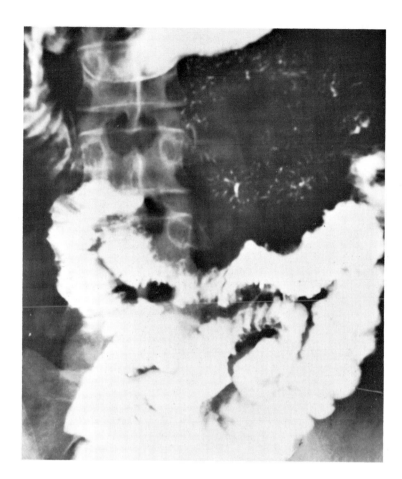

Figure 14-8 Nonstenotic regional enteritis. There is irregularity of the contour of the distal jejunum due to multiple nodular defects which represent skip lesions.

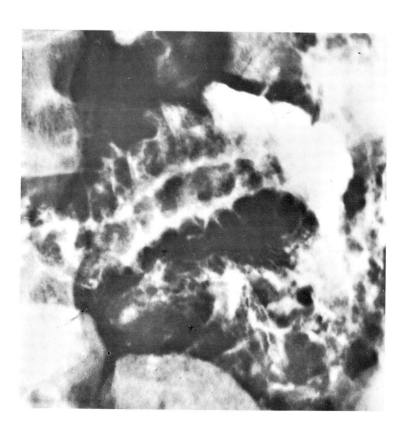

Figure 14-9 Nonstenotic regional enteritis. Longitudinal streaks of barium, indicating ulceration, are seen in association with transverse ulcers. The combination of transverse and longitudinal ulcerations produces an effect which has been called cobblestoning.

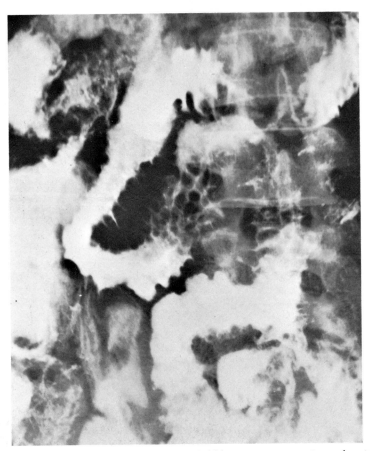

Figure 14-10 *Nonstenotic regional enteritis.* Cobblestone pattern owing to longitudinal and transverse ulcerations is identified. The involved loops are moderately rigid and slightly narrowed. Separation of the involved loops of bowel is also noted.

this region. Ulceration continues at the expense of the intervening islands of mucosa, replacing the cobblestone pattern by an irregular network of interlacing streaks of barium. The appearance at this stage has no uniformity or symmetry and is hazy and reticulated (Figs. 14-13 to 14-15). Denudation of the mucosa is usually incomplete, leaving behind islands of inflamed mucosa (inflammatory polyps) which produce multiple smooth defects of varying size (Fig. 14-16). Their prominence is increased by the narrowing of the bowel lumen, due to beginning cicatricial contraction which occurs at this stage. Finally, one may see the roentgenologic image of a uniform, rigid, castlike tube filled with barium and presenting no mucous membrane pattern. This is similar to the appearance of ulcerative colitis in the colon and represents the stage when scarring and regeneration of an atrophic mucosa are progressing (Figs. 14-17 and 14-18). As scarring proceeds, the transition to the stenotic phase occurs.

Coincident with changes in the mucosa, other characteristic roentgen features appear. The bowel lumen reveals varying degrees of narrowing. Early, the submucosal thickening and spasm, secondary to the marked inflammatory process, are responsible for the narrowing of the lumen. Later, as fibrosis occurs, the narrowing is more marked and leads finally to the stenotic stage. In the early stages, rigidity of the contour and mucosal pattern is incomplete. Some flexibility or dynamic activity is evident from the change in contour and

(Text continued on page 197.)

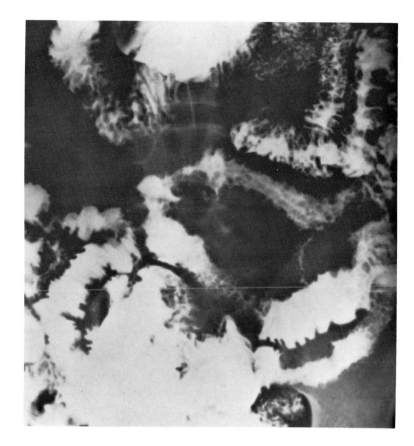

Figure 14-11 Nonstenotic regional enteritis. A cobblestone pattern with transverse and linear ulcerations is seen. The involved segments have a hazy appearance because of increased secretions which are secondary to the inflammatory edema. A fistulous communication is also noted.

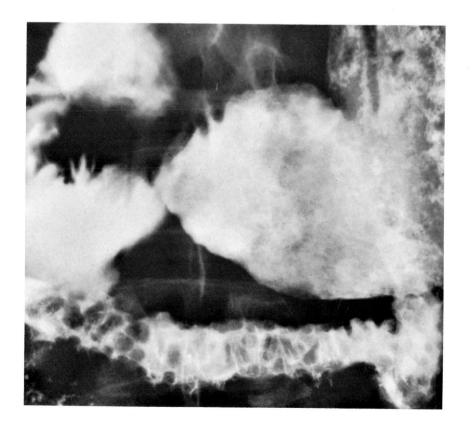

Figure 14-12 Nonstenotic regional enteritis. A cobblestone pattern secondary to longitudinal and transverse ulceration is again seen. The contours are irregular.

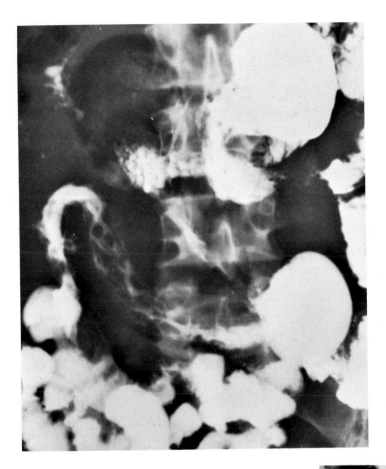

Figure 14-13 *Nonstenotic regional enteritis.* The distal jejunum and proximal ileum are involved. There is an irregular network of interlacing streaks of barium due to ulceration. The radiolucent areas between the streaks of barium represent the edematous mucosa. With continued ulcerations the symmetric cobblestone pattern is no longer identified, and the appearance becomes more reticulated.

Figure 14-14 *Nonstenotic regional enteritis.* There is an irregular reticulated pattern in the terminal ileum from extensive ulceration and edematous mucosa.

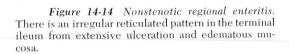

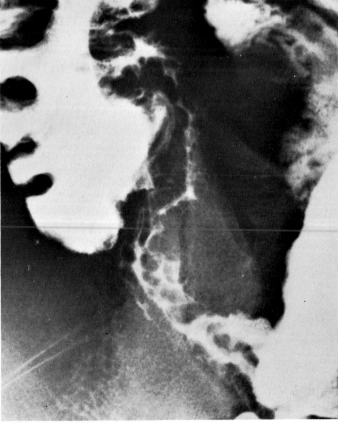

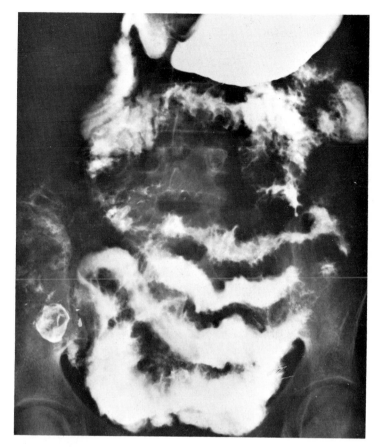

Figure 14-15 *Nonstenotic regional enteritis*. The entire small bowel is involved with thickening and blunting of the folds, which in some areas appear completely effaced because of ulceration. There is narrowing, rigidity, increased secretion, and separation of the loops of bowel.

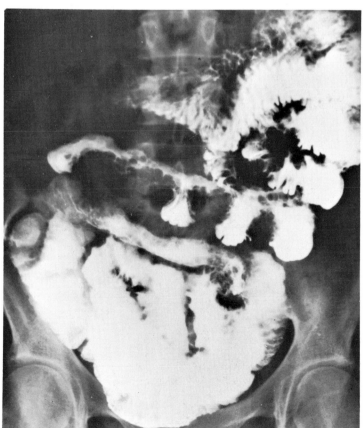

Figure 14-16 *Nonstenotic regional enteritis*. There is rigidity and separation of the distal jejunum and proximal ileum with numerous small filling defects due to inflammatory polyps. Eccentric skip areas are also noted.

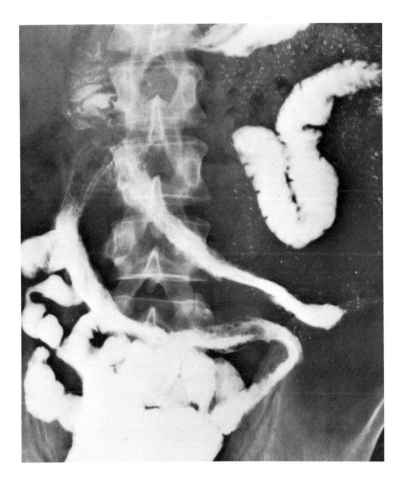

Figure 14-17 Nonstenotic regional enteritis. The distal jejunum and proximal ileum are rigid, moderately narrowed and separated. The mucosal pattern appears castlike due to ulceration and reepithelialization. Several small defects represent inflammatory polyps. This is the late phase of the nonstenotic type of regional enteritis with beginning fibrosis and narrowing.

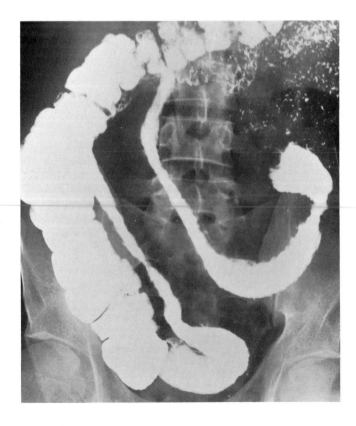

Figure 14-18 Early stenotic regional enteritis. The entire ileum is involved. The findings are similar to those in Figure 14-17 except for more narrowing of the bowel lumen.

mucosal pattern during successive roentgenograms. Later, the roentgen appearance is fixed and unvarying. Pliability is also lost. Furthermore, early in the disease the normal serpentine or coiled pattern of the loops of small intestine disappears. The diseased segments seem to be straightened and rigid. This finding is probably due to loss of flexibility in the intestinal wall and mesentery, as well as longitudinal shortening due to spasm.

Not infrequently, the loops of intestine appear to surround a mass (Fig. 14-19). Although this may be due to an abscess resulting from perforation, more often it is secondary to an indurated mesentery, associated with marked increase in mesenteric fat and enlarged lymph nodes. The silhouette of the intestine may be hazy. This is because the intestine is diffusely ulcerated; it contains exudate and excessive secretions, and the barium does not adhere to the walls. Despite the increase in intestinal content, the barium mixture remains fluid and homogeneous. Neither agglutination, clumping, nor formation of masses of barium is found in regional enteritis in contrast to the findings in the sprue pattern. Segmentation, such as that characteristic of sprue, has not been observed. When unequivocal segmentation occurs, the diagnosis of regional enteritis should be suspect.

Skip areas (Fig. 14-16), that is, segments of normal intestine intervening between diseased segments, represent another characteristic feature. The length of the skip area may vary from a few inches to several feet. The extent of

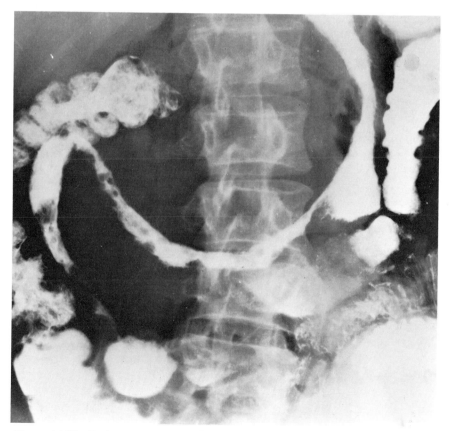

Figure 14-19 Early stenotic regional enteritis. The mucosa is ulcerated and inflammatory polyps are present. The loop is rigid, narrowed, and surrounds an inflammatory mass which consists of indurated mesentery. There is slight proximal dilatation.

involvement on a roentgenogram may be quite accurately determined in most cases, since the transition of disease to the normal intestine is fairly abrupt. In some instances, marked spasm and irritability may be seen in intrinsically normal small bowel because of proximity to diseased segments. Several examinations may be necessary before it can be accurately determined that these spastic and irritable loops of bowel are not involved with regional enteritis. This is important for both surgeon and radiologist in planning a resection in such cases.

An outpouching of the mucosa between the thickened folds (Fig. 14-20) occurs in some cases, creating an appearance much like diverticula. Pseudodiverticula are probably caused by eccentric skip areas affecting one side of the bowel wall and not the other. Ulceration along one wall produces spasm and contraction, and as a result the opposite uninvolved wall becomes folded.

Stenotic Phase

In the stenotic stage, many of the rigid loops described previously become constricted to a remarkable degree. These stenotic segments resemble rigid pipestems (Figs. 14-19, 14-21 to 14-26). This appearance is due to a marked thickening and contraction of the wall of the small intestine. The stenosis may extend through 1 or 2 cm. or over long segments. With severe narrowing, dilatation of the proximal intestine may be marked. In many instances, it is difficult to state whether or not intrinsic disease is present in a dilated segment. Very often disease is present when a loop of dilated intestine exists between two points of constriction. On the other hand, when there is a single area of constriction with proximal dilatation, disease may not be present in the dilated segment (Fig. 14-27). However, because of retained secretions, secondary inflammatory changes, tension ulcers, and muscular hypertrophy, the appearance of the dilated loops may be confused with the alterations seen in regional enteritis. This distinction is of great importance when surgery is considered. Many patients have not undergone operative intervention because the surgeon believed that the entire intestine was involved. Extreme dilatation of long segments of the intestine is rarely associated with intrinsic granulomatous disease. It is not uncommon for foreign bodies to be present in a dilated loop proximal to a stenotic area (Fig. 14-28).

Many of the roentgen phenomena observed in the nonstenotic phase of the disease are again noted in the stenotic phase. The mucosal pattern is usually reticulated or castlike. Small filling defects and inflammatory polyps, irregularly distributed throughout the diseased segments, are noted. Skip areas and wide spacing between the segments of intestine are more striking.

The loops are rigid and maintain a constant position from film to film. The diseased segments of intestine seem to encircle an inflammatory mass. Fistulas, usually involving the distal ileum and adjacent loops of intestine, may be seen. Occasionally, these are difficult to demonstrate, especially when dilated loops of intestine produce overlapping. The fistulas may extend to and penetrate the abdominal wall.

In general, the roentgen findings in regional enteritis are as described; however, there are certain characteristics that are peculiar to the area of involvement.

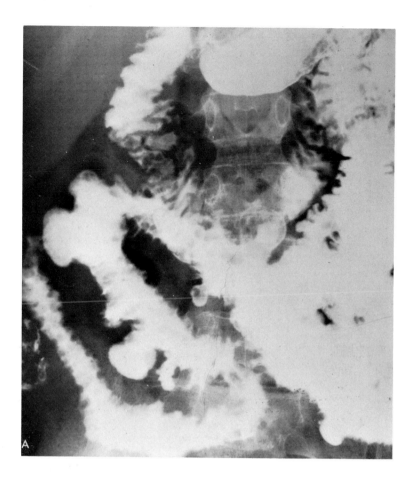

Figure 14-20 *Nonstenotic regional enteritis.* A, Normal bowel protrudes between thickened, blunted folds and suggests the presence of numerous pseudodiverticula. These are due to eccentric skip areas with ulceration on one side of the bowel and pleating on the opposite side.

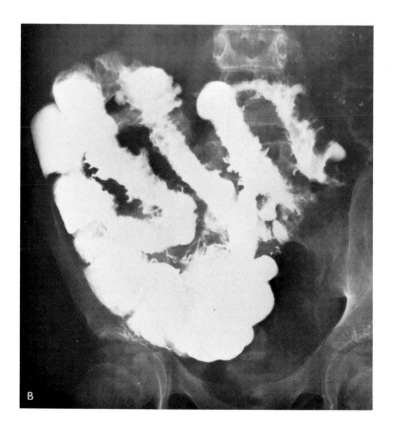

Figure 14-20B Again, multiple pseudodiverticula due to eccentric skip lesions are identified.

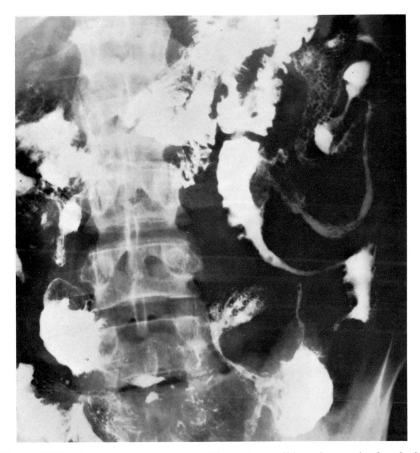

Figure 14-21   Stenotic regional enteritis. The entire small bowel is involved with alternating areas of constriction and dilatation. The patient was a young man who died of an exsanguinating hemorrhage.

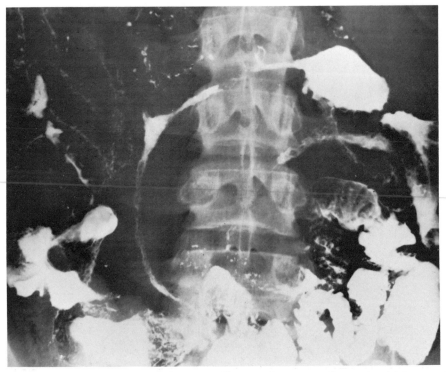

Figure 14-22   Stenotic regional enteritis. There are long areas of stenosis with intervening small areas of dilatation. The stenotic segments have a rigid pipelike configuration.

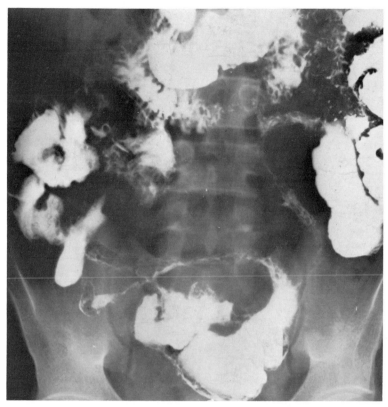

Figure 14-23 *Stenotic regional enteritis.* Long segments of constricted bowel alternate with areas of dilatation. In the constricted segments the mucosa is ulcerated and has a reticulated pattern.

Sites of Involvement

ILEITIS. The most frequent site of involvement of the small bowel with regional enteritis is the terminal ileum. Depending on the degree of involvement, this segment exhibits varying roentgenologic alterations. The early cases may be difficult to detect. There may be only slight disturbance in peristaltic activity, manifested by minimal flattening of the contours or irregular pseudodiverticular contractions, and minimal limitation in distensibility. Spasm and irritability are common and may be so pronounced that the involved segment is difficult to see. Slight spiculation of the contours may be identified with minimal thickening and irregularity of the mucosal folds (Figs. 14-29 and 14-30). Repeat studies are important in minimal cases. If the findings disappear, the diagnosis of regional enteritis should be suspect. Because the ileum remains distensible in early cases, these changes may not be visualized by reflux during barium enema examination (Fig. 14-29B). As ulceration proceeds, there is more spasm and irritability, more coarsening and thickening of the folds, and finally the string sign may be seen.

The string sign has come to be identified as a pathognomonic roentgen manifestation of regional enteritis and is most frequently noted in the terminal ileum. It has been described as a thin, linear shadow, suggesting a frayed cotton string (Fig. 14-31). The string sign is caused by incomplete filling due to irritability and spasm associated with marked ulceration. It may be seen in both the nonstenotic and stenotic phases of this disease. Repeated spot films will

(Text continued on page 205.)

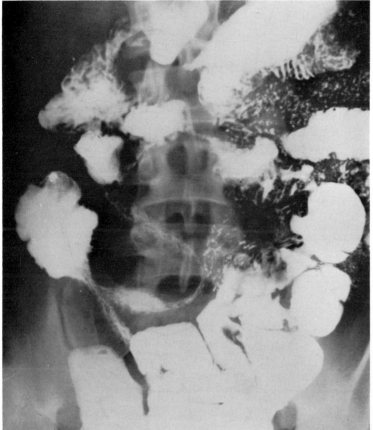

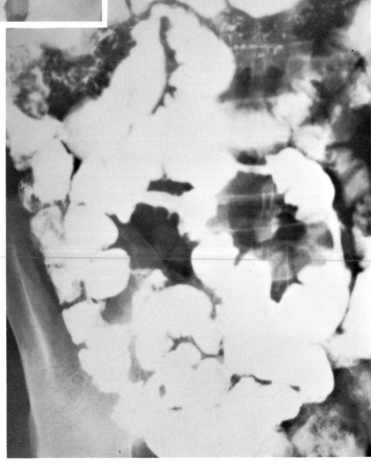

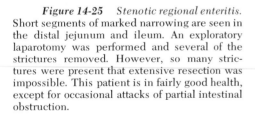

Figure 14-24 *Stenotic regional enteritis* with alternating areas of constriction and dilatation.

Figure 14-25 *Stenotic regional enteritis.* Short segments of marked narrowing are seen in the distal jejunum and ileum. An exploratory laparotomy was performed and several of the strictures removed. However, so many strictures were present that extensive resection was impossible. This patient is in fairly good health, except for occasional attacks of partial intestinal obstruction.

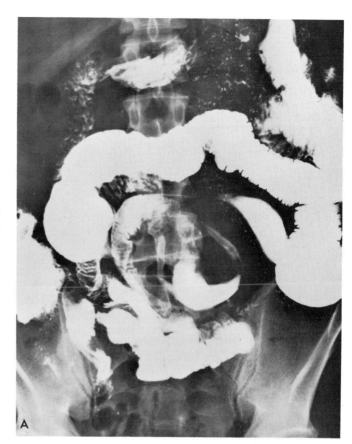

Figure 14-26 *Stenotic regional enteritis.* A, Rigid narrowed segments are noted in the distal jejunum and ileum with proximal dilatation.

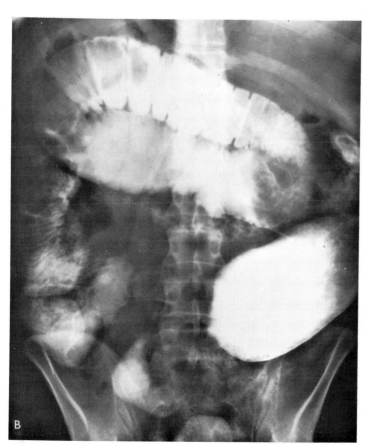

Figure 14-26B The same patient nine years later. Considerable dilatation is now present in the proximal loops of bowel. The constricted segments are poorly visualized because of incomplete filling.

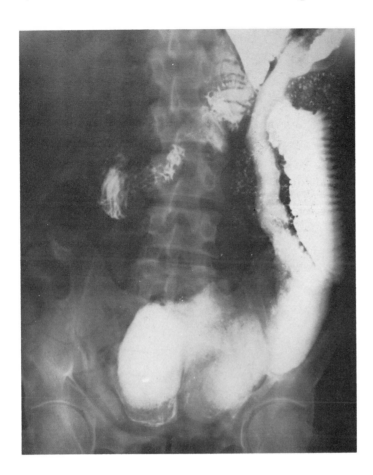

Figure 14-27 Stenotic regional enteritis. There are markedly dilated segments of jejunum proximal to areas of narrowing in the distal jejunum which were visualized on subsequent films.

Figure 14-28 Stenotic regional enteritis. Multiple areas of narrowing and dilatation are identified. Foreign bodies are noted in several of the dilated loops. This is not uncommon in the stenotic phase of regional enteritis.

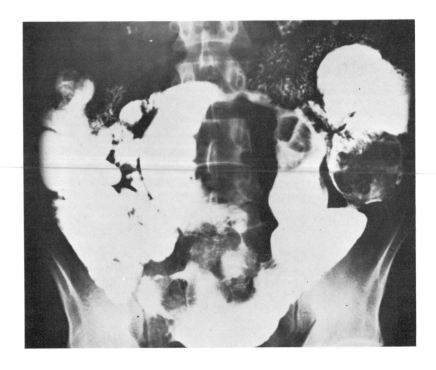

demonstrate that some distensibility is present in this segment (Fig. 14-32). The bowel proximal to the string sign may or may not be dilated, depending on the stage of the disease. In the nonstenotic phase, the proximal intestinal lumen is generally not dilated despite the marked narrowing associated with the string sign, indicating the importance of spasm in producing this characteristic appearance (Fig. 14-33). This spasm is usually inconstant. When persistent, however, temporary proximal dilatation may occur with symptoms of obstruction. In the stenotic phase there is constant proximal dilatation, which may be accentuated by spasm secondary to ulceration. Despite the narrowing, complete intestinal obstruction is rare. It is important to recognize that the string sign does not always indicate marked fibrosis and stenosis, for operations performed during the stage of marked ulceration and activity are often followed by high rates of recurrence.

Because of the marked ulceration, fistulas and perforation (Figs. 14-34 to 14-37), thickening of the mesentery, and separation of the loops of bowel are all more frequent in the distal ileum than in the remainder of the small bowel. A possible explanation of marked ulceration in the distal ileum may be the higher bacterial content in this area.

Fistulas may be numerous, producing multiple overlapping tracks of barium. These are usually associated with abscesses, so that removal of the diseased segment is difficult or impossible (Fig. 14-38). Multiple fistulas may sometimes produce an appearance of segmentation, with many globular pockets of barium (Fig. 14-39). Rectal filling during small bowel examination without visualization of the rest of the colon indicates the presence of a fistula from small bowel to colon (Fig. 14-40). In some of these cases the fistula may not be identified because of overlapping loops of small bowel (Fig. 14-41).

Deformities of the cecum and ascending colon are not unusual with involvement of the terminal ileum. This may vary from a concavity in the mesial aspect of the cecum at the ileocecal region (Figs. 14-31 and 14-32) to marked narrowing of the cecum. This is an especially important sign if at the time of the first examination by barium enema the terminal ileum cannot be filled with barium because of marked spasm and irritability. The presence of this sign is suggestive of regional enteritis, and reexamination with filling of the terminal ileum is important. This deformity of the mesial aspect of the cecolic region is most often due to the pressure on the colon by the thickened terminal ileum with its inflamed mesentery and by the heavy pad of mesenteric fat. In some cases it is due to fistulas or intramural sinus tracts arising from the terminal ileum and extending into the right side of the colon.

JEJUNOILEITIS.   The distal half of jejunum and proximal half of ileum are characteristically involved (Fig. 14-42). Skip areas are frequent, and large inflammatory polyps may be noted (Fig. 14-42A). Ulceration is not as marked as in the terminal ileum, and fistula formation is less frequent. Because of the extent of involvement, operative intervention until recently has been rare and long follow-up of the natural course of the disease has been possible. The transition from the nonstenotic to the stenotic stage can be observed, and in the average case the interval varies from four to 16 years.

JEJUNITIS.   Regional jejunitis is that variety of regional enteritis in which the initial manifestations are mainly or exclusively in the jejunum. Regional jejunitis has a roentgenographic pattern which differs somewhat from that of disease localized in the ileum.[10, 11] The most common site of granulomatous

(Text continued on page 210.)

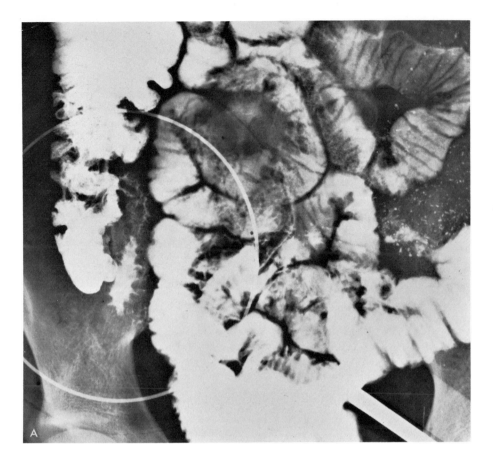

Figure 14-29 *Early regional enteritis.* A, There are minimal changes involving the distal third of ileum, characterized by spasm, irritability, and slight thickening and irregularity of the mucosal folds.

Figure 14-29B In the same patient, a barium enema examination performed at the time of the original examination demonstrates minimal thickening of the folds of the terminal ileum. Early regional enteritis can be missed on a barium enema examination with reflux.

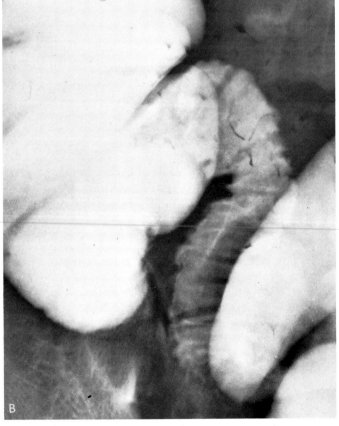

(Illustration continued on opposite page.)

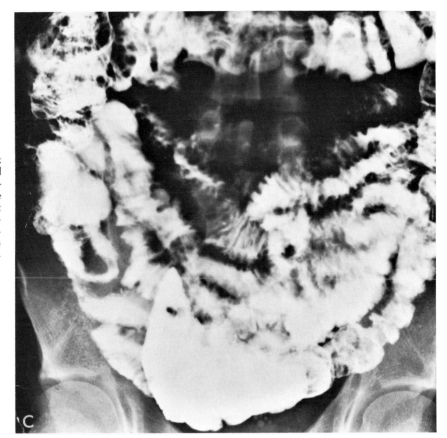

Figure 14-29 Continued C, Six months later the findings in the terminal ileum are more marked, with more narrowing and rigidity. At this time the entire ileum appears to be involved with slight narrowing, rigidity, thickening of the valvulae conniventes, and increased secretions. This case is unusual in that there appears to be an extension of the inflammatory process.

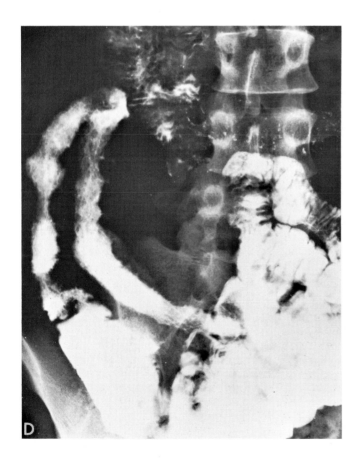

Figure 14-29 Continued D, One year later there is further involvement of the loops of ileum with more ulceration of the mucosa. Numerous small inflammatory polyps are seen.

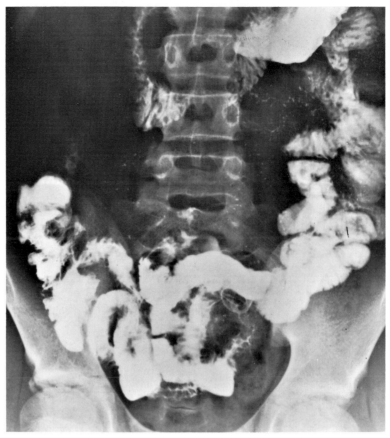

Figure 14-30   *Nonstenotic regional enteritis* with involvement of the distal ileum in a 12 year old boy. The loop proximal to the terminal ileum reveals cobblestoning of the mucosa.

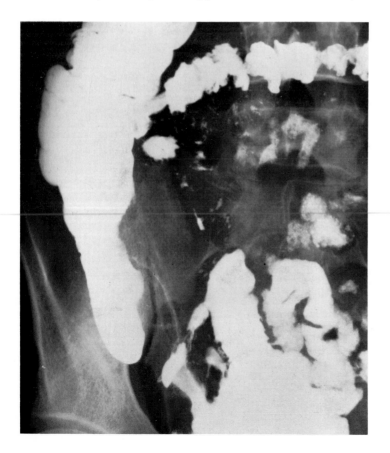

Figure 14-31   *String sign in regional enteritis.* The findings in the ileum are due to marked ulceration with secondary spasm. The cecum and ascending colon have a conical configuration. This is not unusual with any inflammatory process in the right lower quadrant.

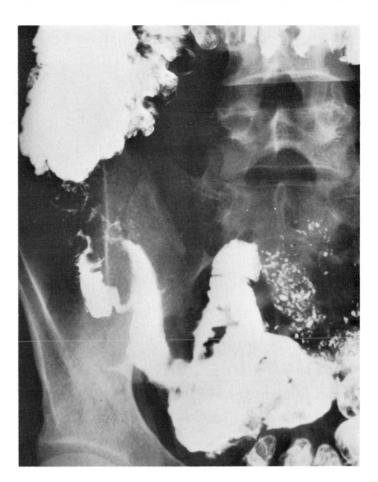

Figure 14-32 The same patient as in Figure 14-31 a few minutes later. There is more distensibility of the distal ileum. The narrowing and rigidity of the cecum and ascending colon are due to multiple sinus tracts, extending from the distal portion of the terminal ileum to the colon.

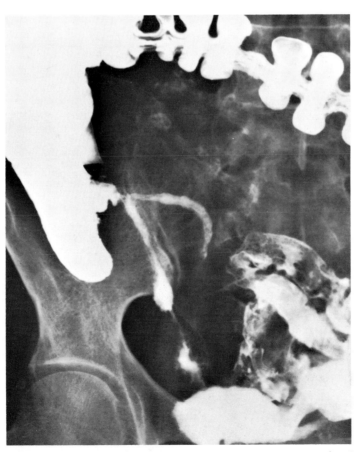

Figure 14-33 String sign in regional enteritis. The characteristic string sign due to marked ulceration of the ileum is present. The proximal bowel is not dilated. The appendix is visualized.

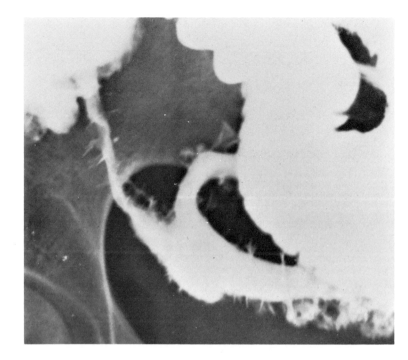

Figure 14-34 *Regional enteritis.* Numerous fistulas extend from the terminal ileum into the mesentery and toward the urinary bladder.

involvement is the distal portion of the ileum, and the frequency progressively diminishes in the more proximal and distal portions of the gastrointestinal tract. Practically all our patients with jejunitis appeared to have long-standing disease. However, early cases of jejunitis are being recognized with increasing frequency. Most of these proceed to the more chronic form. On the other hand, there have been reports of isolated instances of acute regional jejunitis that

Figure 14-35 *Regional enteritis.* There is a large fistula between the terminal ileum and the ascending colon.

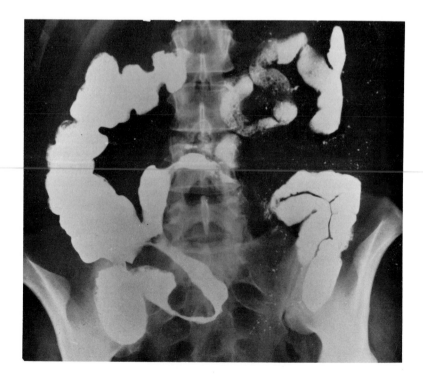

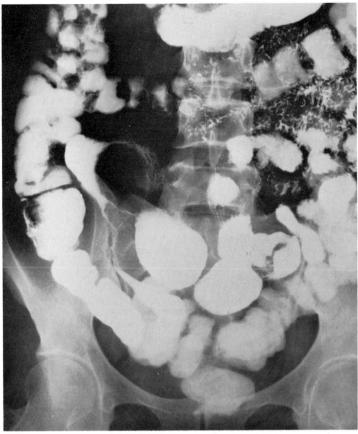

Figure 14-36 *Regional enteritis.* There is a short fistulous communication between the distal loops of ileum.

have healed completely without sequelae. In these instances, the diagnosis has arisen from observations made at laparotomy, not necessarily with pathologic or roentgenographic confirmation.

Roentgenographically, the prestenotic phase of the disease has been demonstrated on a number of occasions and is similar to the changes previously described. Some of these cases have been followed until the actual development of stenosis. However, since none of our patients has been operated upon in the prestenotic period, the pathologic signs of that phase have not been observed. It would seem that this stage of the disease would be encountered when long segments of jejunum are resected for multiple areas of involvement. However, it has been our experience that such resected specimens show all the involved areas to be in the cicatrizing stenotic phase. This observation suggests that the disease appears in different segments at approximately the same time and progresses in them at the same rate.

In distal ileitis the roentgenographic picture is dominated by the appearance of diseased segments of bowel per se. In regional jejunitis, on the other hand, the sequelae of the diseased stenotic segments, namely, markedly dilated, chronically obstructed loops, are the striking findings (Figs. 14-43 and 14-44). The retention of food and secretions and the inflammatory reaction which frequently develops in these chronically obstructed loops produce roentgenographic features that are characteristic of prolonged obstruction. It is often impossible in this situation to determine roentgenologically whether there is

(Text continued on page 215.)

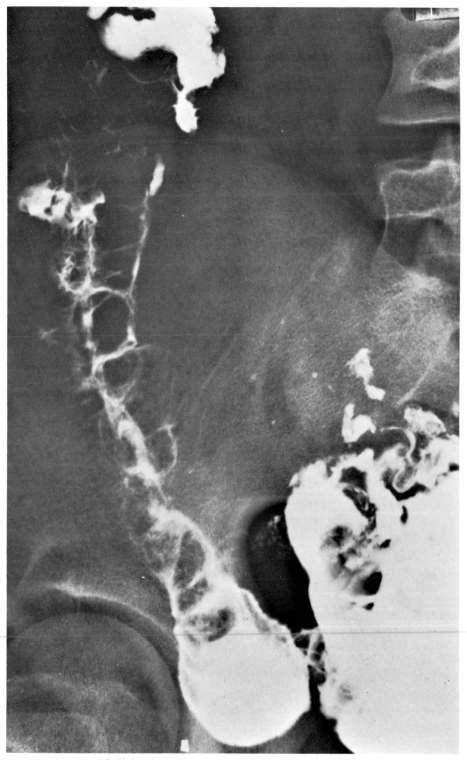

Figure 14-37 *The terminal ileum is markedly involved with regional enteritis.* There are numerous sinus tracts and fistulas extending through the wall of the bowel into the mesentery producing a stepladder configuration.

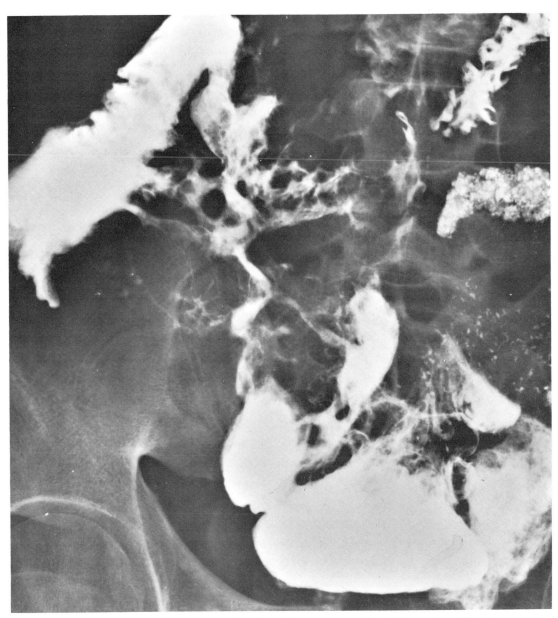

Figure 14-38 *Granulomatous ileocolitis.* There are a considerable number of fistulas extending from a markedly involved terminal ileum into the right side of the colon. A cobblestone pattern is noted in the proximal transverse colon. The prognosis in this type of ileocolitis is poor.

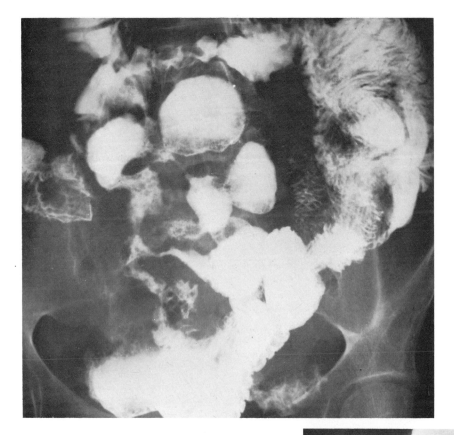

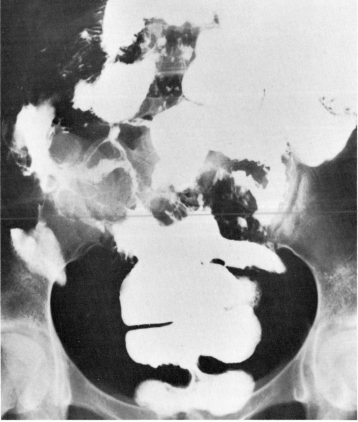

Figure 14-39   Regional enteritis. Multiple fistulous communications extend between amorphous globular sacs of barium. The failure to recognize the fistulous communications may lead to an incorrect diagnosis of sprue.

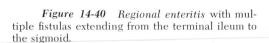

Figure 14-40   Regional enteritis with multiple fistulas extending from the terminal ileum to the sigmoid.

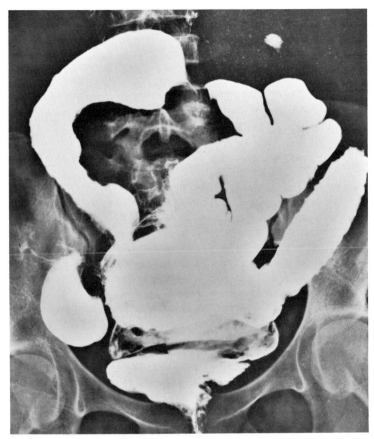

Figure 14-41 *Regional enteritis.* The inflammatory process in the ileum is easily recognized. The rectum is also filled with barium without visualization of the remainder of the large bowel. This is pathognomonic of a fistulous communication from ileum to rectum. It is not unusual for the fistulous communication to be overlooked because of overlapping intestinal loops.

intrinsic involvement or whether changes are produced by the long-standing obstruction. The diameter of the loops obstructed proximally and distally may attain the proportions of a markedly distended colon (Fig. 14-45).

In most instances, the stenotic segments are easily visualized (Figs. 14-46 and 14-47). However, when numerous overlapping dilated intestinal loops are present, a single short stricture, or even multiple strictures, may be difficult to delineate. A lateral projection in these cases may be helpful (Figs. 14-48 and 14-49).

Although the stenotic segments indicate a considerable degree of fibrosis, the narrowing may be further enhanced by superimposed edema and spasm resulting from the inflammation. The contours of the narrowed segments generally are smooth. The lumen is concentrically located. The mucosa may be castlike or reveal numerous pseudopolyps and ulcerations. The stenotic segments are rigid. They may be single or multiple and vary in length. If there is only a single area of constriction, a more or less uniform dilatation of the proximal bowel may be seen. The presence of a skip lesion may result in a "hammock" or "sausage link" type of deformity (Fig. 14-48). When obstruction occurs near the ligament of Treitz, duodenal and even gastric dilatation may be evident (Fig. 14-47). Ulceration, perforation, and their sequelae are much less common in regional jejunitis than in ileitis.

(Text continued on page 221.)

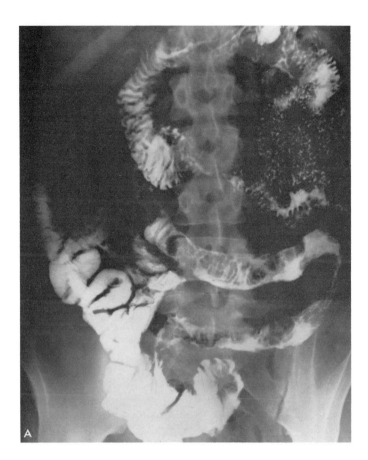

Figure 14-42 *Jejunoileitis.* A, There is involvement of the distal half of jejunum and proximal half of ileum. Unusually large inflammatory polyps are noted.

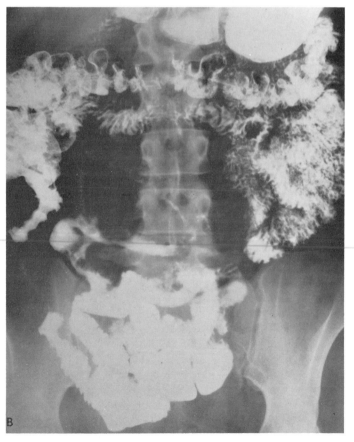

Figure 14-42 B, The same patient ten years later. At this time the lumen of the bowel is narrowed. The filling defects previously described are not as prominent. There has been no proximal or distal extension of the inflammatory process.

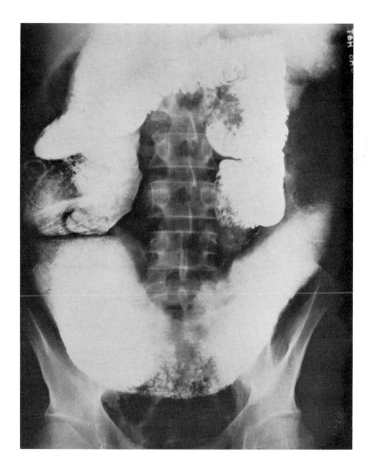

Figure 14-43 Jejunitis. The mid-jejunum is considerably dilated. Constricted segments are not identified because of the marked distention of the overlying loops of bowel.

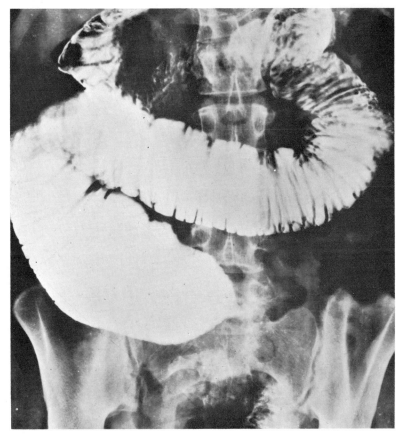

Figure 14-44 Jejunitis. There is a short constricted segment with marked dilatation of the proximal jejunum. At laparotomy there was only a single area of stenosis which revealed the pathologic changes associated with regional enteritis. A single area of stenosis is uncommon in regional enteritis.

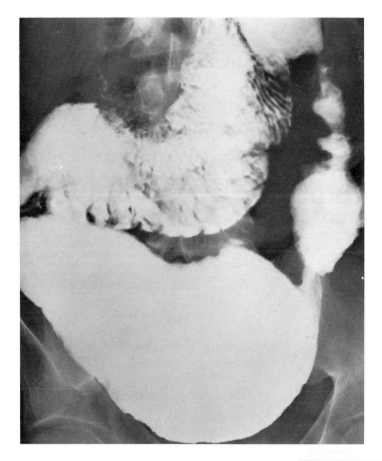

Figure 14-45 *Jejunitis.* There is a huge dilated loop of jejunum enclosed by two short strictures. Additional narrowed segments are also identified. At operation the disease was confined to the jejunum.

Figure 14-46 *Jejunitis.* Starting at the ligament of Treitz alternating areas of constriction and dilatation are seen. The duodenum is dilated.

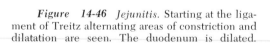

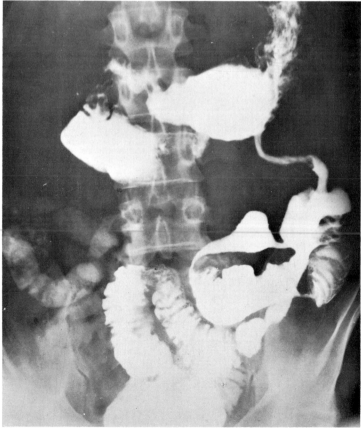

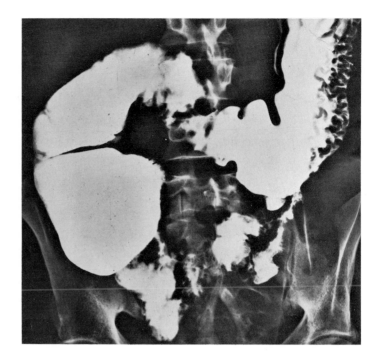

Figure 14-47 *Jejunitis* with marked dilatation of the second and third portions of the duodenum, secondary to stenosing jejunitis of the proximal jejunum.

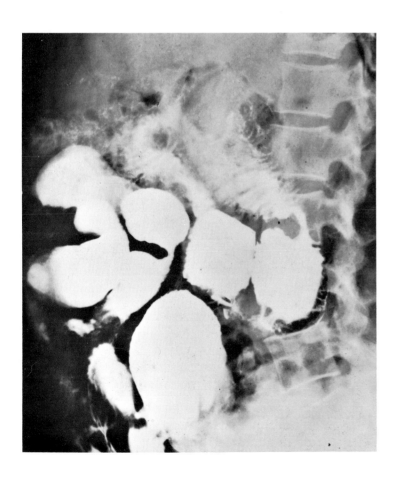

Figure 14-48 *Jejunitis* with alternating areas of stenosis and dilatation. These are best identified on the lateral projection.

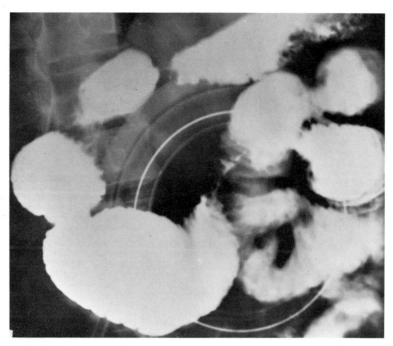

Figure 14-49 *Jejunitis*. A diagnosis of sprue was incorrectly made in this case because of dilatation and the failure to identify the stenotic segments. These, however, were well seen after compression.

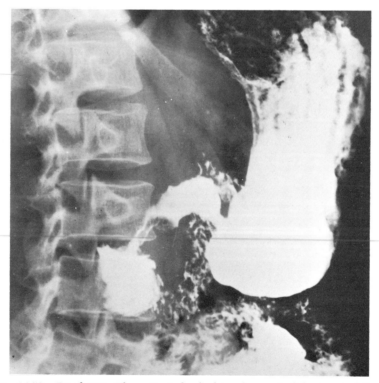

Figure 14-50 *Duodenitis*. The patient also had involvement of the terminal ileum. In the absence of other segments of regional enteritis the diagnosis of regional enteritis of the duodenum may be difficult.

DUODENITIS. Duodenitis is more common than had previously been considered and may occur with or without involvement of distal small bowel (Figs. 14-50, 14-51). The conspicuous feature is varying degrees of stenosis. Discrete ulcerations are usually not identified and fistulas are uncommon. Early cases are not easy to recognize because spasm and irritability commonly accompany inflammation in adjacent jejunum or other parts of the bowel. The use of anticholinergic drugs or glucagon in these cases helps to differentiate narrowing due to spasm from that due to intrinsic inflammatory disease. Granulomatous duodenitis should be considered in the differential diagnosis of stenotic lesions of the duodenum. In fact, when the lesion involves most of the duodenum and is not associated with overhanging edges, the most likely cause is regional enteritis.

GASTRITIS. In the cases that we have studied, the roentgen alterations have been limited to the antrum of the stomach and have consisted of an area of narrowing with fairly smooth margins and no evidence of discrete ulceration. Again, the diagnosis of regional enteritis involving the stomach is difficult when there is no involvement of other portions of the intestinal tract (Fig. 14-53). On occasion, the antrum, pylorus, and duodenum form a continuous tubular channel with no anatomic landmarks. Regional enteritis involving the esophagus has not been observed in our series of cases.

Long-term Follow-up in Regional Enteritis

The natural history of regional enteritis can be studied by a long-term follow-up of unoperated cases. Another approach is to follow serial x-rays obtained in the months or years following surgery to search for the earliest roentgen changes in recurrent disease and the subsequent progression of these changes.

In our experience almost every patient who has sinus tracts, fistulas, or abscess formation is eventually operated upon, so that there are few cases in this group available for follow-up without surgery. Some of these patients, however, because of extensive disease or medical contraindications to surgery, are not operated upon. The course of their disease tends to be one of progressive debility, with death usually occurring because of infection. Systemic amyloidosis has been the cause of death in some patients with regional enteritis.[12]

The patients most suitable for long-term follow-up have been those in whom the disease has been low-grade, confined to the distal ileum, or in whom the disease has been extensive but without sinus tracts or fistulas. In these patients linear extension of the disease has been rare on follow-up roentgen examinations, but stenosis with varying degrees of obstruction invariably occurs (Figs. 14-42, 14-54, and 14-55).

The natural history of the disease would seem to be in the direction of healing, with fibrosis and stenosis (Figs. 14-10, 14-56 to 14-59). In most cases, however, sinus tracts, fistulas, or abscess formation eventually occur. Even in the absence of these complications operation is usually necessary after an interval of time because of obstruction. This may not occur, however, for periods as long as five to 15 years. It is surprising that many patients with evidence of severe stenosis may be relatively asymptomatic for many years.

(Text continued on page 226.)

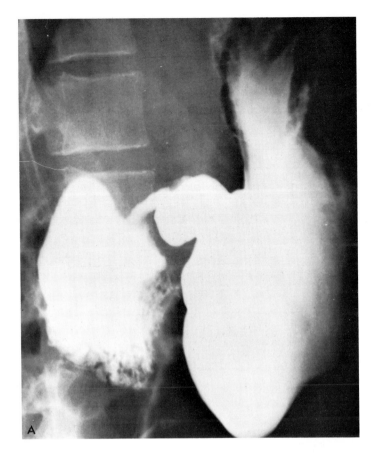

Figure 14-51 *Regional enteritis. A,* The proximal part of the second portion of the duodenum is involved. There is considerable dilatation of the third portion of the duodenum. This was due to an inflammatory process adjacent to the ligament of Treitz in the mesentery.

Figure 14-51 *B,* In the same patient following gastroenterostomy, there is recurrent disease at the stoma. Biopsy after subtotal gastric resection revealed the presence of granulomatous disease at the stoma.

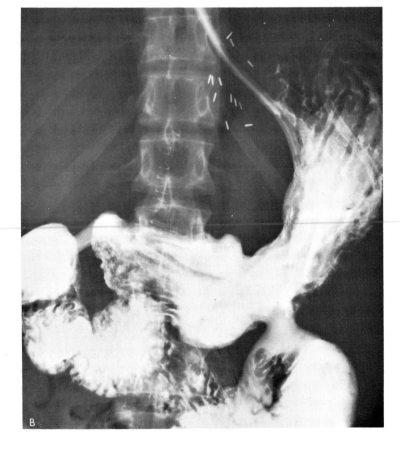

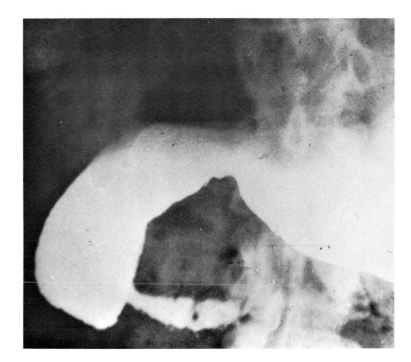

Figure 14-52 Regional enteritis. Involvement of the third portion of the duodenum with proximal dilatation.

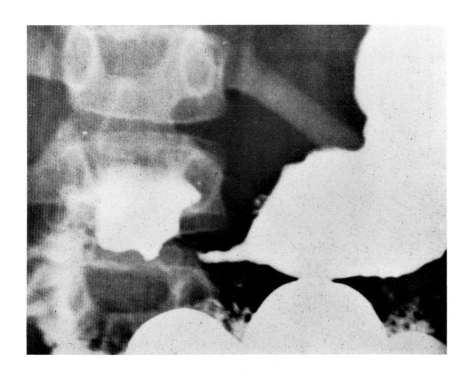

Figure 14-53 Gastritis. Narrowing and rigidity of the prepyloric region of the stomach. In the absence of regional enteritis elsewhere, a diagnosis of granulomatous gastritis would be difficult. When regional enteritis involves the stomach it usually is confined to its distal half. Other forms of granulomatous gastritis are more diffuse.

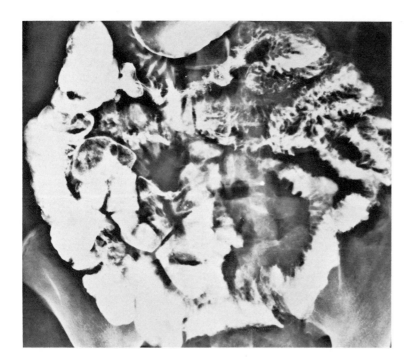

Figure 14-54 Long-term follow-up in *regional enteritis.* There is involvement of the distal jejunum and proximal ileum, characterized by thickening and blunting of the folds with rigidity and separation of the loops of intestine. Patient was explored for findings of an acute abdomen. No surgical procedure was performed when regional enteritis was found.

Figure 14-55 Same patient as in Figure 14-54. Six years later there are alternating areas of constriction and dilatation. The patient is in the stenotic stage of the disease. Two years after this examination, resection was performed because of continuing attacks of partial intestinal obstruction.

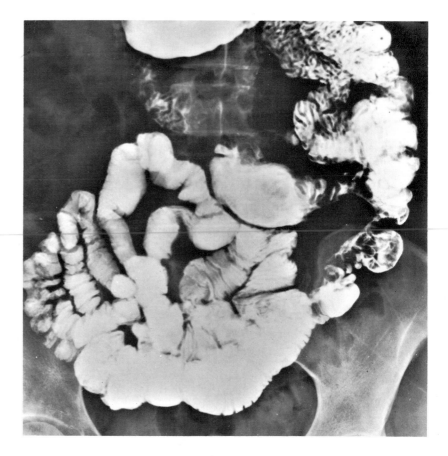

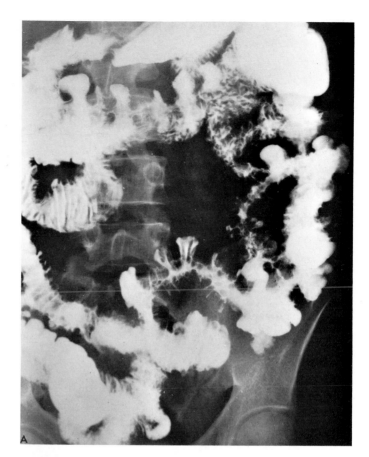

Figure 14-56 A. Same patient as in Figure 14-10, six years later. There has been a considerable change in the appearance of the involved segments. There is more narrowing and rigidity and multiple pseudodiverticula are identified.

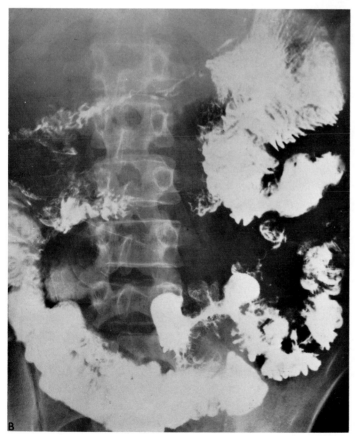

Figure 14-56 B, Three years later more narrowing and rigidity are identified and the jejunum is more dilated.

Recurrent Regional Enteritis

Following operation, recurrent granulomatous disease is common (Fig. 14-60). The recurrence occurs most frequently during the first two years, but many years may elapse before new involvement is seen. Many patients with early recurrent lesions may be asymptomatic for long periods of time. Recurrences appear more frequently in those patients in whom the original disease is most active and in whom there are sinus tracts and fistulas. If operation is performed in the more chronic and stenotic phase of the disease and in the absence of fistulas, the recurrence rate is less.

In general, the recurrent lesions are similar to the original disease. The

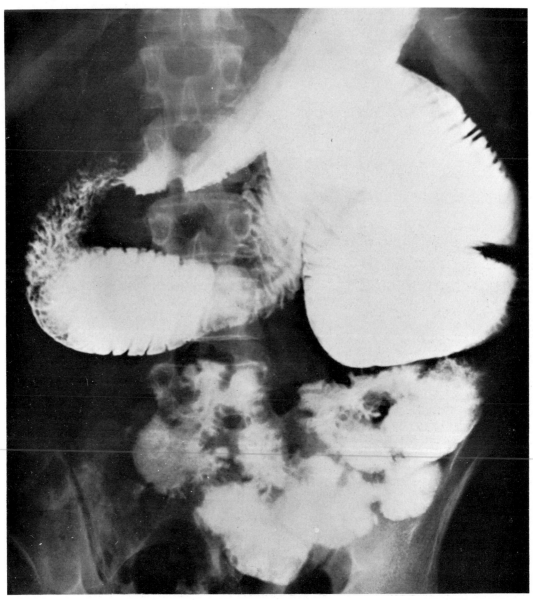

Figure 14-57 Same patient as in Figure 14-56. There is considerable dilatation of the proximal jejunum. The areas of constriction are not well seen on this film. During the period of 15 years of observation there has been more stenosis and proximal dilatation but no longitudinal extension. This is the usual sequence in patients with regional enteritis.

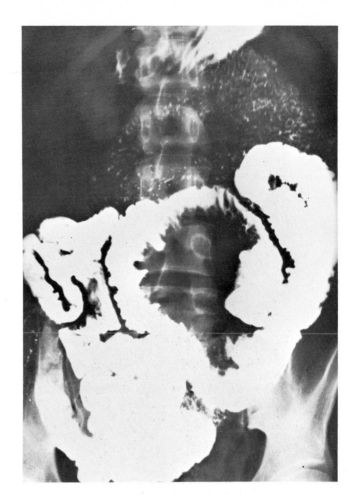

Figure 14-58 *Nonstenotic phase of regional enteritis* involving the distal jejunum and proximal ileum. There is irregularity of the contour, and thickening and blunting of the folds.

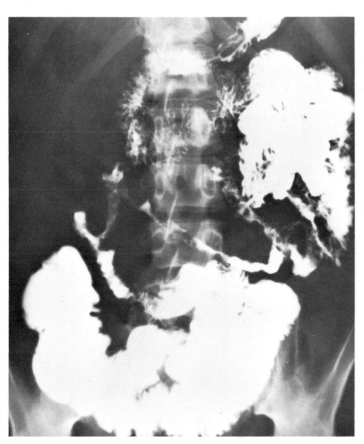

Figure 14-59 Same case as in Figure 14-58, six years later. Stenosis is present. There has been no proximal or distal extension of the inflammatory process.

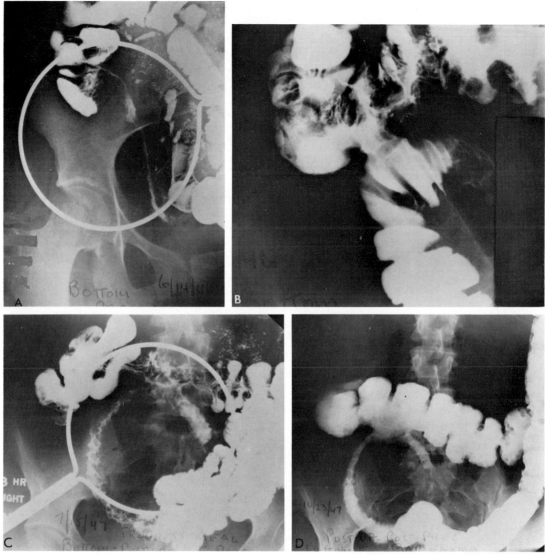

Figure 14-60 *A*, The original terminal regional ileitis in a young female, age 22. *B*, Barium enema examination six weeks after resection and proximal ileotransverse colostomy. *C*, One year later examination shows nodular, rigid terminal ileum, characteristic of recurrent terminal ileitis. *D*, Three months later increased shortening, narrowing, and rigidity of the involved segments are seen. (Reproduced with permission from Bockus, H. L.: Gastroenterology, Volume II. Philadelphia, W. B. Saunders Co., 1964.)

earliest roentgen findings are thickening and blunting of the folds progressing through the nonstenotic to the stenotic phase. Fistula formation appears less frequently. The length of the original lesion has no effect on the recurrence rate. A remarkable feature of this disease is that the recurrences in regional enteritis are practically always at the site of the new terminal ileum (Figs. 14-61 to 14-66). Extension into the colon has also been seen.

Healing in Regional Enteritis

Roentgenologic demonstrations of improvement without operation are rare in our experience. However, cases have been observed in which re-

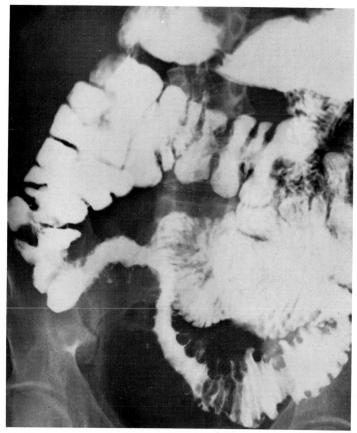

Figure 14–61 Recurrent regional enteritis. Status post ileoascending colostomy. This patient had two previous resections of regional enteritis involving the terminal ileum. This is a second recurrence. There is thickening and blunting of the folds with some narrowing and rigidity.

Figure 14–62 Recurrent regional enteritis. Status post ileotransverse colostomy with end to end anastomosis and recurrent disease adjacent to the stoma. Recurrent disease in our experience has usually developed in the new terminal ileum.

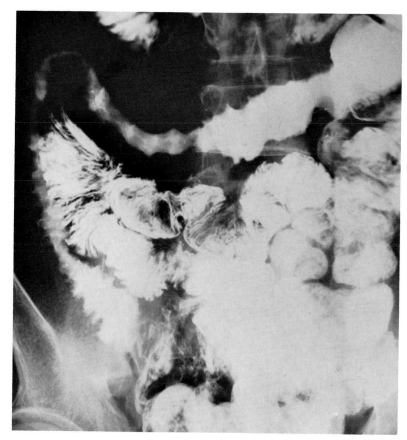

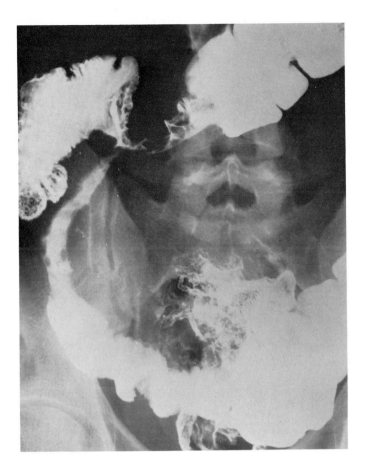

Figure 14–63 *Recurrent regional enteritis.* Status post ileotransverse colostomy with recurrent disease in the new terminal ileum.

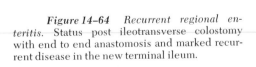

Figure 14–64 *Recurrent regional enteritis.* Status post ileotransverse colostomy with end to end anastomosis and marked recurrent disease in the new terminal ileum.

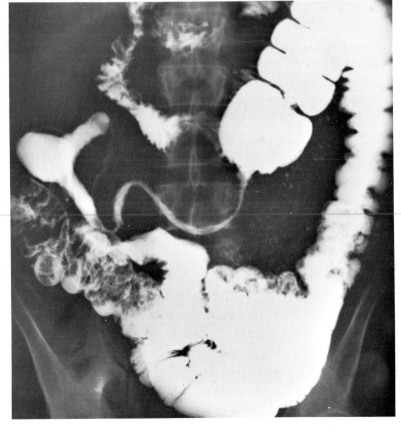

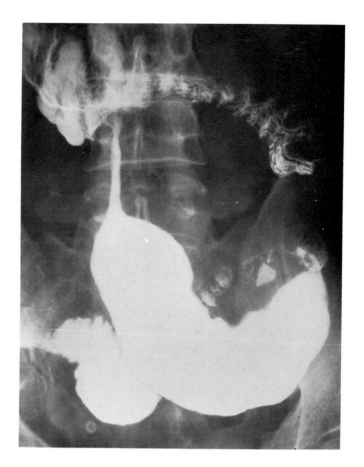

Figure 14-65 Recurrent regional enteritis. Status post ileotransverse colostomy. There is marked narrowing of the ileum adjacent to the stoma for a distance of 6 cm. and considerable dilatation proximal to the narrowed segment. Other alternating areas of constriction and dilatation are seen proximal to this loop.

markable changes indicating healing occurred (Figs. 14-67 and 14-68). Despite these instances of improvement, a large majority of cases demonstrate the disease to be continuous. Many years may elapse, however, before stenosis supervenes. It should be pointed out that in patients who show clinical improvement, secondary changes may occur, notably stenosing lesions and permanent loss of the normal small intestinal structure. These changes are due to healing with scar formation.

Regional Enteritis in Children

The roentgen findings in children are essentially the same as described in adults[13] (Figs. 14-30, 14-69 to 14-71). The children we have seen have ranged in age from two to 15 years. The anatomic distribution of the disease was the same as in adults. Most cases were of the nonstenotic variety, reflecting the relatively short duration of the illness. As in adults, fistulas usually occurred in the distal ileum.

In recent years there has been an increasing number of reports of so-called acute ileitis occurring in children. The condition is clinically indistinguishable from acute appendicitis. At operation the terminal ileum is found to be congested, thickened, and possibly rigid, and in most cases there is an associated mesenteric adenitis. The majority of such patients recover spontane-

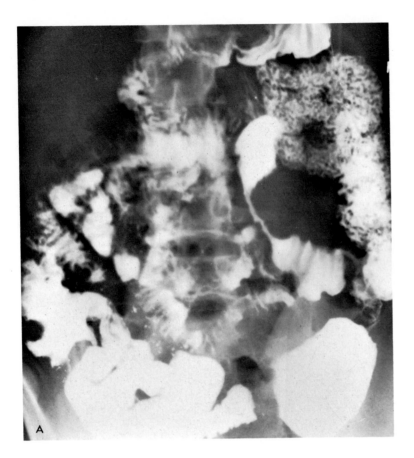

Figure 14-66 A, *Stenosing jejunitis.*

ously and there is no progression to the chronic stage. The condition is considered by some clinicians to be a distinct, nonrecurring, nonsclerosing form of acute ileitis, essentially unrelated to chronic cicatrizing granulomatous enteritis. A number of such cases, however, apparently develop into regional enteritis, and a clear distinction between the two forms of the acute disease has not

(*Text continued on page 235.*)

Figure 14-66 B, Drawing of removed specimen, demonstrating alternating areas of constriction and dilatation, thickened bowel, and enlarged lymph nodes.

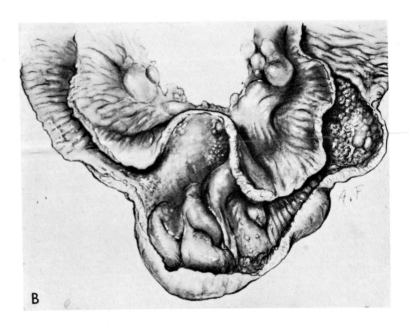

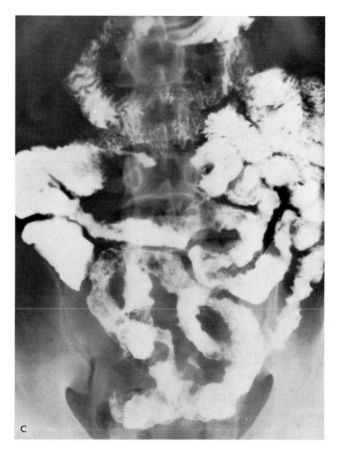

Figure 14-66 Continued   C, Recurrent disease in the same patient, six months following operation.

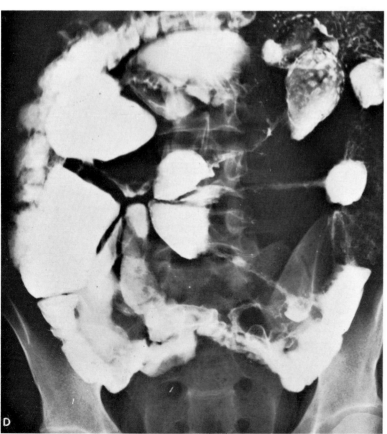

Figure 14-66   D, The same patient, four years following surgery. Extensive areas of stenosis, alternating with areas of dilatation, are now noted. The rapidity with which stenosis developed in this case is remarkable.

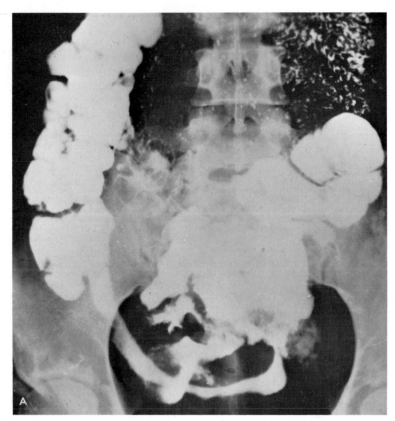

Figure 14-67   A, Regional enteritis involving the distal 18 inches of ileum.

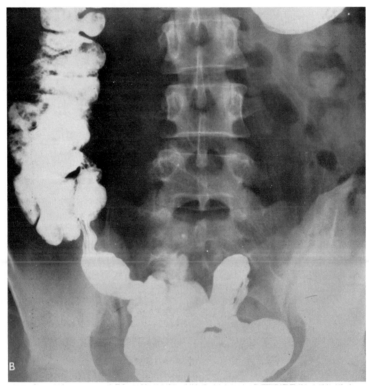

Figure 14-67   B, Eighteen months later there is resolution in the appearance of the inflammatory process. Despite the apparent healing of the mucosal ulceration, fibrosis continued with partial intestinal obstruction requiring surgical intervention. It is of interest that between these examinations, the patient delivered a normal infant.

been satisfactorily established in the current literature. The roentgen findings in so-called acute ileitis are similar to the early changes of regional enteritis and consist of slight spiculation of the contours of the bowel with minimal thickening and irregularity of the mucosal folds. The roentgenologic alterations in the few cases of acute ileitis that were studied did not persist and disappeared in a few weeks (Fig. 14-72).

Carcinoma with Regional Enteritis

Primary carcinoma of the small intestine is an uncommon lesion. Thus several reports[14, 15] in recent years of adenocarcinoma of the small bowel in association with longstanding regional enteritis or in surgically excluded loops have aroused much interest and concern that regional enteritis may be a premalignant lesion. Such an inference is not yet warranted in view of the few cases reported relative to the overall incidence of regional enteritis. Further studies and follow-up for malignancy are clearly indicated, however, in all patients with inflammatory bowel disease.

When carcinoma does complicate regional enteritis the diagnosis is difficult to establish because the presence of multiple strictures with intervening segments of dilated bowel tends to obscure the associated malignancy on small bowel examination (Fig. 14-73). Moreover, the clinical features of the carcinoma mimic those of the obstructing inflammatory disease.

Similar concern about a possible relationship to carcinoma has been expressed in granulomatous colitis. In one study[15] the incidence of colorectal cancer in patients with granulomatous disease of the bowel was found to be 20 times greater than in a control population.

Lymphoid Hyperplasia

The terminal ileum in children and young adults sometimes contains sufficient lymphoid tissue to produce small filling defects within the lumen. These are usually symmetric and fairly sharply demarcated, with no evidence of an inflammatory process. At the present time we do not understand the exact significance of this lymphoid tissue; however, resolution usually occurs (Fig. 14-74).

Differential Diagnosis

In most instances, the roentgen alterations in regional enteritis are sufficiently characteristic that differential diagnosis is not difficult. The following diseases may, on occasion, simulate the roentgen findings described previously.

LYMPHOSARCOMA. Lymphosarcoma (Figs. 14-75 and 14-76) can simulate the nonstenotic phase of regional enteritis. Thickening and blunting of the folds, irregularity of the contour, ulceration, intraluminal nodules, and fistulas are features that are common to both. In regional enteritis there is more inflammation, producing spasm and narrowing of the bowel lumen. Irregular nodules that can be identified as tumors are an uncommon feature of regional enteritis but a frequent finding in lymphosarcoma. Although narrowing of the bowel

(Text continued on page 239.)

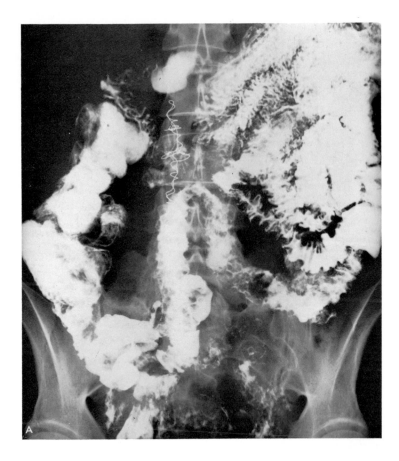

Figure 14–68 Regional enteritis. A, Moderately extensive regional enteritis involving the distal two-thirds of jejunum and proximal two-thirds of ileum, characterized by spasm, irritability, thickening of the folds and increased fluid.

Figure 14-68 B, Three years later there is minimal dilatation of the distal jejunum and proximal ileum with no definite evidence of an inflammatory process. This type of healing has been unusual in our experience.

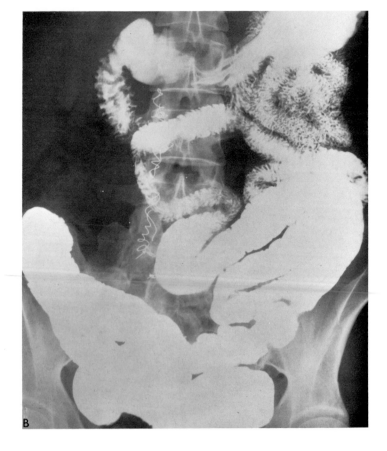

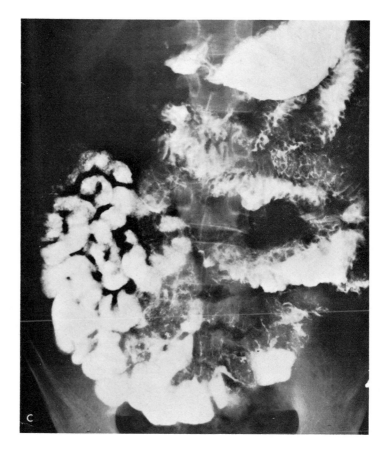

Figure 14-68 Continued   C, A different patient: Extensive and severe regional enteritis involving the distal two-thirds of jejunum and proximal half of ileum. This patient is a 17 year old boy who appeared emaciated and underdeveloped.

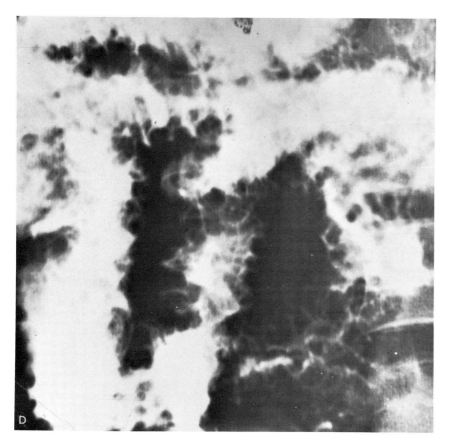

Figure 14–68   D, Spot film of distal jejunum in the same patient as 14-68 *C*, revealing marked cobblestoning secondary to severe ulceration.

(Illustration continued on following page.)

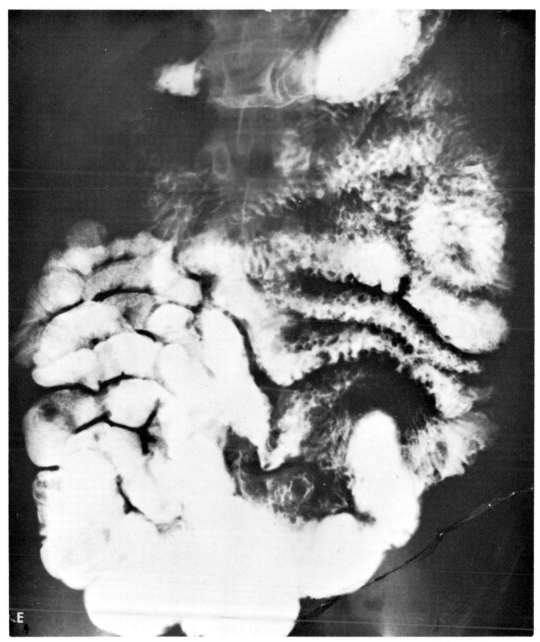

Figure 14-68 *Continued   E,* Same patient six months later. The patient has been on moderate intermittent doses of steroids. There is considerable healing of the inflammatory process. These cases are of considerable interest, since long follow-up study has revealed the development of partial intestinal obstruction. In the interim the patient may have a paucity of symptoms.

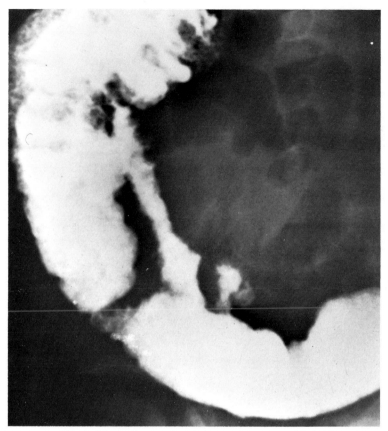

Figure 14-69   Regional enteritis in a two year old child.

lumen can be seen in lymphosarcoma, owing to tumor encroachment, the bowel as a rule is of normal caliber or slightly dilated. Ulcerations in lymphosarcoma are usually discrete or multiple and do not have the linear configuration seen in regional enteritis. Separation of the loops of bowel in regional enteritis is more marked than in lymphosarcoma.

HODGKIN'S DISEASE. Hodgkin's disease (Fig. 20-45) can produce all the roentgen alterations described in lymphosarcoma. In addition, however, marked fibrosis of the bowel can be seen, with constriction of the lumen. The features that distinguish this disease from a single stenotic lesion of regional enteritis are the eccentric lumen, the presence of a tumor nodule, and the absence of chronic intestinal obstruction. In regional enteritis, multiple areas of stenosis are more frequent and the proximal dilated loops of bowel are usually longer, with evidence of considerable secretion and chronic obstruction.

SEGMENTAL INFARCTION OF THE SMALL INTESTINE. (Fig. 14-77.) An infarcted small bowel may show fairly rapid progressive changes leading to stricture formation. An individual segment may completely mimic a stenotic segment in regional enteritis, but the evidence of chronic proximal intestinal obstruction is less marked and the history is usually characteristic.

CARCINOMA. Lesions are usually short with an eccentric rigid lumen; the mucosa shows destruction and occasionally ulceration. Proximal dilatation and overhanging edges are frequent roentgen findings.

(Text continued on page 245.)

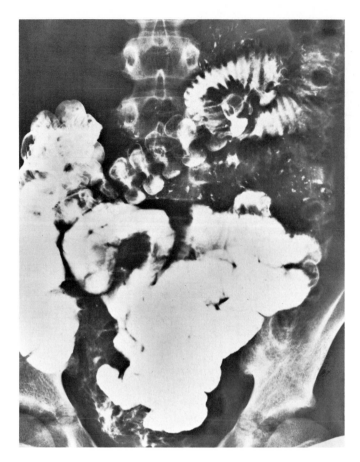

Figure 14–70   Regional enteritis. There is a string sign in the distal ileum secondary to marked ulceration. A small fistulous tract is seen extending from the distal ileum into the adjacent loop of small bowel.

Figure 14-71   Regional enteritis with considerable narrowing of the ileum and dilatation of the proximal bowel. Involvement of the cecum is seen as a result of a fistula from the ileum.

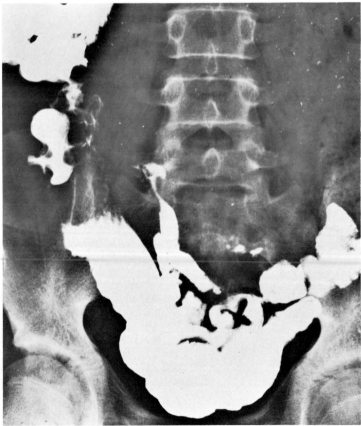

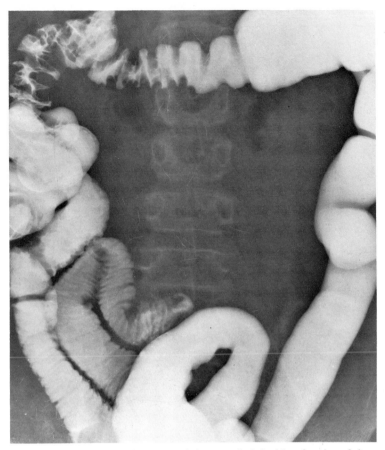

Figure 14–72 Acute ileitis. The terminal ileum is slightly dilated with nodular indentations along its contour and within the lumen. These alterations completely disappeared in one month. The relationship of this entity to regional enteritis has not been established.

Figure 14–73 Carcinoma of the small bowel in a patient with regional enteritis. There are alternating areas of narrowing and slight dilatation involving the jejunum. There is an associated carcinoma of the jejunum in the left upper quadrant immediately below the stomach. The arrows point to multiple skip lesions.

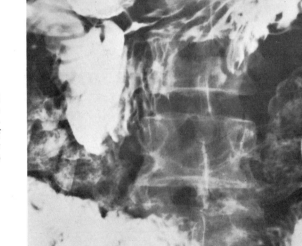

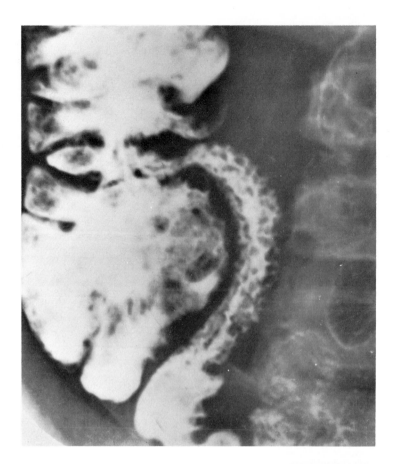

Figure 14–74 Lymphoid hyperplasia. Numerous small fairly sharply demarcated radiolucent filling defects due to lymphoid hyperplasia. This finding has no relationship to regional enteritis.

Figure 14–75 Lymphosarcoma of the jejunum simulating regional enteritis. The recognition of nodular defects along the contours helps in differentiating the two lesions.

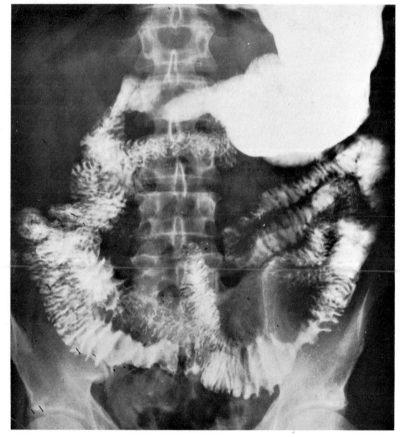

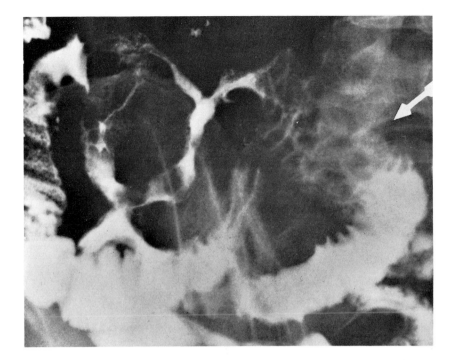

Figure 14-76 *Endoexoenteric lymphosarcoma of the distal ileum simulating fistulous tracts in regional enteritis.* The normal bowel lumen is replaced by many intercommunicating tortuous tracts through the tumor. The arrow points to the nodular mucosal pattern proximal to the mass. The lumen in this segment is not narrowed. A mass developed in the neck of this patient and on biopsy a diagnosis of lymphosarcoma was made.

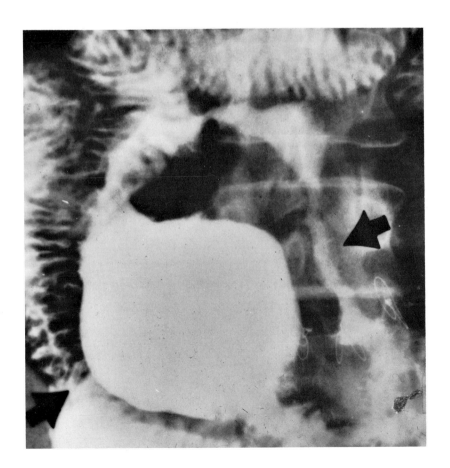

Figure 14-77 *Infarction of the small bowel secondary to a strangulating incisional hernia.* Note the resemblance to regional enteritis.

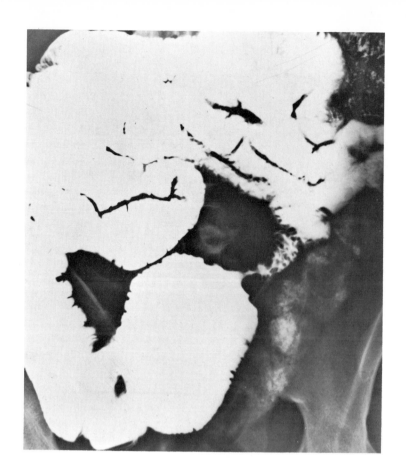

Figure 14-78 Tuberculosis of the small intestine. A single diagnosis in this type of case is impossible. See Figure 20-45. Note the resemblance to Hodgkins disease.

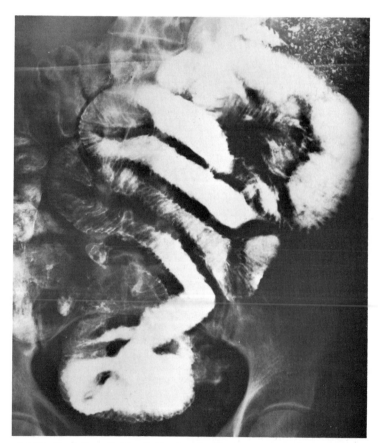

Figure 14-79 Radiation ileitis. Following irradiation, various degrees of necrosis of the small intestine may occur, producing changes that are indistinguishable from regional enteritis.

MALABSORPTION SYNDROME. Although the clinical features of both may be similar, the roentgen features are entirely different. In the spruelike states ulceration and stenosis are rare. Evidence of an inflammatory process is either minimal or completely absent. Dilatation, segmentation, and increased secretions are the prominent roentgen features in sprue.

TUBERCULOSIS. (Fig. 14-78). Tuberculosis can completely mimic the findings associated with regional enteritis. There is generally more marked involvement of the colon than of the terminal ileum. The lesion has a tendency to be associated with more irregular contours, and the mucosal markings are coarser. This is due to the large irregular ulcerations frequently seen in tuberculosis. Tuberculosis of the small intestine is not necessarily associated with involvement of the lungs, and this can make the problem of differential diagnosis extremely difficult.

AMEBIASIS. Amebiasis involving the small bowel rarely has been observed in this country. A cone-shaped appearance of the cecum is frequently mentioned as a pathognomonic feature of ameboma. We have seen this configuration much more often with regional enteritis, appendicitis, and ulcerative colitis.

CARCINOID. On rare occasions multiple carcinoid tumors of the small bowel may simulate regional enteritis. (Fig. 17-9, Chapter on Carcinoid).

RADIATION ILEITIS. (Fig. 14-79). Following irradiation, various degrees of necrosis of the small intestine may occur, producing changes indistinguishable from regional enteritis.

References

1. Crohn, B. B., Ginzburg, L., and Oppenheimer, G. D.: Regional ileitis: a pathological and clinical entity. *J.A.M.A.*, 99:1323-1328, 1932.
2. Wilks, S., and Moxon, W.: Lectures on Pathological Anatomy, 2nd Ed. London, Churchill Livingstone, 1875, pp. 408 and 672.
3. Shapiro, R.: Regional ileitis: a summary of the literature. *Amer. J. Med. Sci.*, 198:269-292, 1939.
4. Moschcowitz, E., and Wilensky, A. O.: Non-specific granulomata of the intestine. *Amer. J. Med. Sci.*, 166:48-66, 1923.
5. Colp, R.: Case of nonspecific granuloma of terminal ileum and cecum. *Surg. Clin. N. Amer.*, 14:443-449, 1934.
6. Mitchell, D. N., and Rees, R. W.: Agent transmissible from Crohn's disease tissue. *Lancet*, 2:168-171, 1970.
6a. Sachar, D., Taub, R. N., and Janowitz, H. D.: A transmissible agent in Crohn's disease? New pursuit of an old concept. *New Eng. J. Med.*, 293:354-355, 1975.
7. Slaney, G.: Hypersensitivity granulomata and the alimentary tract. *Ann. Roy. Coll. Surg. Eng.*, 31:249-267, 1962.
8. Gray, B. K., Lockhart-Mummery, H. E., and Morson, B. C.: Crohn's disease of the anal region. *Gut*, 6:515-524, 1965.
9. Rosman, M., and Bertini, J. R.: Azathioprine. *Ann. Int. Med.*, 79:694-700, 1973.
10. Ginzburg, L., Marshak, R. H., and Eliasoph, J.: Regional jejunitis. *Surg. Gynec. Obstet.* 111:1-7, 1960.
11. Marshak, R. H., and Wolf, B. S.: Chronic ulcerative granulomatous jejunitis and ileojejunitis. *Amer. J. Roentgen.*, 70:93-112, 1953.
12. Werther, J. L., Schapira, A., Rubenstein, O., and Janowitz, H. D.: Amyloidosis in regional enteritis. *Amer. J. Med.* 29:416-423, 1960.
13. Moseley, J. E., Marshak, R. H., and Wolf, B. S.: Regional enteritis in children. *Amer. J. Roentgen.*, 84:532-539, 1960.
14. BenAsher, H.: Adenocarcinoma of the ileum complicating regional enteritis. *Amer. J. Gastroenterol.*, 55:391-398, 1971.
15. Weedon, D. D., Shorter, R. G., Ilstrup, D. M., et al.: Crohn's disease and cancer. *New Eng. J. Med.*, 289:1099-1103, 1973.

15

Granulomatous Colitis and Ileocolitis

The unusual nature of granulomatous disease of the intestine requires that this volume, otherwise restricted to diseases of the small bowel, include a chapter on inflammation of the colon. We have noted in the chapter on regional enteritis (page 180) that when this disease was first described by Crohn, Ginzburg, and Oppenheimer, it was thought to be an inflammation confined to the terminal ileum. Subsequently it became apparent that the same nonspecific granulomatous inflammatory process can involve any portion of the gastrointestinal tract, from the stomach to the anus. Commonly the disease involves both small bowel and colon (granulomatous ileocolitis), and our discussion must therefore include granulomatous colitis and its very important distinctions from ulcerative colitis.[1]

The slow and sometimes hesitant development of an awareness that granulomatous disease can involve the colon is of considerable historical interest. In 1934, only two years after the description of regional enteritis, Colp[1] reported the first case of granulomatous colitis in a patient who had involvement of the terminal ileum and cecum. This case demonstrated that the ileocecal valve is no barrier to the development of granulomatous disease of the colon.

Rappaport, Burgoyne, and Smetana[2] reviewed, in 1951, 100 cases of histologically proved regional enteritis and found that approximately half had similar, although less severe, disease in the colon. These authors concluded, however, that colonic pathology was probably sufficiently different from regional enteritis to be considered another disease process. Wells,[3] in 1952, was the first to note that some patients who were thought to have ulcerative colitis demonstrated on careful pathological examination features closely resembling those of regional enteritis. In 1954, Warren and Sommers[4] found that in approximately 10 per cent of patients with regional enteritis, skip lesions could be identified in the colon.

Despite great familiarity with granulomatous disease at Mount Sinai Hospital, pathologists at that institution refused for many years to recognize that regional enteritis can involve the colon. Resected specimens of inflamma-

246

tory disease of both ileum and colon were consistently reported as regional enteritis of the small bowel—and ulcerative colitis.

As early as 1951, the senior author, who worked with Dr. Crohn as his radiologist, had noted that from a roentgen point of view some patients with so-called ulcerative colitis seemed to have in the colon an appearance which resembled regional enteritis, and other patients with definite regional enteritis had concomitant radiologically identical disease in the colon. He presented these observations at a meeting of the Inter-American Association of Radiologists in 1951. In 1955, at a meeting of the American Gastroenterological Association, he presented some roentgen distinctions between ulcerative and granulomatous colitis. In 1959 his findings on granulomatous colitis were published in a paper[5] entitled "Segmental Colitis," which described the roentgen alterations in both ulcerative and granulomatous colitis.

It was Morson and Lockhart-Mummery,[6] in 1959, who clearly defined the features of granulomatous colitis and separated this entity from ulcerative colitis. A series of subsequent papers described the clinical and pathological features of granulomatous disease of the colon. The radiological features of granulomatous colitis were summarized by Wolf and Marshak,[7] and Marshak, Janowitz, Lindner, and Wolf[8, 9, 9a, 9b, 9c] reviewed clinical and radiological findings as seen in the United States.

The manner in which the colon becomes involved in the granulomatous process may have a great bearing on the clinical manifestations and the prognosis of the disease. Four types of involvement may be considered:

1. The colon alone may be the site of granulomatous disease.

2. Both the colon and the small bowel may be involved in granulomatous disease. In such patients the disease seems to begin at about the same time in the two areas, for both small bowel and colon are involved when the patient is first examined radiologically. It is uncommon to be able to document the spread of granulomatous disease from ileum to colon or colon to ileum in the absence of surgery.

3. The colon may become involved with granulomatous disease only after an ileocolic anastomosis has been performed for treatment of regional enteritis of the small bowel. The diseased segment of colon is usually immediately adjacent to the anastomosis, but the process may extend to include any or all of the colon.

4. Finally, the colon may be involved directly by fistula formation from an adjacent loop of diseased small bowel. Such fistulas, in our experience, do not lead to granulomatous colitis. The lesion does not appear to spread, and the colonic lesion heals when the diseased small bowel has been removed and the fistula closed.

It is only in the past decade and a half that substantial progress has been made in distinguishing granulomatous from ulcerative colitis. Much of the data concerning ulcerative colitis derived from studies made prior to this time must be reassessed, for these series surely included a significant number of patients with granulomatous disease. In our experience the incidence of granulomatous colitis has been increasing greatly in recent years, whereas that of ulcerative colitis has declined. In part this change may simply represent a greater awareness of granulomatous disease, but we suspect that it reflects either the referral nature of our hospitals or a true increase in the incidence of the disease.

Not all inflammatory disease of the colon can be characterized as either ulcerative or granulomatous colitis. Intermediate forms defying classification sometimes occur, and other now unidentified inflammatory processes may in time become apparent. It is now recognized, for example, that ischemic vascular disease of the colon may present a picture resembling granulomatous colitis.[10] Nevertheless, we are convinced that a diagnosis of granulomatous colitis can be made with confidence most of the time when current clinical, radiologic, and pathologic criteria are carefully applied. When a definite diagnosis cannot be made, we prefer to classify the case for the time being as "colitis, type unknown," with a description of the salient features, rather than to force the case into the category of either ulcerative or granulomatous colitis or to add intermediate classifications. Although some common etiology may in time become apparent, it seems to us that ulcerative and granulomatous disease are distinct entities and that subsequent investigations will more likely be advanced by maintaining the two groups separate than by attempting to unify them.

Although regional enteritis and ulcerative colitis tend to occur in the same populations and genetic studies have shown both diseases to occur in different members of the same family,[11] we have never observed regional enteritis of the small bowel and ulcerative colitis in the same patient. We believe that such an association does not occur. Thus when definite regional enteritis is present in the small bowel, concomitant inflammatory disease in the colon will prove to be granulomatous.

Clinical Features

Many of the clinical features of granulomatous colitis are shared by the other chronic nonspecific inflammatory diseases of the gut, regional enteritis and ulcerative colitis. Thus patients complain, with an onset that is acute in some but quite low grade and subtle in others, of abdominal cramps, diarrhea, fever, malaise, anorexia, and weight loss. Most patients develop their disease in young adult life, in their teens or twenties, but the age of onset in itself is of little diagnostic value, since granulomatous colitis can present at any age. Anemia is common and usually of the iron deficiency type. Three clinical features of granulomatous colitis help to distinguish it from ulcerative colitis (although not from regional enteritis): a normal sigmoidoscopy, the absence of gross blood in the stools, and the presence of fistulas.

Granulomatous colitis tends to be segmental and right-sided in its distribution, sparing the rectum. Since rectal involvement is an outstanding characteristic of ulcerative colitis, the finding of a normal rectal mucosa in a patient with clinical features of inflammatory bowel disease immediately alerts the physician to the possibility of granulomatous colitis. In our series of patients, the rectum was involved in only about 20 per cent of all cases of granulomatous disease of the colon. The rectum is usually involved in those cases in which the lesion is diffuse. Granulomatous disease confined to rectum and sigmoid alone is infrequent. On sigmoidoscopy we have noted two types of lesions. In one, which is the less common, the disease is severe and resembles ulcerative colitis. In the other, the findings are more chronic, unassociated with friability or with blood in the lumen, and on occasion there is a cobblestone appearance; it is not always easy to distinguish this stage from that of chronic ulcerative colitis on the basis of sigmoidoscopic appearance alone.

Gross blood may be absent from the stools of patients with granulomatous colitis even when diarrhea is severe and the course of the illness prolonged. The consistent absence of blood is thus a valuable point of distinction from ulcerative colitis, a disease in which bleeding is virtually always a prominent feature. More often, however, patients with granulomatous colitis do have some episodes of blood in the stool during the course of their disease; as a rule bleeding is small in amount and intermittent in occurrence. In a minority of patients, gross rectal bleeding is a major part of the history. In our experience it is in this last group that involvement of the rectum in the inflammatory process is found.

Despite the absence of gross blood, the stools are often positive on testing for occult blood, and chronic blood loss is probably the principal cause of the anemia which commonly occurs in granulomatous disease.

Fistulas, so characteristic a feature of regional enteritis, are also common in patients with granulomatous disease of the colon. They occur at some time during the course of the illness in about half the patients with granulomatous colitis and ileocolitis. Most of these fistulas are perianal in location. When internal fistulas are present, they usually arise from matted and adherent loops of diseased small bowel and may extend into the colon. Colonic fistulas are less common.

Extracolonic manifestations, such as uveitis, arthritis, erythema nodosum, and pyoderma gangrenosum, are less common in granulomatous than in ulcerative colitis, although they do occur. In contrast to the well-known malignant potential of ulcerative colitis, we have rarely observed the development of carcinoma of the colon in patients with granulomatous colitis. A possible explanation is that because of persistent symptoms and an unremitting course, the patient with granulomatous colitis tends to be operated upon and to have the diseased portions resected sooner than the patient with ulcerative colitis.

A number of case reports have recently appeared concerning colon carcinoma arising in association with granulomatous disease of the small bowel and colon. In one series[12] the incidence of carcinoma was 20 times greater than in a control population. Further studies will be required to determine whether the association of carcinoma and granulomatous disease is a valid one and, if so, how great a risk it presents for the individual patient.

In further contrast to ulcerative colitis, free perforation of the large bowel and toxic dilatation of the colon are much less frequent.[13] The pathology of the disease, with gross thickening of the bowel wall by edema and fibrosis, would seem to militate against these acute complications.

Pathology

The pathologic features of granulomatous colitis are identical to those of regional enteritis. The wall of the involved bowel is greatly thickened and rigid, and the lumen is narrowed, sometimes even strictured. The mesenteric attachments are thick, and regional lymph nodes are often enlarged. When the bowel is opened, the mucosa is found to be red and swollen, with long longitudinal and transverse ulcers intersecting islands of edematous mucosa to give a cobblestone appearance (Fig. 15-1). Sinus tracts and fistulas may be present, sometimes extending to adjacent viscera or to the body wall. Skip lesions may

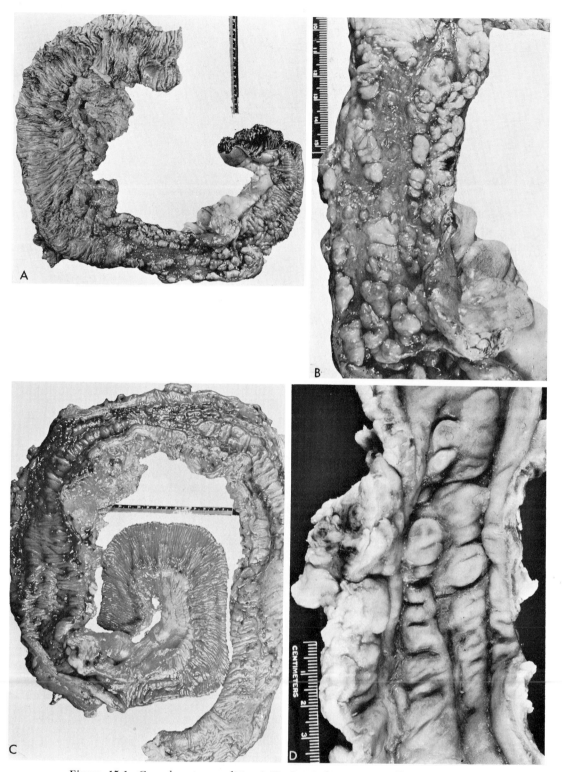

Figure 15-1 *Granulomatous colitis.* A–D, Surgical specimens illustrating characteristic pathologic features of granulomatous colitis. Cobblestoning, longitudinal ulcerations, transverse ulcers, skip lesions, stricturing, and thickening of the bowel wall are seen.

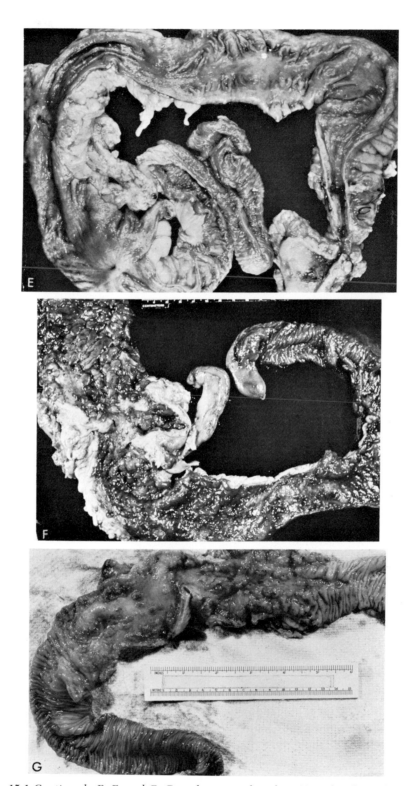

***Figure 15-1** Continued E, F, and G, Granulomatous ileocolitis.* Note that the pathologic findings in the terminal ileum and the right side of the colon are identical.

be seen as areas of disease in the bowel, separated by lengths of normal-appearing gut.

On histologic examination there is a chronic granulomatous inflammatory reaction with edema and fibrosis involving all layers of the colonic wall, although changes are usually most pronounced in the submucosa. The deep ulcers seen on the mucosal surface extend into the submucosa and muscularis as fissures. The most useful diagnostic histologic feature of granulomatous colitis is the presence in the bowel wall or in regional lymph nodes of noncaseating granulomas containing multinucleated giant cells, epithelioid cells, and mononuclear cells.

Not many pathologic specimens from patients with early or minimal disease have been available to us, because surgical intervention is usually deferred until the disease is advanced. In several patients who were operated upon early in their course, the resected specimens showed mucosal and submucosal edema, with scattered irregular ulcers. In many areas the mucosa was intact. Inflammatory cells were present in all layers of the gut wall, and typical granulomas were seen.

Prognosis

The prognosis in granulomatous colitis seems to be dictated in part by the status of the small bowel. Patients who have granulomatous disease confined to the colon do better than those with ileocolitis.[9] In comparison to patients with ulcerative colitis, those with granulomatous colitis often come to surgery earlier, and the course of their disease may be more chronic and unremitting. Desperate acute episodes such as toxic dilatation and free perforation occur less frequently. The indication for surgery is usually intractability to a medical program, less frequently stenosis. Patients may do well following segmental resection of the colon. Recurrences appear to be less frequent in the colon than in the small bowel. When ileostomy and total colectomy must be performed for granulomatous colitis, spread of the disease into previously normal small bowel is less common.

When the ileum is involved in the disease process—that is, in granulomatous ileocolitis—a different prognosis is encountered.[10] The disease tends to be more severe than when only the colon is involved, and the greater the degree and extent of ileal disease, the more severe the illness and the worse the prognosis.

Two groups of patients with ileocolitis can be distinguished, largely on the basis of the nature and extent of the ileal involvement. When sinus tracts, fistulas, and abscesses are present, the clinical course is unremitting, early surgery is required, recurrences are frequent, and disability is chronic. When the ileal disease is less marked and incomplete obstruction rather than infection is the predominant feature of the illness, the response to a medical regimen is better, disability is less, surgery can be deferred, and when it is required, can be performed with less risk of recurrence.

Medical Treatment

The goal of medical treatment in granulomatous colitis and ileocolitis is to induce full clinical remission. Unfortunately, sustained remissions are uncommon in granulomatous disease, and most often the physician finds that his task is to make the patient as comfortable as possible, functioning in daily life despite the activity of a chronic illness.

The medical treatment of granulomatous colitis, not surprisingly, does not differ from that of regional enteritis or ulcerative colitis in any important respect. Supportive treatment, appropriate for all patients, includes dietary manipulation to avoid foods to which the patient in his own experience is intolerant; adequate rest; sedation; antidiarrheal agents, such as the opiates; correction of anemia, which usually can be accomplished with iron; and—perhaps as important as any of these—supportive psychotherapy by the internist or gastroenterologist.

Antibiotics appear to be of limited value in the treatment of granulomatous colitis itself and usually are reserved for acute management of such infectious complications as abscess formation. Salicylazosulfapyridine (Azulfidine) is sometimes employed in treatment, in the same manner as in ulcerative colitis. Studies are now underway to evaluate the effectiveness of azathioprine (Imuran) in the treatment of granulomatous colitis and regional enteritis. The insoluble sulfa drugs such as sulfathalidine are sometimes employed in treatment; we are not convinced that these drugs actually are of value.

It is our experience that adrenocorticotropic hormone and the adrenal corticosteroids are in general less effective in granulomatous than in ulcerative colitis and are less likely to induce a remission. Jones and Lennard-Jones,[14] in a retrospective study of 105 patients with granulomatous disease admitted to London's Central Middlesex Hospital from 1954 to 1964, concluded that steroids are beneficial in some cases, but that treatment must often be continued for long periods of time, and that steroids do not obviate the need for surgical intervention in most cases. We have found steroids useful in the management of symptoms, even though we have no evidence that the drugs alter at all the natural history of the disease. We have tended therefore to withhold steroids as long as possible in the course of the illness and to rely upon combinations of the supportive measures indicated previously. Steroids are employed when the clinical condition is deteriorating or when symptoms persist for prolonged periods or worsen. It seems reasonable to us to undertake a trial of steroid therapy before resorting to surgical treatment of granulomatous disease when the indications for surgery are obstructive symptoms or inflammation. Steroids are not likely to forestall surgery when the indications are the infectious complications of granulomatous disease, such as fistulas or abscess formation. Occasionally, reversibility of the roentgen alterations to a normal pattern is observed. This has been seen both spontaneously and following steroid therapy.

In considering the type of steroid therapy to be undertaken, both the severity and the location of the disease should be taken into account. When the illness is of a moderate degree, prednisone or related oral compounds are administered. When the patient is severely ill, intravenous adrenocorticotropic hormone may be the treatment of choice, just as in severe ulcerative colitis. If the rectum is involved, rectal instillation of steroids, either alone or in conjunction with systemic steroids, may be of benefit.

Surgical Treatment

Surgery is indicated for treatment of the complications of granulomatous colitis. The indications include obstruction, fistulas which are symptomatic or causing debility, abdominal masses and abscesses, and the very rare complications of perforation or massive hemorrhage. Usually obstruction and infection with abscess formation are the complications which require surgical intervention. "Intractability" to a medical regimen, without development of complications, is a difficult surgical indication to define, but it is a real one. It embraces patients who, despite good medical management, simply do not do well; they have progressive disability with diarrhea, abdominal pain, fever, and chronic illness. In this group, one must consider treating the disease surgically.

The consideration of surgery in granulomatous disease is complicated by the threat of recurrences, for the contemplated surgery may not be curative. It is an interesting but unexplained observation that recurrences appear to be less common when only the colon is diseased. In ileocolitis, however, with disease in both small bowel and colon, development of granulomatous disease in what appeared to be normal small bowel or colon often occurs following resection of the involved gut. As a general rule in the management of granulomatous disease, we believe that surgery should be deferred in favor of medical treatment as long as possible. Nevertheless, surgery is ultimately required, or deemed desirable, in many patients during the course of their illness. Recurrent disease is managed on the same principles as the original inflammatory process, with medical treatment employed as long as possible and re-resection reserved for complications.

When surgical intervention is required, the choice of the procedure may be influenced by the location of the disease. If only a portion of the colon is involved in granulomatous disease and the small bowel is normal, segmental resection and end to end anastomosis may be successful. When all or most of the colon is involved, ileostomy with total or subtotal colectomy may be required. Since the rectum is often spared, subtotal colectomy with ileoproctostomy may prove feasible. In some cases of granulomatous disease confined to the rectum and sigmoid, it has been possible to resect the diseased area and construct a "dry" left-sided colostomy rather than an ileostomy.

We believe that patients with ileocolitis, because they are highly susceptible to recurrent disease, and because long segments of small bowel are often involved, are best managed supportively on medical programs. When surgical intervention is mandatory, we believe the minimum resection possible should be performed.

Roentgen Features

Granulomatous Colitis[15]

Among the patients with granulomatous disease involving the colon that we have studied, 85 per cent had disease in both ileum and colon, and in 15 per cent the disease was confined to the colon. Total involvement of the large bowel, including the rectum, was noted in 20 per cent of the series. In those patients with universal granulomatous colitis, the ileum was usually involved. This finding is of help in differentiating granulomatous from ulcerative colitis, especially when the ileum displays characteristic features of regional enteritis. The roentgen findings characteristic for granulomatous colitis and ileocolitis are listed in Table 15-1.

Table 15–1. Roentgen Findings in Granulomatous Colitis and Ileocolitis

Universal distribution in colon usually associated with involvement of terminal ileum.
Nodular, irregular pattern after evacuation.
Transverse ulcerations.
Longitudinal ulcerations.
Combination of transverse and longitudinal ulcerations with cobblestoning.
Strictures.
Irregularity of contour with asymmetric involvement and pseudodiverticula.
Skip lesions, and contour defects.
Fistulas, frequent in ileum, less common in colon.
Intramural abscesses.
Tiny discrete ulcers in early cases, associated with small irregular nodules.

There has been some discussion in the literature concerning the technical method which best illustrates the roentgenologic findings in this disease. We prefer the barium-filled colon to double contrast studies. However, air studies are routinely employed immediately after the evacuation films, primarily for confirmation. We do not perform any contrast studies in very sick or toxic patients. We have frequently found the evacuation film to be superior to the barium-filled or air-filled colon film for determining the extent of the disease and the presence of skip lesions, and for the detection of tiny ulcerations and the nodular configuration, which are so typical of granulomatous colitis. Of course, it is not necessary to restrict the examination to one procedure. An optimal evaluation is achieved by utilizing the filled colon, double contrast, and postevacuation films.

The roentgen features characteristic of granulomatous colitis are essentially the same as those seen in regional enteritis. They include skip lesions, contour defects, longitudinal ulcerations, transverse fissures, deep ragged ulcerations, eccentric involvement and pseudodiverticula, narrowing or stricture formation, pseudopolypoid changes that produce a coarse cobblestone pattern, internal fistulas, and sinus tracts.

The earliest roentgen features we have observed are small, irregular nodules along the contours of the bowel, sometimes associated with tiny ulcerations. Slight rigidity and thickening of the haustral markings may be evident (Fig. 15-2). These minimal alterations usually extend over a short segment or are seen in the form of skip lesions. On occasion the process is diffuse.

Spasm and irritability are present, but are less marked than in ulcerative colitis, and the bowel is more easily filled. Secretions are noted within the lumen of the bowel as a consequence of the mucus, edema, and exudate (Fig. 15-3A). The usual homogeneous barium mixture has a granular, flocculent quality. These findings depend on the extent of involvement and are usually noted when long segments of bowel are involved.

Overfilling and distention of the colon may obscure the slight irregularity of the contour described (Fig. 15-3B). The mucosal pattern after evacuation is helpful in these cases, as it may reveal thickening or nodularity of the mucosa with an irregular ropelike appearance (Figs. 15-4 and 15-5). Involvement is frequently more extensive on the evacuation film than is apparent in barium- or air-filled colon films. This observation is important in planning operative procedures and accounts for discrepancies in reports concerning linear spread of the disease. Although small areas of ulceration may be difficult to identify, their presence may be suggested by straightening or rigidity of a segment or by the presence of pseudodiverticula on the opposite wall. This is

(Text continued on page 259.)

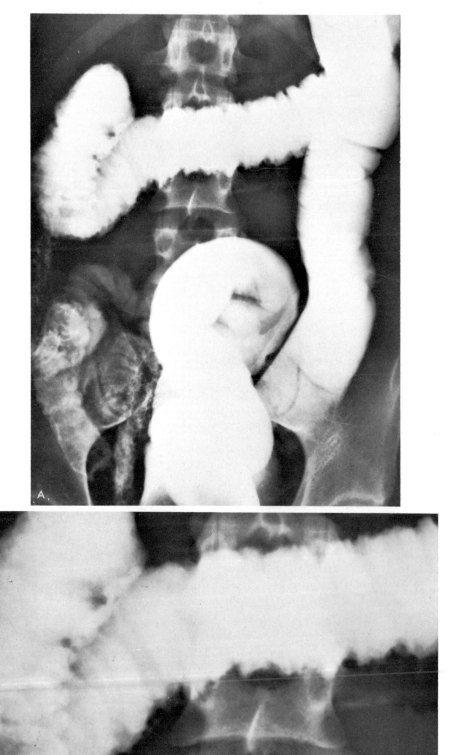

Figure 15-2 Granulomatous colitis. A, There are numerous small irregular nodular defects along the contour of the transverse colon associated with minimal rigidity. The cecum and ascending colon are spastic and irritable. The terminal ileum reveals the early changes of regional enteritis. The folds are hazy and thickened, and there are small nodular defects. *B*, Magnified view of the transverse colon in *A*. The irregular nodular defects are seen along the contour of the transverse colon.

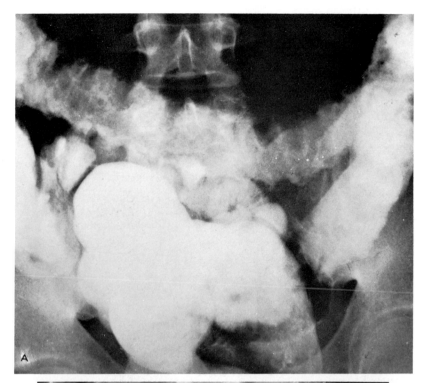

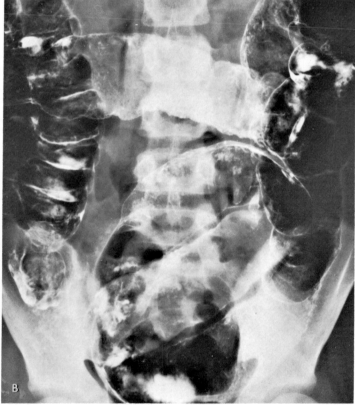

Figure 15-3 *Granulomatous colitis. A,* Numerous irregular nodules are seen along the contour of the bowel from the cecum to the proximal descending colon. The findings are most marked in the transverse colon. The barium has a granular quality due to an admixture of secretions, mucus, and pus. The haustral markings are absent. The bowel was easily filled. *B,* Granulomatous colitis involving the transverse colon. There is minimal involvement of the inferior aspect of the transverse colon characterized by irregularity and nodular filling defects. The findings are partially obscured by overfilling of the colon with air. These minimal findings are frequently better identified on a motility film or an evacuation film.

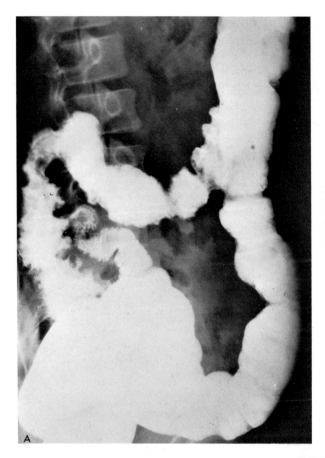

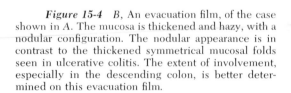

Figure 15-4 Granulomatous colitis. A, The colon is involved from cecum to sigmoid. The findings are most marked on the right side of the colon, where multiple irregular nodules are seen. There is a moderate degree of narrowing and rigidity, and the haustral markings are absent. There is minimal lack of distensibility of the left side of the colon.

Figure 15-4 B, An evacuation film, of the case shown in A. The mucosa is thickened and hazy, with a nodular configuration. The nodular appearance is in contrast to the thickened symmetrical mucosal folds seen in ulcerative colitis. The extent of involvement, especially in the descending colon, is better determined on this evacuation film.

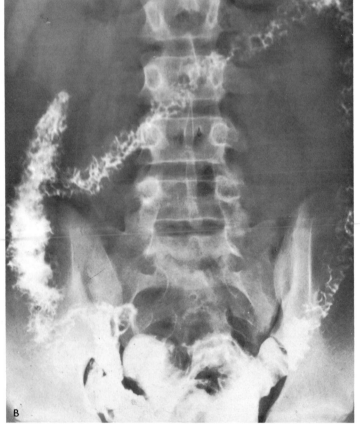

because ulceration produces spasm and contraction and the opposite uninvolved wall becomes folded.

On occasion, tiny ulcers are seen extending perpendicularly from the contour of the colon or as tiny specks within the lumen (Fig. 15-6). In contrast to the ulcers in ulcerative colitis, these are surrounded by the small irregular nodules described previously. Pathologic examination of tissue at this stage reveals mucosal edema, submucosal infiltration, and small, irregular ulcerations. The small ulcers combine to produce large longitudinal ulcerations or gutters, which are frequently multiple. When this is associated with transverse linear ulcerations, it produces the characteristic cobblestone pattern (Figs. 15-7 to 15-10).

Ulcers may penetrate beyond the contour of the bowel, presenting in profile as numerous long spicules, perpendicular to the long axis of the bowel, or as sinus tracts (Fig. 15-11*A* and *B*). At times they ultimately lead to intramural abscesses, which may be large, producing a marked irregularity of the contour of the bowel (Fig. 15-11*C* to *I*). When they penetrate into adjacent loops, a fistula is formed (Fig. 15-12*A, B, C, D, E*). In later stages of the disease, the entire mucosa may be sloughed off because of diffuse ulceration. In those cases in which the bowel is diffusely and symmetrically involved and there are no typical features of granulomatous disease, differentiation from ulcerative colitis may be impossible, especially in the absence of characteristic features in the small intestine (Figs. 15-13 and 15-14).

In some instances, larger, irregular, nodular contour defects with hazy margins are seen. These are primarily due to mucosal and submucosal edema. Although ulceration is frequently present at this time on pathologic examination, ulcers usually cannot be demonstrated roentgenologically in these defects (Fig. 15-15). When the ulcers are large, circumferential narrowing of the bowel wall due to spasm occurs, and a carcinoma is simulated.

Marked thickening of the bowel secondary to intramural fibrotic changes is common in granulomatous colitis, producing irregular, stenotic segments and strictures (Figs. 15-16, 15-17, and 15-18). Occasionally, granulomatous colitis presents as a single stricture of the colon (Fig. 15-19). When this stricture is eccentric and associated with overhanging edges, differentiation from a carcinoma may be impossible. In most cases, however, there is further evidence of involvement of the bowel in the form of skip lesions, strictures, or other identifying features of granulomatous disease.

Linear extension of the disease in granulomatous colitis, as in regional enteritis, is uncommon in the absence of surgery (Fig. 15-20), but normal areas between skip lesions may become involved. A minimally involved colon with multiple skip lesions may become severely and diffusely ulcerated in a short period of time.

Granulomatous Ileocolitis

There are no specific roentgen features of granulomatous ileocolitis except for the anatomic distribution. In the small bowel, the characteristic findings of regional enteritis are not affected by concomitant inflammatory disease of the colon (Figs. 15-21 and 15-22). In the majority of these cases, the inflammatory process in the small bowel is confined to the distal ileum, but at times long segments of small bowel are involved.

Granulomatous ileocolitis must be distinguished from so-called back-

(Text continued on page 268.)

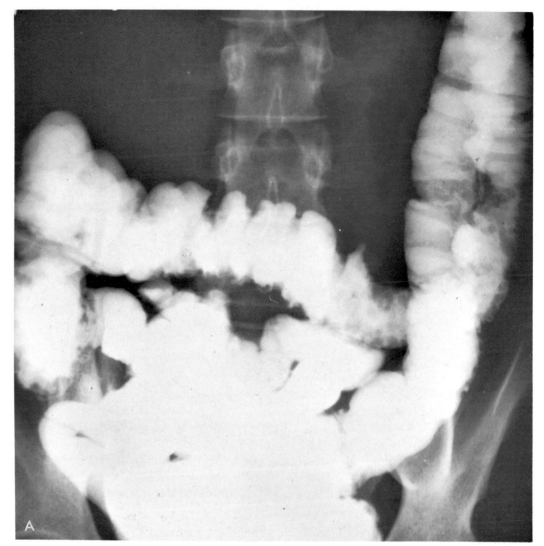

Figure 15-5 *Granulomatous colitis.* A, There is minimal involvement of the colon from cecum to the splenic flexure, characterized by irregularity of the contour as a result of multiple small nodular defects. The findings are most marked in the distal transverse colon. There is some rigidity and lack of distensibility. B, Evacuation film of A. The mucosal pattern has an irregular cobblestone appearance. Several small skip lesions indicated by pseudodiverticula are identified. Involvement of the left side of the colon, which was not appreciated in A, is well demonstrated on this film, again showing the value of the evacuation film in granulomatous colitis. C, Spot film of B. The nodular, cobblestone, ropelike configuration of the mucosal pattern, associated with multiple small pseudo-diverticula, is again identified.

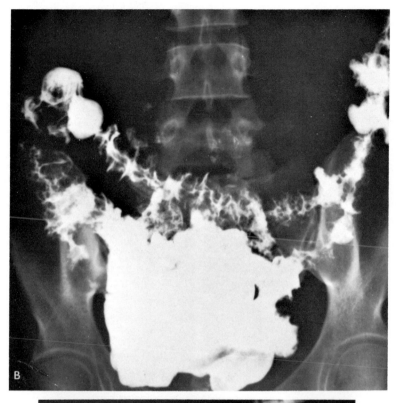

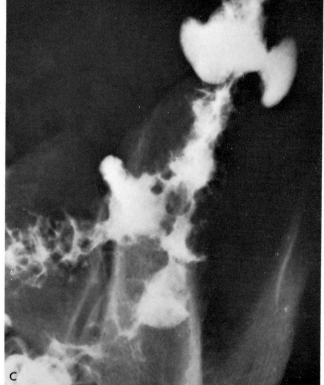

Figure 15-5 Continued   See legend on opposite page.

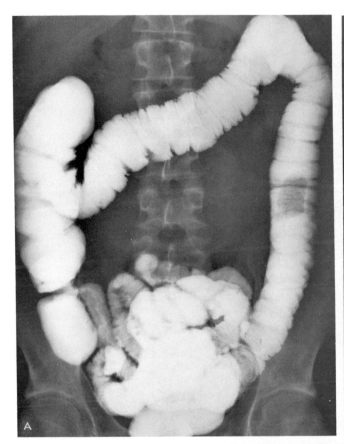
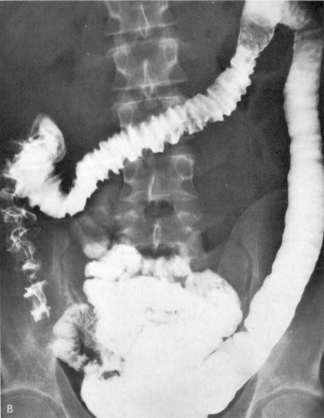
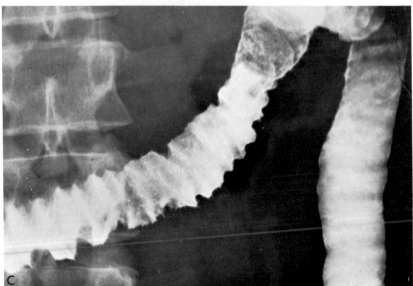

Figure 15-6 Granulomatous ileocolitis. A, There is moderate narrowing of the cecum and the ileocecal valve. The remainder of the colon appears within normal limits. The terminal ileum is moderately narrowed, rigid, with effacement of the mucosa.

B, Evacuation film. On this film involvement of the colon extends as far as the sigmoid. The haustral markings in the transverse colon are thickened and there are small nodular defects along the contours.

C, Magnified view of the distal transverse colon, demonstrating numerous tiny spicules, due to small ulcerations, extending from the contour of the bowel. Again note the nodular defects.

This case is of significance because it demonstrates that the filled colon may completely obliterate the early manifestations of granulomatous colitis. Also, the demonstration of tiny ulcers is unusual in granulomatous colitis. These are undoubtedly the precursors of the larger transverse ulcerations. Note the granular quality of the barium and the thickened haustra.

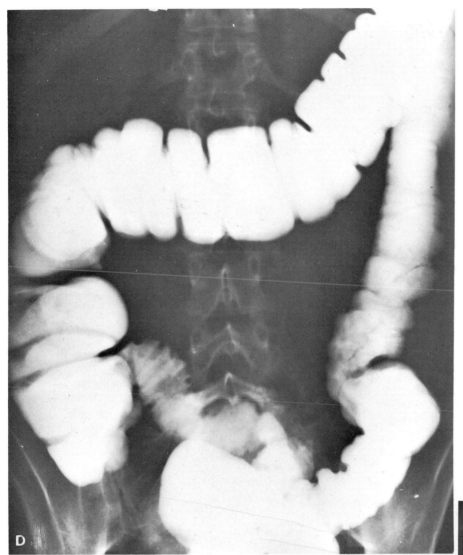

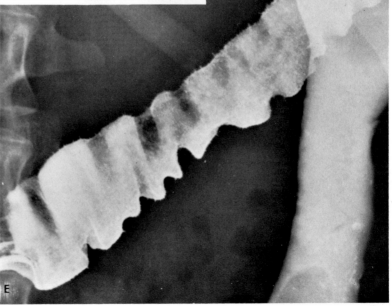

Figure 15-6 Continued D, Early roentgen signs of granulomatous ileocolitis. The full colon is normal except for minimal thickening of the haustral markings of the descending colon. The folds of the terminal ileum are slightly thickened.

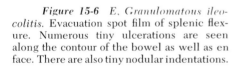

Figure 15-6 E, Granulomatous ileocolitis. Evacuation spot film of splenic flexure. Numerous tiny ulcerations are seen along the contour of the bowel as well as en face. There are also tiny nodular indentations.

(Illustration continued on following page.)

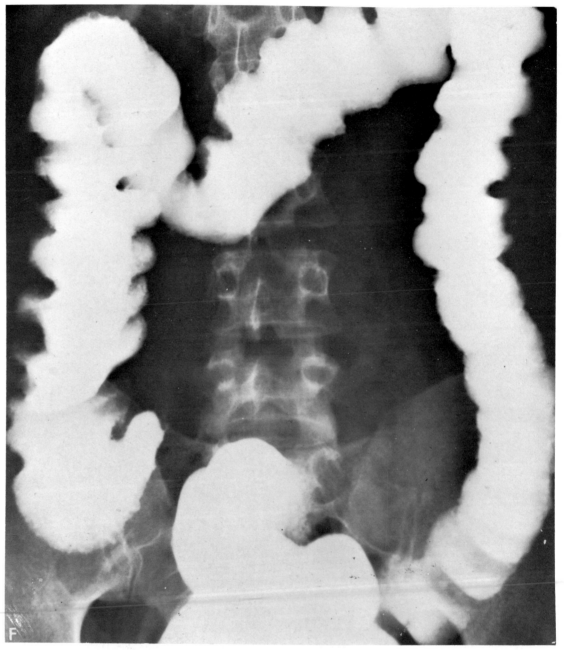

***Figure 15-6** Continued   F, Granulomatous colitis.* The entire colon except the rectum is involved with numerous small ulcers associated with tiny nodular defects. The haustral markings are thickened or absent. The colon is moderately spastic and irritable.

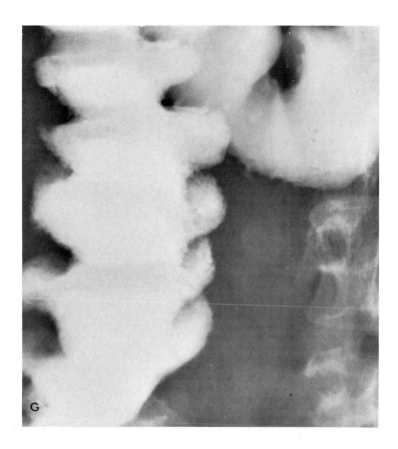

Figure 15-6 Continued G, Magnified view of right side of colon shown in *F*, revealing the small ulcers associated with the tiny nodular defects.

Figure 15-6 H, Magnified view of left side of colon revealing the small ulcers and tiny nodular defects.

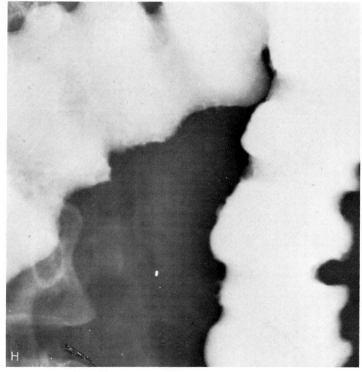

(Illustration continued on following page.)

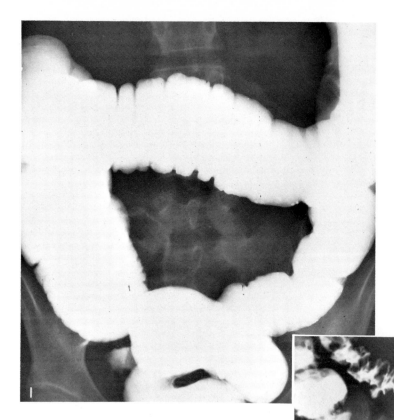

Figure 15-6 Continued I, Early granulomatous ileocolitis. There is minimal flattening of the contours of the distal transverse colon. The haustral markings are not as distinct as usual. There is slight narrowing of the upper rectum. A diagnosis of an inflammatory process involving the colon would be difficult from this film. The air study revealed similar minimal changes.

Figure 15-6 J, The evacuation film of the same patient reveals nodularity of the entire mucosa of the colon. The terminal ileum is now visualized and is extensively involved.

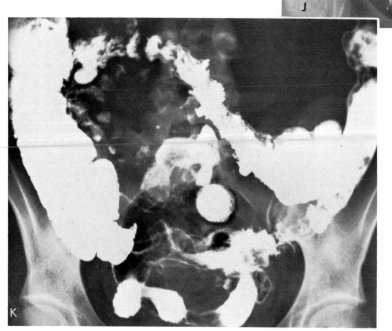

Figure 15-6 K, A motility film of the same patient better demonstrates the changes, especially those in the left side of the colon and distal ileum.

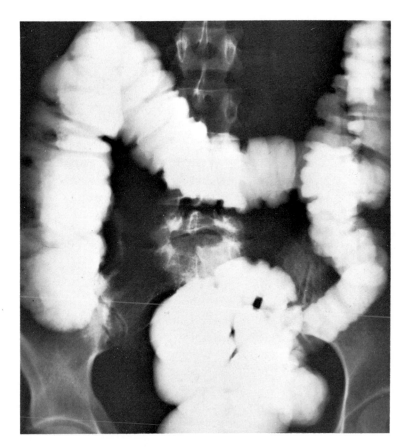

Figure 15-7 Granulomatous ileocolitis. There is minimal irregularity of the contours of the right side of the colon and transverse colon. The haustra in the transverse colon are not as distinct as usually seen.

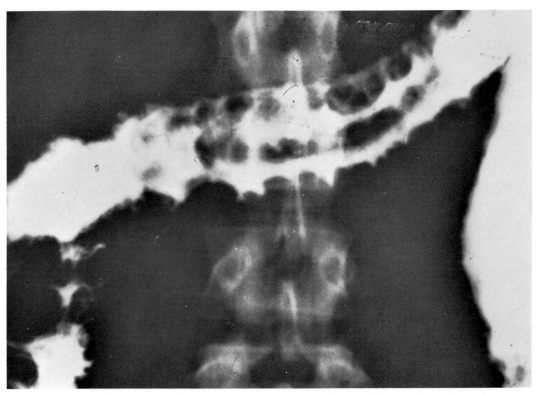

Figure 15-8 Same patient as in Figure 15-7. Six months later there are longitudinal ulcerations and numerous transverse ulcerations.

wash ileitis (ulcerative colitis with involvement of the terminal ileum). In the latter cases, narrowing of the intestinal lumen is usually minimal and the length of ileum involved is small (Fig. 15-23A). Sinus tracts, skip areas, and fistulas are not seen, and the mucosa is only slightly altered with minimal thickening of the folds. In a rare case differentiation is impossible (Fig. 15-23B). Involvement of the colon in patients with ileocolitis is most frequently continuous with the disease in the ileum. Segmental involvement of the colon is more common than diffuse involvement of the entire large bowel.

In those cases in which the radiologic findings of granulomatous disease of the colon are subtle (Fig. 15-22), a motility follow-through film of the colon, performed as part of a small bowel examination, may be helpful.

Inflammatory Disease of the Stoma

Since ileostomy and colectomy are performed for both ulcerative and granulomatous colitis, the appearance of postoperative inflammatory disease in the ileum proximal to the stoma is important. Such prestomal ileitis is of two varieties. One is secondary to obstruction of the stoma—ileostomy dysfunction—and is a mechanical problem relating to narrowing of the stoma. The other is secondary to extension of the granulomatous process. Ileostomy dysfunction may be seen following surgery for both ulcerative colitis and granulomatous colitis. Development of the granulomatous process in the region of the new stoma is seen only if surgery was performed for granulomatous disease. As noted previously, recurrent disease at the stroma is less common if the small bowel was initially *un*involved in the disease process.

The roentgen findings in ileostomy dysfunction and granulomatous prestomal ileitis differ. In ileostomy dysfunction, the ileum is dilated, with considerably increased secretions. The folds are slightly thickened, and ulcerations are minimal and difficult to identify. When prestomal granulomatous ileitis develops, however, the roentgen findings are identical to those described previously for regional enteritis (Figs. 15-24A and B).

Diverticulitis and Granulomatous Colitis

Diverticulitis may be confused with granulomatous colitis, especially when granulomatous disease is confined to the sigmoid. Granulomatous colitis is not uncommon in middle-aged and elderly patients, an age group in which diverticulosis and diverticulitis are also often found. On occasion, granulomatous disease and diverticula may coexist.

In granulomatous colitis the involved segment tends to be long—usually 10 cm. or more—whereas in diverticulitis the segment is short, perhaps 3 to 6 cm. in length. The abscesses of granulomatous colitis often have a triangular shape, but at times they may be difficult to distinguish from coexistent diverticula. In the ulcerating mucosa of granulomatous colitis the folds are straightened, perpendicular, and associated with a thick wall and intraluminal secretions; in a perforated diverticulum the abscess usually creates an extramural defect or an arcuate configuration of the folds that stretch over the abscess. The transverse fissures and marked mucosal edema of granulomatous colitis produce a step-ladder configuration; in diverticulitis there are no transverse fissures and the folds tend to be arcuate rather than straightened.

In 1970 the senior author[16] described a sign throught to be pathognomonic

(Text continued on page 300.)

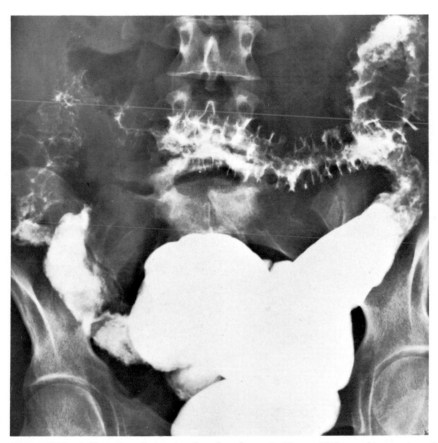

Figure 15-9 A film taken 6 months after that shown in Figure 15-8 reveals extensive ulceration of the colon from cecum to mid descending colon. In the transverse colon, there are marked transverse ulcerations. The terminal ileum is also involved. The rectum, sigmoid, and lower descending colon are normal.

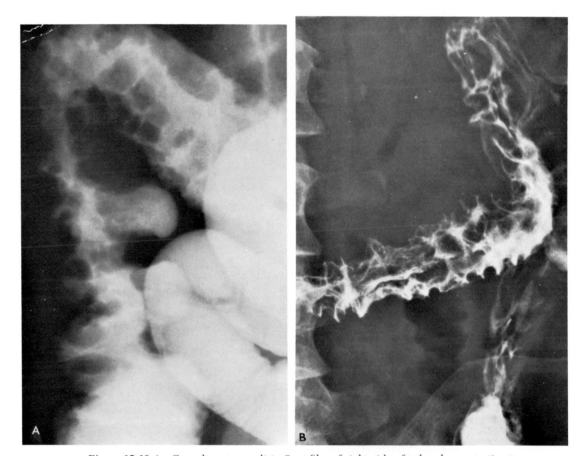

Figure 15-10 *A Granulomatous colitis*. Spot film of right side of colon demonstrating transverse and linear ulcerations, large inflammatory polyps, narrowing, rigidity, and irregular contours.
    B, Granulomatous ileocolitis. Evacuation film demonstrating the irregular nodular, thickened mucosal pattern seen in granulomatous colitis.

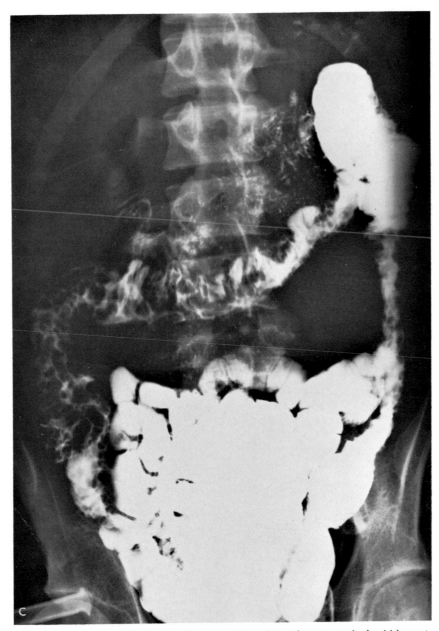

Figure 15-10 *Continued   C, Granulomatous ileocolitis.* There is marked cobblestoning produced by the longitudinal and transverse ulcerations, with narrowing and rigidity of the colon. The rectum and sigmoid are normal. The involvement of the ileum was seen simultaneously with the involvement of the colon. This has been true in most of our cases.

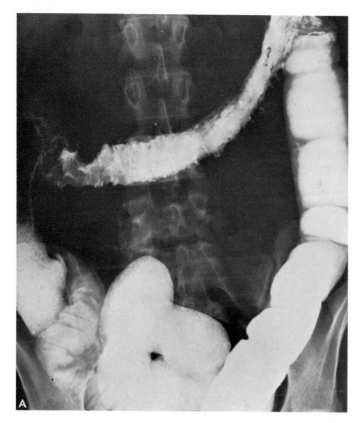

Figure 15-11 Granulomatous colitis. **A,** The right side of the colon is markedly involved with numerous spike-like ulcerations extending from the contour of the transverse colon.

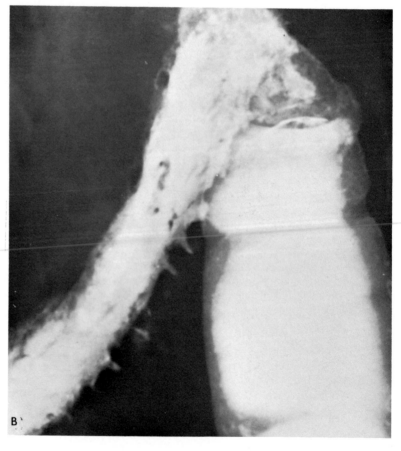

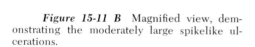

Figure 15-11 B Magnified view, demonstrating the moderately large spikelike ulcerations.

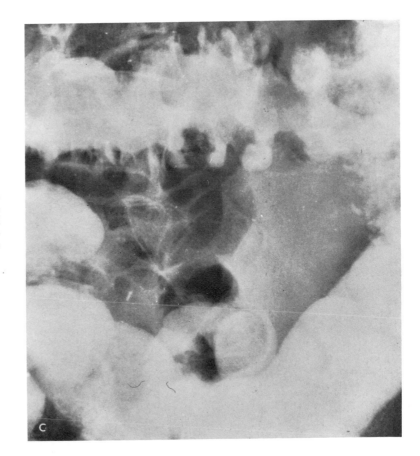

Figure 15-11 Continued C, Granulomatous colitis. Numerous saclike ulcerations simulating diverticula extend from the contour of the transverse colon and are associated with marked irregularity of the contour. The segmental distribution of the granulomatous colitis is again seen.

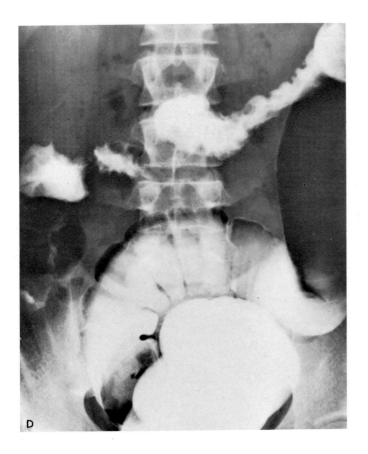

Figure 15-11 D, Granulomatous colitis. Marked involvement of the transverse colon is noted. There is a large irregular ulcer crater in the middle of the transverse colon.

(Illustration continued on following page.)

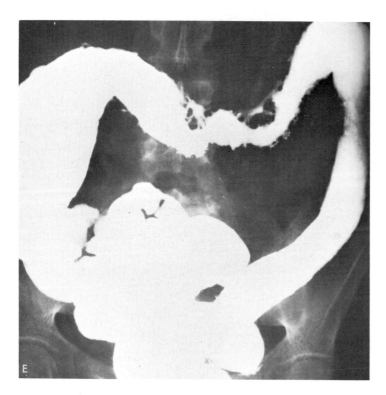

Figure 15-11 Continued E, Two large ulcers associated with radiating folds and surrounded by thickened mucosa are identified in the midportion of the transverse colon. Smaller ulcerations are seen throughout the remainder of the transverse colon.

Figure 15-11 F, Magnified view of two large ulcers shown in Figure 15-11E. Collar-button ulcers are also seen in the inferior portion of the distal third of the transverse colon. This type of collar-button ulceration may be seen in both ulcerative and granulomatous colitis, and in amebiasis and ischemic colitis as well.

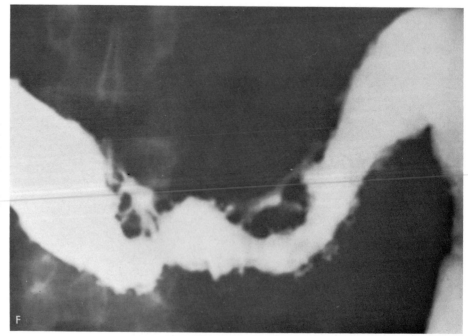

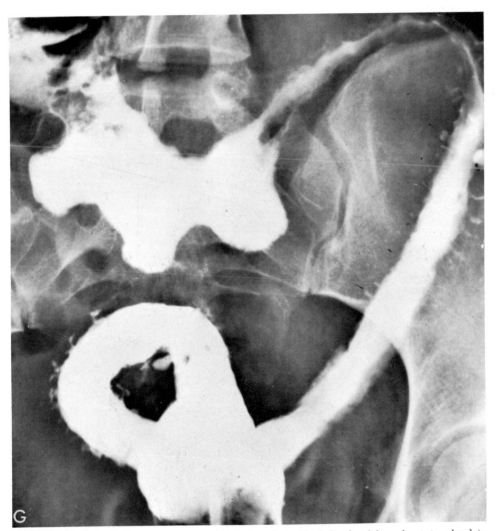

Figure 15-11 Continued *G, Granulomatous colitis.* The left side of the colon is involved, including the rectum. Numerous collar-button and transverse ulcers are identified. Pseudodiverticula are seen in the transverse colon. This is an unusual distribution for granulomatous colitis.

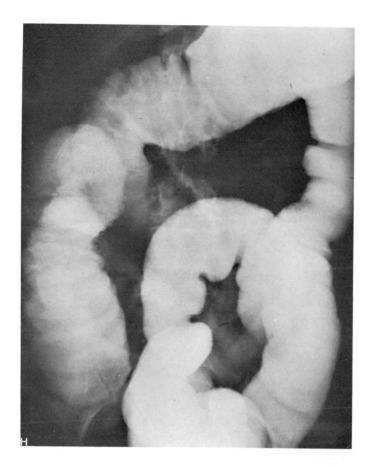

Figure 15-11 Continued *H,* The right side of the colon is involved with granulomatous colitis. The right side of the colon is slightly dilated and the contours are irregular. Haustral markings are thickened or absent. Marked dilatation as seen in ulcerative colitis has not been identified in our series of patients with granulomatous colitis.

Figure 15-11 *I,* In a magnified view numerous moderately large ulcers are seen along the superior segment of the proximal transverse colon.

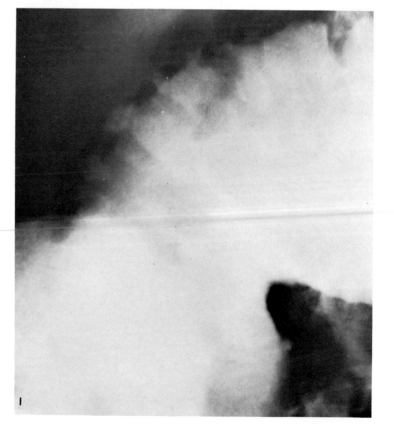

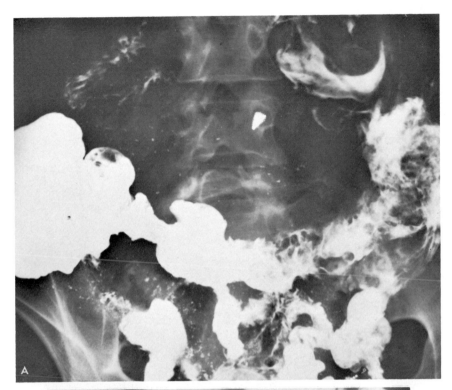

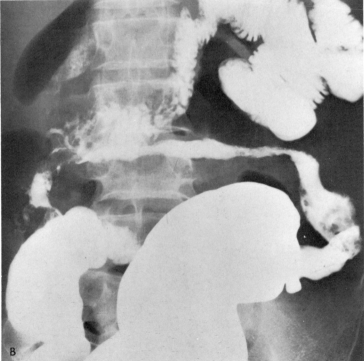

Figure 15-12 *Granulomatous ileocolitis.* The same case as shown in Figures 15-7, 15-8, and 15-9, two years after the original study. There is more extensive involvement of the colon with a fistulous communication between the splenic flexure and the stomach. The distal transverse colon is markedly ulcerated with gross irregularity of the contours.

B, Granulomatous colitis. There is a fistulous communication between the narrowed transverse colon and the duodenum. Fistulas are a feature of granulomatous rather than ulcerative colitis.

(Illustration continued on following page.)

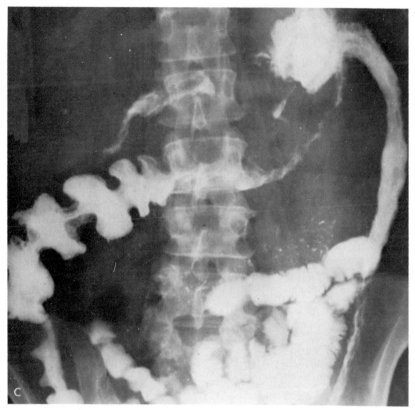

Figure 15-12 *Continued   C, Granulomatous ileocolitis.* There is a fistula between the distal transverse colon and the stomach.

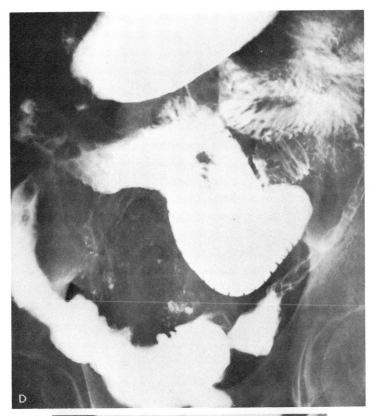

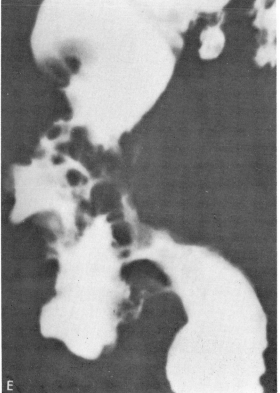

Figure 15-12 Continued D, Granulomatous ileocolitis. Multiple fistulas extend from the colon to the stomach and small intestine.

E, Fistulas in granulomatous ileocolitis. Characteristic intramural sinus tracts and fistulas extend from the terminal ileum to the right side of colon. These tracts are typical of granulomatous disease.

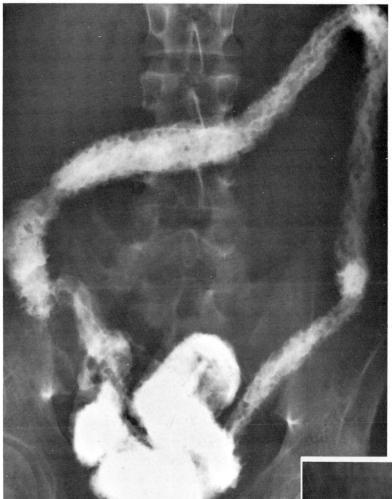

Figure 15-13 There is a moderate degree of narrowing and rigidity of the entire colon with ulceration of the mucosa and numerous small inflammatory polyps. This type of diffuse involvement is more commonly seen with ulcerative colitis, but can also be identified in granulomatous colitis. The involvement of the terminal ileum in this case with typical regional enteritis enables the radiologist to make a diagnosis of granulomatous ileocolitis.

Figure 15-14 A   The findings in the colon could be those of ulcerative or granulomatous colitis. The findings in the ileum with fistula formation, marked narrowing and rigidity are those of regional enteritis, and therefore the process is granulomatous ileocolitis.

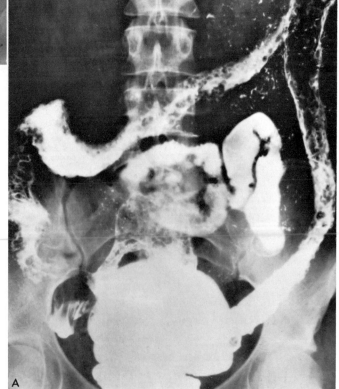

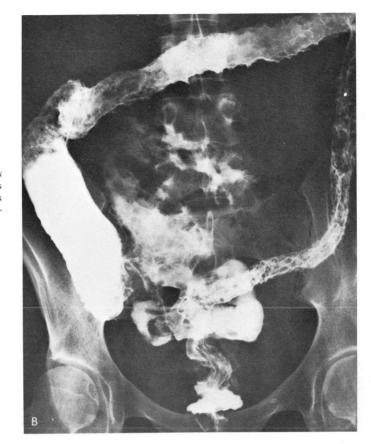

Figure 15-14 Continued   B, Diffuse granulomatous ileocolitis. Diffuse ulceration of the entire colon. There is a perforation of the terminal ileum with a large fistulous communication. This finding is associated with granulomatous disease rather than ulcerative colitis.

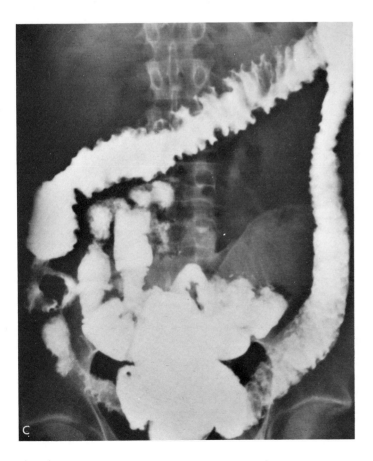

Figure 15-14   C, Granulomatous ileocolitis. The distal ileum and entire colon are involved. The findings in the transverse colon are suggestive of granulomatous disease but the typical involvement of the terminal ileum with regional enteritis permits an accurate diagnosis.

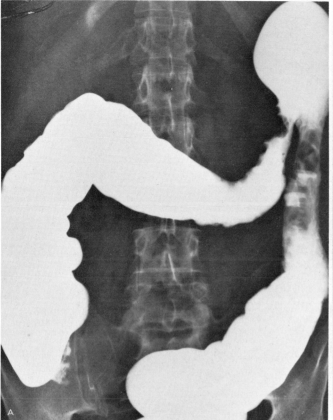

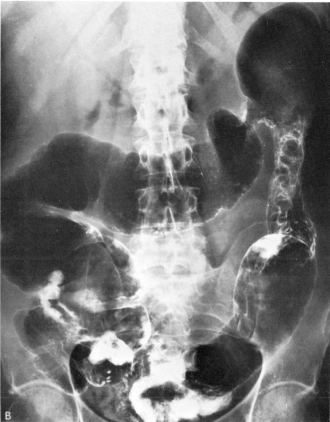

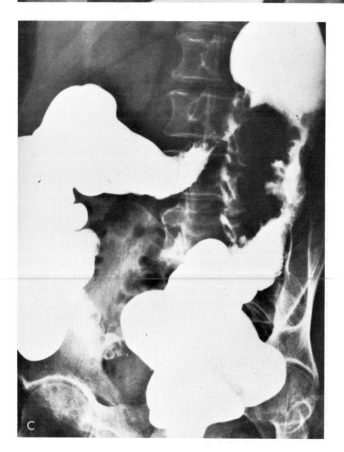

Figure 15-15 Granulomatous colitis. A, There are two skip lesions, one in the distal transverse colon and the second in proximal descending colon, with normal intervening bowel. The remainder of the colon is also within normal limits. There is marked irregularity of the contour of the superior surface of the transverse colon. This type of contour defect is frequently associated with a moderately larger ulcer. Inflammatory polyps are identified in the proximal descending colon, associated with transverse ulceration. The terminal ileum is normal.

B, An air study of the same patient. One year later.

C, Same case as *A* and *B.* The two skip lesions are again identified. There has been no linear extension of the disease process. This is the usual situation in granulomatous disease. At this time pseudodiverticula are seen in the descending colon, reflecting the asymmetric involvement.

Figure 15-15 Continued   D, Granulomatous colitis. Spot film of rectum and sigmoid. Large submucosal nodules are associated with irregularity of the contour, narrowing and rigidity. The nodules probably represent ulcerations with surrounding edema. The thickening of the submucosa also plays a role in the genesis of these nodules.

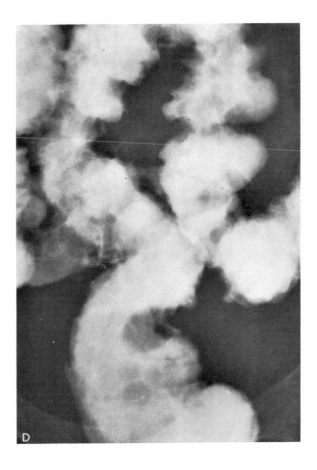

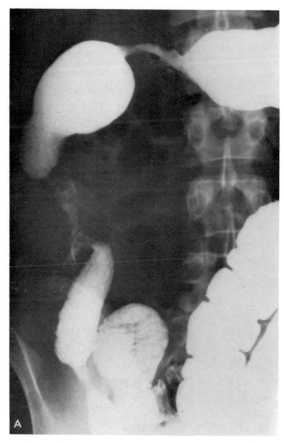

Figure 15-16 A, Multiple strictures characteristic of granulomatous colitis.

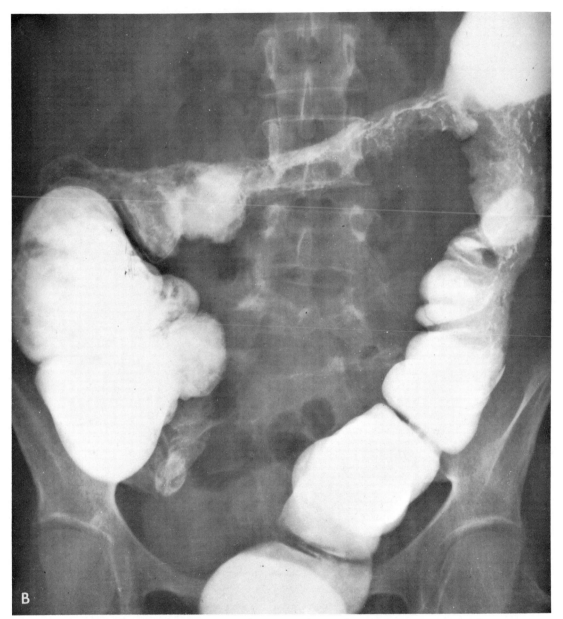

Figure 15-16 *Continued* **B,** *Granulomatous colitis* with strictures, narrowing, and irregularity of the transverse and proximal descending colon. Pseudodiverticula and pleating of the folds are seen along the medial aspect of the proximal transverse colon. Flattening and rigidity of the opposite contour are noted.

(Illustration continued on following page.)

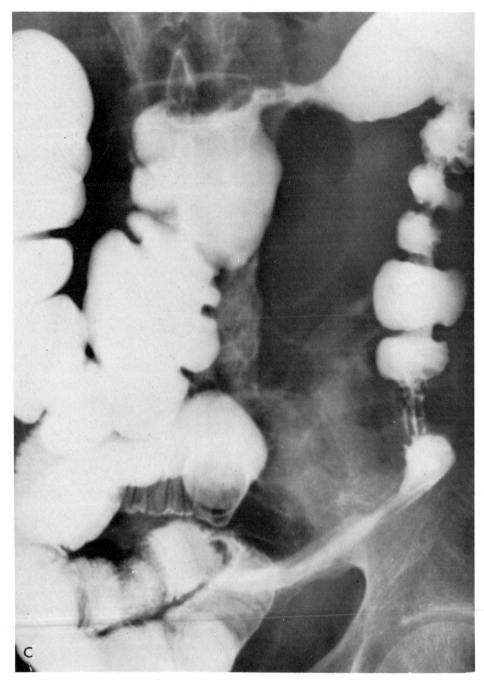

Figure 15-16 *Continued C,* Multiple smooth strictures are identified in granulomatous ileocolitis.

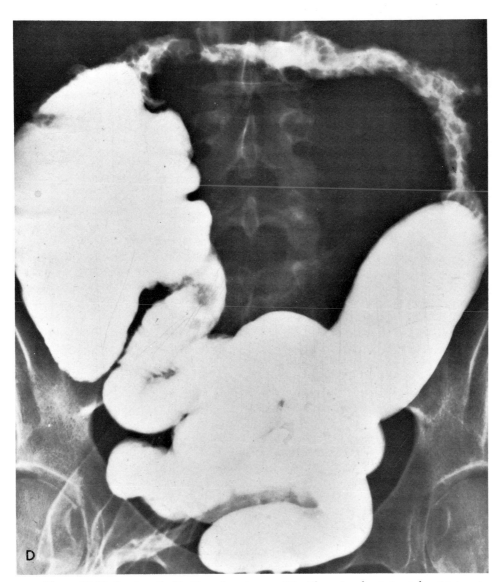

Figure 15-16 Continued D, Granulomatous colitis. There is a long, irregular stricture involving the entire transverse colon and proximal descending colon associated with shortening of the bowel in this region.

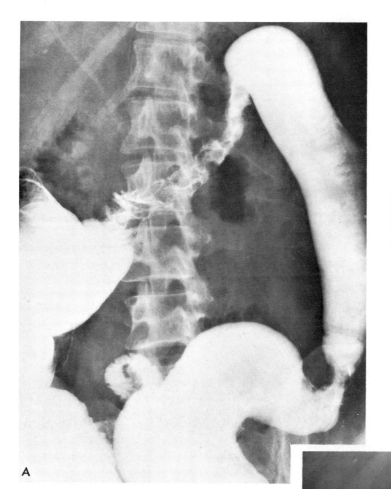

Figure 15-17 Granulomatous colitis. A, The distal half of the transverse colon is narrowed. Another short segment of narrowing is seen in the mid descending colon. In the absence of granulomatous disease elsewhere, differentiation of the latter lesion from a carcinoma would be difficult.

Figure 15-17 B A similar case of granulomatous colitis. In the absence of the lesion in the descending colon the diagnosis of granulomatous colitis would be uncertain.

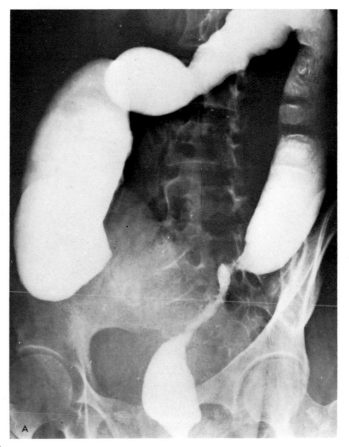

Figure 15-18 A Granulomatous ileocolitis. Minimal involvement of the entire colon with an inflammatory process and a stricture in the sigmoid. Differentiation of this case from a carcinoma in ulcerative colitis is difficult. The evacuation film, however, revealed definite involvement of the terminal ileum with granulomatous disease, indicating that the stricture is probably benign. Clinical features were those of granulomatous colitis.

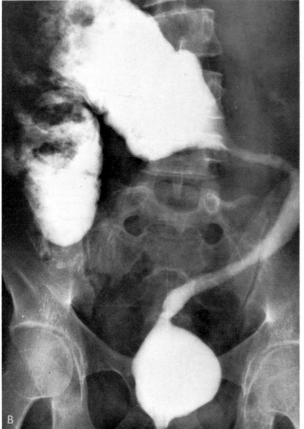

Figure 15-18 B Granulomatous colitis. Marked shortening and narrowing of the left side of the colon are noted. The rectum is also involved.

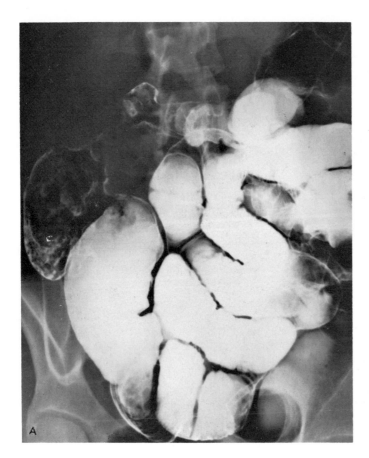

Figure 15-19 *A Granulomatous colitis.* There is a single stricture involving the right side of the colon. Differentiation of this lesion from a carcinoma is impossible.

Figure 15-19 *B* There is a single long stricture in the transverse colon with mild chronic inflammatory disease involving the remainder of the colon. The differentiation between a carcinomatous stricture with chronic, burnt-out ulcerative colitis or a single stricture with granulomatous colitis is difficult in this case. At operation the stricture proved to be a carcinoma with ulcerative colitis.

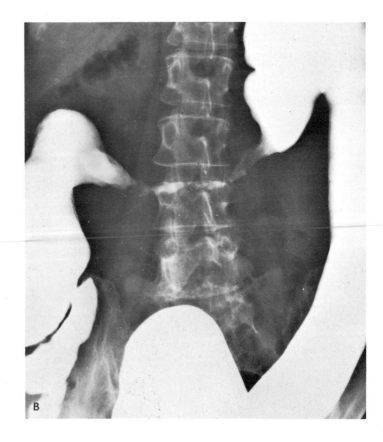

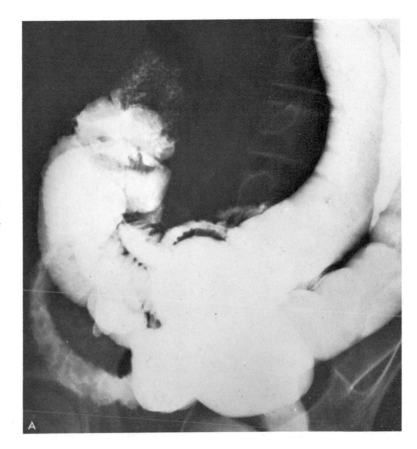

Figure 15-20 Regional enteritis with extension into the colon. A, The terminal ileum is involved with the characteristic findings of regional enteritis. The colon appears normal.

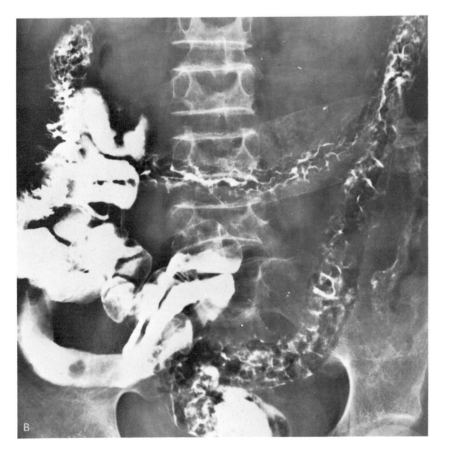

Figure 15-20 B An evacuation film of the same patient one year later shows marked involvement of the entire colon with a sinus tract extending lateral to the descending colon. The mucosa has a cobblestone appearance with numerous and longitudinal ulcerations. In granulomatous disease, extension in the absence of surgery is uncommon.

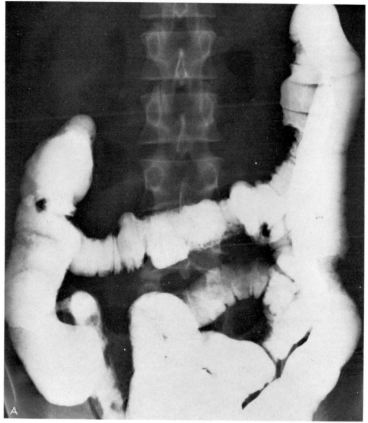

Figure 15-21 A   The ileum and colon to the splenic flexure are involved with typical granulomatous ileocolitis, characterized by narrowing, rigidity and irregularity of the contour. A small skip lesion is identified on the lateral aspect of the mid-descending colon.

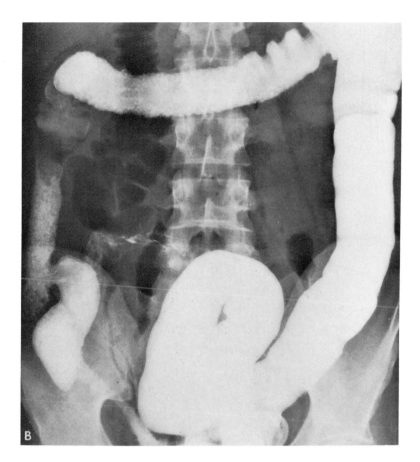

Figure 15-21 *Continued* *B, Granulomatous ileocolitis.* The inflammatory process involves primarily the right side of the colon. There is a skip lesion in the terminal ileum.

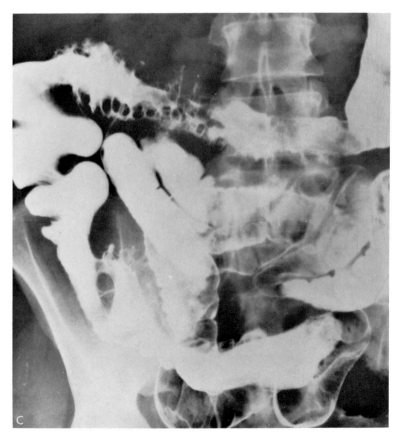

Figure 15-21 *C, Granulomatous ileocolitis.* In this case the ileum and right side of the colon are involved. Transverse ulcerations and inflammatory polyps are seen in the proximal transverse colon. A small fistulous communication from the ileum to the cecum is noted. The left side of the colon is normal.

(Illustration continued on following page.)

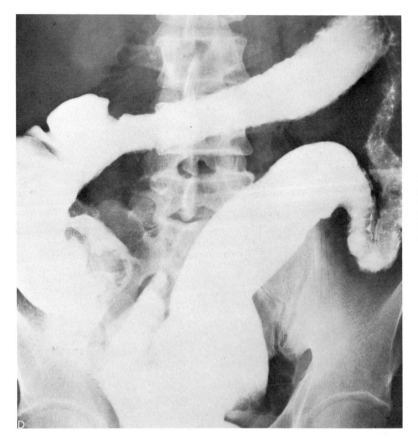

Figure 15-21 Continued   D, Granulomatous ileocolitis. Here the findings are severe in the descending colon, where there is narrowing, rigidity, and marked ulceration. The inflammatory process is segmental. The unevenness of involvement is another characteristic feature of granulomatous disease.

Figure 15-21   E, Granulomatous ileocolitis. In this case the entire colon is involved through the sigmoid and the rectum is normal. The terminal ileum is also involved. The findings on the left side of the colon are minimal.

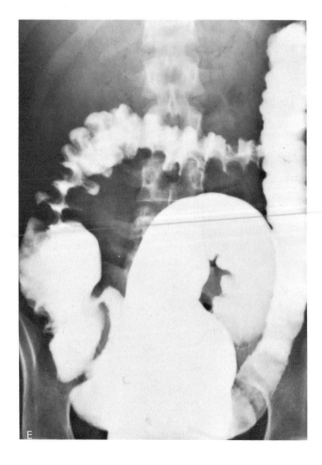

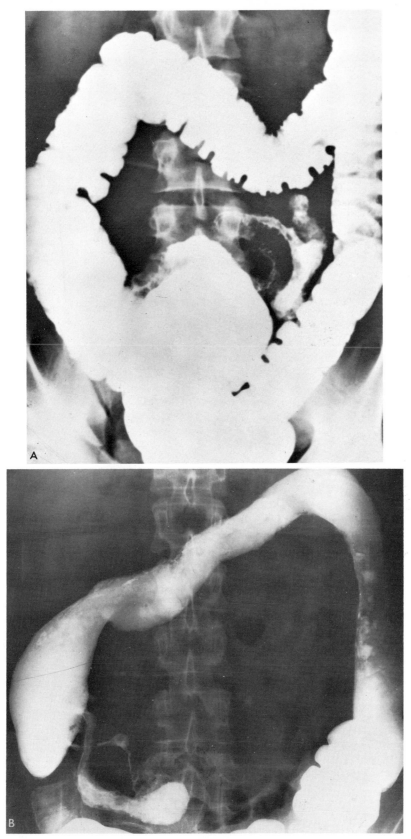

Figure 15-22 *Granulomatous ileocolitis.* A, Roentgen findings in the ileum are due to regional enteritis. In the colon the findings are minimal and characterized by slight flattening of the contours and minimal distortion of the haustral markings. The findings in terminal ileum indicate that the subtle findings in the colon are due to granulomatous colitis. *B,* In this case the alterations in the colon simulate burnt-out ulcerative colitis. Presence of a fistula in the terminal ileum, however, is characteristic of regional enteritis. The findings in the colon therefore are due to granulomatous disease. This appearance is uncommon in granulomatous colitis.

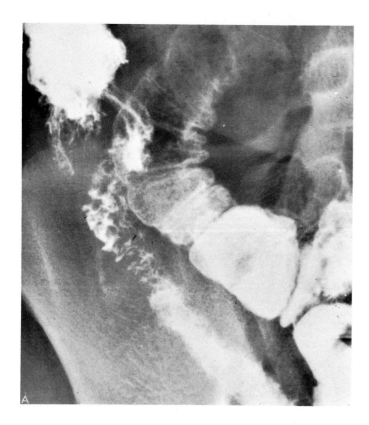

Figure 15-23 *Diffuse ulcerative colitis with backwash ileitis.* A, The backwash ileitis in this case is unusually extensive and mimics regional enteritis. There is a moderate degree of narrowing and rigidity with slight irregularity of the contour and thickening of the mucosal folds. The more marked involvement of the ileum in this case suggests granulomatous disease. At operation, however, the findings were those of ulcerative colitis and backwash ileitis.

Figure 15-23 B *Ulcerative colitis with backwash ileitis.* Terminal ileum is distensible, associated with minimal irregularity of contour and increased secretions. The narrowing and rigidity usually associated with regional enteritis are absent. Inflammatory process involving the colon is evident.

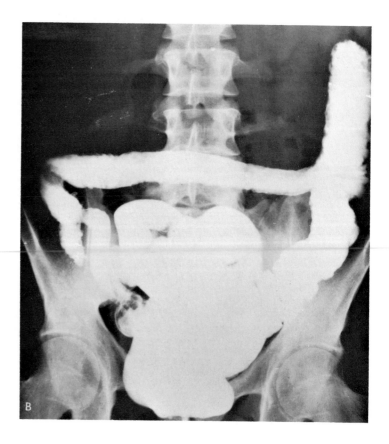

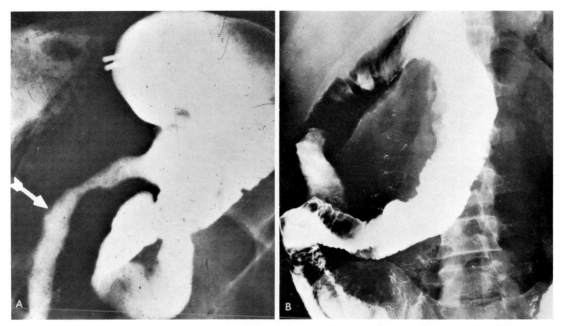

Figure 15-24   A, *Granulomatous ileitis* following ileostomy for granulomatous ileocolitis. The ileum adjacent to the ileostomy is narrowed and rigid (arrow). The findings here are in contrast with the findings seen in ileostomy dysfunction and are due to extension of the granulomatous process. B, *Ileostomy dysfunction*. The ileum is dilated, with increased secretions. The folds are slightly thickened.

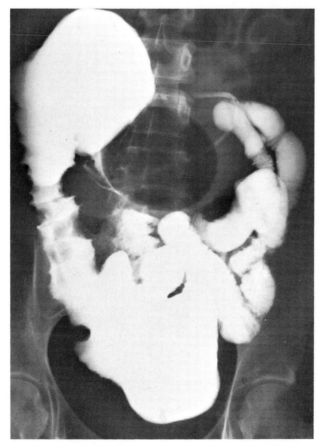

Figure 15-25   Status after a distal transverse colostomy for granulomatous colitis involving only the left side of the colon. Three years later there is recurrent disease of the right side of the colon proximal to the colostomy.

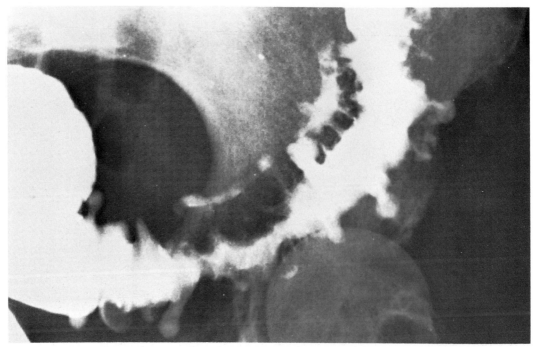

Figure 15-26 There is a long fistulous tract extending parallel to the sigmoid. Multiple transverse fissures producing a stepladder configuration are seen in the proximal part of the sigmoid. The multiple sacs are due to abscesses as the result of transverse fissures. A few tiny diverticula are noted in the distal sigmoid. The fistulous tract is in the wall of the colon, probably in the submucosa.

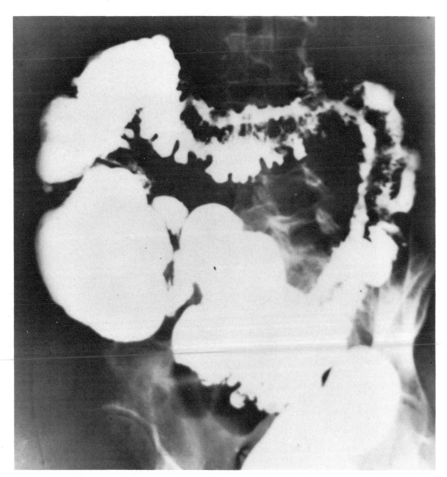

Figure 15-27 Granulomatous colitis. There is a long fistulous tract extending from hepatic flexure to sigmoid. Multiple diverticula are also present. At autopsy this patient had severe granulomatous colitis and the long fistulous tract was located in the submucosa and muscular layers. This is the longest fistulous tract we have encountered.

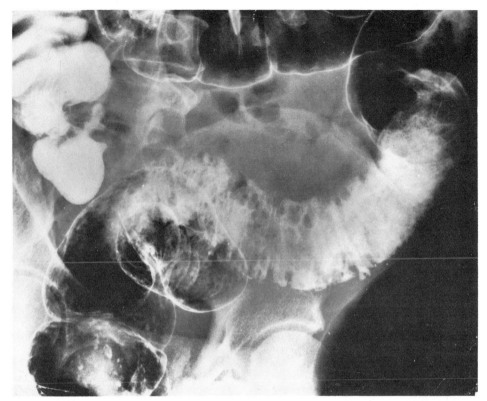

Figure 15-28 *Granulomatous colitis.* There are multiple abscesses on both contours of the sigmoid, simulating diverticula. The absence of fecaliths is noteworthy. The mucosa is thickened.

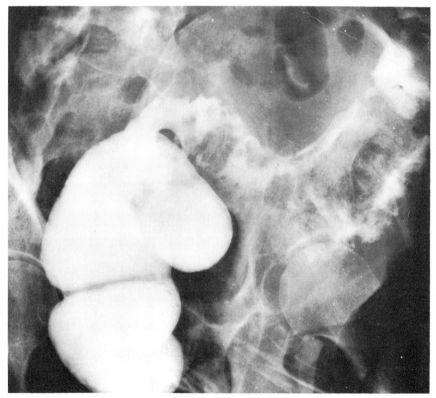

Figure 15-29 *Granulomatous colitis.* Same patient as Figure 15-28, three months later. A long fistulous tract is identified on the mesial border of the sigmoid. At laparotomy the characteristic findings of granulomatous colitis were present.

of granulomatous colitis. This finding is the presence of a long fistulous tract in the submucosa or the muscular layers, parallel to the lumen of the bowel (Figs. 15-27, 15-28, and 15-29). This tract, which had been noted for many years in patients with inflammatory disease of the colon, has previously been attributed to diverticulitis with multiple perforations of diverticula and development of tracking in the bowel wall. Pathologic examination of most resected specimens containing the long fistulous tract has revealed the typical lesions of granulomatous colitis. A few cases have now been reported in which the disease is clearly diverticulitis and not granulomatous colitis, and thus the fistulous tract cannot be considered pathognomonic of granulomatous disease.[17] Nevertheless, the majority of patients in whom the long fistulous tract can be demonstrated will prove to have granulomatous colitis.

References

1. Colp, R.: Case of nonspecific granuloma of terminal ileum and cecum. *Surg. Clin. N. Amer.,* 14:443-449, 1934.
1a. Kirsner, J. B., and Shorter, R. G. (Ed.): Inflammatory Bowel Disease. 1975, Philadelphia, Lea and Febiger.
2. Rappaport, H., Burgoyne, F. H., and Smetana, H. F.: The pathology of regional enteritis. *Milit. Surg.,* 109:463, 1951.
3. Wells, C.: Ulcerative colitis and Crohn's disease. *Ann. Royal Coll. Surg. Eng.,* 11:105-120, 1952.
4. Warren, S., and Sommers, S. C.: Pathology of regional ileitis and ulcerative colitis. *J.A.M.A.,* 154:189-193, 1954.
5. Marshak, R. H., Wolf, B. S., and Eliasoph, J.: Segmental colitis. *Radiology,* 73:706-716, 1959.
6. Morson, B. C., and Lockhart-Mummery, H. E.: Crohn's disease of the colon. *Gastroenterologia,* 92:168-172, 1959.
7. Wolf, B. S., and Marshak, R. H.: Granulomatous colitis (Crohn's disease of the colon): Roentgen features. *Amer. J. Roentgen.,* 88:662-670, 1962.
8. Lindner, A. E., Marshak, R. H., Wolf, B. S., and Janowitz, H. D.: Granulomatous colitis. *New Eng. J. Med.,* 269:379-385, 1963.
9. Marshak, R. H., Lindner, A. E., and Janowitz, H. D.: Granulomatous ileocolitis. *Gut,* 7:258-264, 1966.
9a. Marshak, R. H., and Lindner, A. E.: Ulcerative and granulomatous colitis. *J. Mount Sinai Hosp. N.Y.,* 33:444-502, 1966.
9b. Marshak, R. H., and Lindner, A. E.: Granulomatous colitis and ileocolitis, with emphasis on the radiologic factors. *In* Progress in Gastroenterology, Vol. I. G. B. Jerzy Glass (Ed.), New York, Grune and Stratton, Inc., 1968, pp. 357-390.
9c. Marshak, R. H., and Lindner, A. E.: Roentgen features of Crohn's disease. Clinics in Gastroenterology 1:2 (May, 1972). London, W. B. Saunders Company, pp. 411-432.
10. Marston, A., Pheils, M. T., Thomas, M. L., et al.: Ischemic colitis. *Gut,* 7:1-15, 1966.
11. McConnell, R. B.: Genetics of Crohn's disease. *In* Crohn's Disease, Bryan Brooke (Ed.). Clinics in Gastroenterology. Vol. 1, No. 2 (May), 1972. London, W. B. Saunders Company, pp. 321-334.
12. Weedon, D. D., Shorter, R. G., Ilstrup, D. M., et al.: Crohn's disease and cancer. *New Eng. J. Med.,* 289:1099-1103, 1973.
13. Buzzard, A. J., Baker, W. N. M., Needham, P. R. G., et al.: Acute toxic dilatation of the colon in Crohn's colitis. *Gut,* 15:416-419, 1974.
14. Jones, J. H., and Lennard-Jones, J. E.: Corticosteroids and corticotrophin in the treatment of Crohn's disease. *Gut,* 7:181-187, 1966.
15. Marshak, R. H., and Lindner, A. E.: Roentgen features of granulomatous colitis and ileocolitis. *In* Ulcerative and Granulomatous Colitis. 1973, Springfield, Illinois, Charles C Thomas, pp. 105-175.
16. Marshak, R. H., Janowitz, H. D., and Present, D. H.: Granulomatous colitis in association with diverticula. *New Eng. J. Med.,* 283:1080-1084, 1970.
17. Loeb, P. M., Berk, R. N., and Saltzstein, S. L.: Longitudinal fistula of the colon in diverticulitis. *Gastroenterology* 67:720-724, 1974.

16

Benign Small Bowel Tumors and Their Malignant Counterparts

Tumors of the small bowel are uncommon. They constitute less than five per cent of all neoplasms found in the gastrointestinal tract. It is unclear why tumors are so much more frequently found in the stomach and in the colon, at either end of the small intestine. Recent studies[1] have suggested several possible explanations, although proof for all is lacking: the fluid content of the small bowel may dilute potential carcinogens; rapid transit may decrease contact time with the small bowel mucosa; the small bowel is relatively sterile in comparison with the colon and bacteria may facilitate production of carcinogens; and finally local immune responses in the small intestine may protect against development of tumor.

It has been frequently stated that the accuracy rate for the detection of small bowel tumors is low. Since benign tumors are often submucosal, they usually do not produce roentgen findings until they distort the wall or become intraluminal. It is easy to understand why early symptoms of intestinal obstruction or intussusception caused by small bowel tumors could be ascribed to functional complaints. A small bowel study may not be performed in these instances. Moreover, small intestinal loops are pliable and may overlap, especially in the distal ileum, and unless the clinician and radiologist keep in mind the entity of small bowel tumors, these may be overlooked on a single examination. Compression studies are important, and every loop of small bowel must be visualized. In contrast to obstruction or intussusception, the other clinical manifestation of small bowel tumor—intestinal bleeding—is more likely to lead to an early, careful examination of the small bowel.

Intestinal obstruction from small bowel tumors may be sudden and severe in onset or low grade and chronic in development. Often obstruction is intermittent and the patient is asymptomatic between bouts of pain. Benign small bowel tumors commonly cause pain by intussusception, and thus quite small lesions can be responsible for severe symptoms. Larger tumors obstruct the lumen by their bulk or by causing kinking of the bowel. The pain of small bowel obstruction is characteristically crampy and may be associated with nausea and vomiting. Pain of small bowel origin is frequently periumbilical in location. Experimental studies in which balloons were distended at levels along the intestinal tract have confirmed the tendency of mesenteric small bowel pain to be localized around the umbilicus.[2]

Small bowel tumors may cause intestinal bleeding because they intussuscept or because they ulcerate. Although bleeding may present as melena or massive hemorrhage, blood loss may be slow and chronic, causing iron deficiency anemia and stools positive on testing for occult blood.

BENIGN TUMORS

Benign small bowel tumors are more common in the ileum than in the duodenum or jejunum. The relative frequency of tumor types varies in the reported series and is somewhat affected by differences in histologic classification. The study of River et al.[3] included almost 1500 cases. Adenoma was the most common tumor, followed, in decreasing incidence, by lipoma, myoma, fibroma, and hemangioma. Other reported tumors included myxoma, cystadenoma, hemangiopericytoma, and teratoma. Good,[4] in a series of 328 benign small bowel tumors collected at the Mayo Clinic, reported 119 leiomyomas, 67 adenomas, 53 lipomas, 43 hemangiomas, and 46 other tumors, including fibromas and neurogenic tumors. Darling and Welch[5] point out that five histologic types make up 95 per cent of all small bowel tumors: adenomas, lipomas, myomas, fibromas, and hemangiomas.

Adenomas, lipomas, myomas, and fibromas have many pathologic and roentgen features in common. They may be single or multiple, intraluminal, lobulated, ulcerated, or pedunculated, and they may intussuscept. In addition to these features, myomas and fibromas may be intramural, both intraluminal and intramural, or completely extramural. It can readily be seen that differentiation of these four lesions and rare tumors such as myxomas and cystadenomas may be impossible. Despite their apparent similarity, there are some differential points, and therefore these lesions will be described separately.

Adenomas are usually small and may be asymptomatic, being demonstrated only at incidental laparotomy or biopsy. Most commonly they occur in the duodenum and jejunum. Since adenomas arise from the mucosa, they are intraluminal and may be sessile or polypoid (Figs. 16-1 to 16-3). They tend to be vascular, are frequently lobulated, and bleed readily. Despite the bleeding, ulcerations are superficial and difficult to find. As with adenomatous polyps elsewhere in the intestinal tract, it is controversial whether benign adenomas become malignant. It seems likely that the malignant potential of adenomas of the small intestine is negligible. When the lesion becomes pedunculated it frequently intussuscepts (Figs. 16-4 and 16-5).

Villous adenomas, unlike adenomatous polyps, have the same general appearance noted in the colon. The contours are lobulated and irregular, and the interior appears cystic (Fig. 16-6). Because they contain a minimal amount of stroma they sometimes are compressible and conform to the lumen of the bowel. They are frequently large. Pedicles are uncommon. Unless the surface of the tumor is covered with barium, they can be mistaken for other small intestinal lesions.

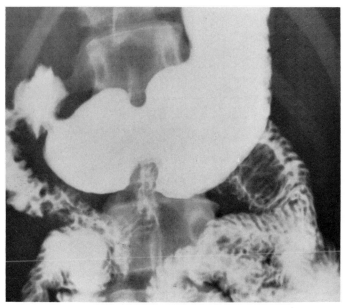

Figure 16-1   Adenoma. There is a sharply demarcated filling defect in the proximal jejunum.

Lipomas are fatty tumors which are always intraluminal. Despite their origin from the submucosal layers, the stronger muscular layer displaces the lipoma intraluminally. Also, because they are fatty and soft, they frequently conform to the lumen of the bowel and sometimes change in shape (Figs. 16-7 to 16-9). They can be pedunculated (Fig. 16-10), and therefore intussusception is common (Fig. 16-11). Ulcerations are deep enough to be recognized on roentgen study (Fig. 16-12).

Leiomyomas are among the most common benign tumors of the small

(Text continued on page 309.)

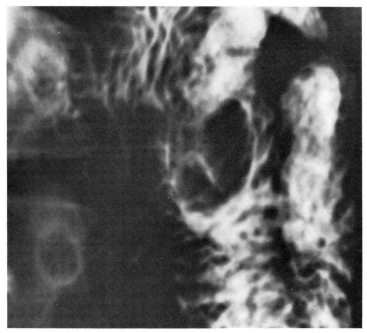

Figure 16-2   Spot film of case shown in Figure 16-1.

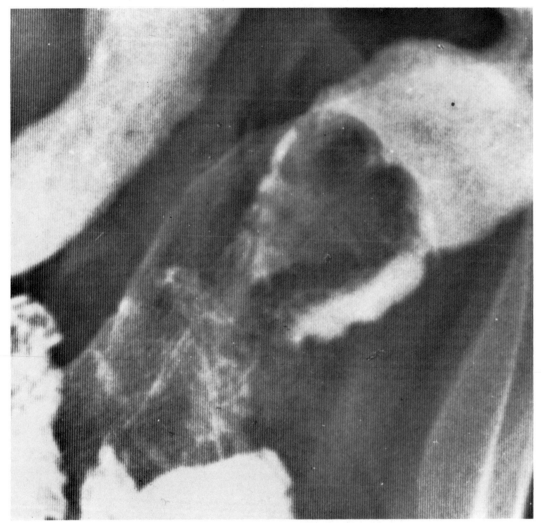

Figure 16-3 Adenoma. A slightly lobulated but sharply demarcated filling defect in the distal jejunum is noted. This lesion produced intussusception on many occasions.

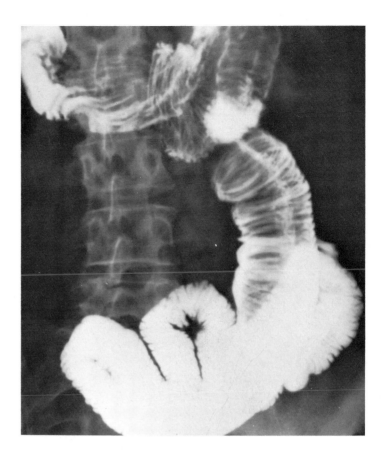

Figure 16-4 *Adenoma* producing intussusception.

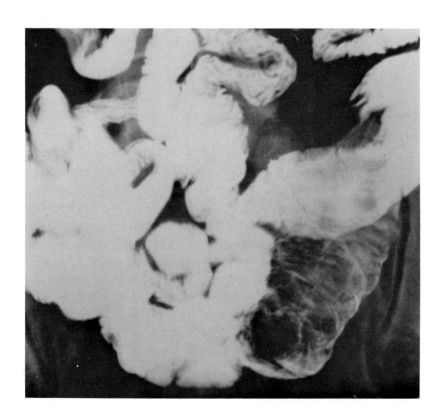

Figure 16-5 *Adenoma* producing intussusception.

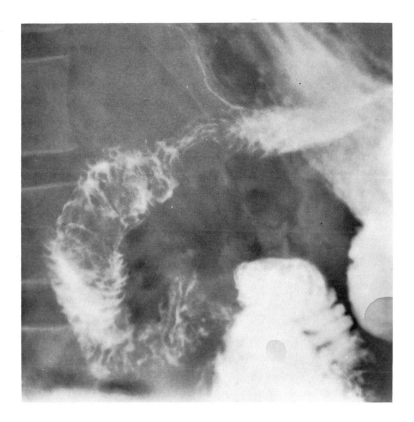

Figure 16-6 *Villous adenoma* (Courtesy of Dr. Harold Izard, Philadelphia). There is a moderately large, slightly irregular filling defect in the second portion of the duodenum. The tumor has a cystic appearance characteristic of a villous adenoma.

Figure 16-7 *Lipoma.* A sharply demarcated, dumbbell-shaped tumor is identified in the second portion of the duodenum. The tumor conforms to the lumen of the bowel, suggesting a soft lesion such as a lipoma.

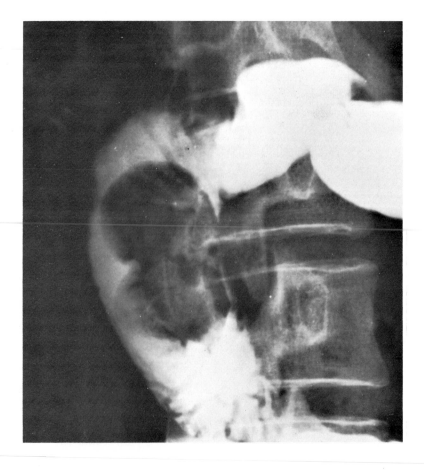

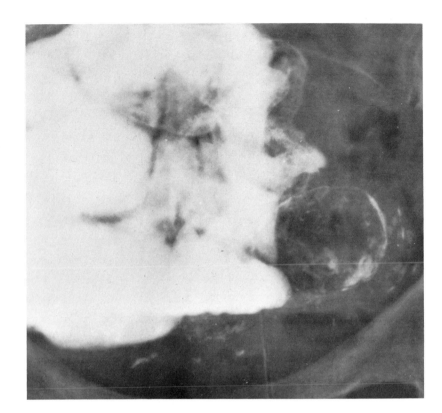

Figure 16-8 Lipoma. There is an elliptical, sharply demarcated filling defect in the distal jejunum.

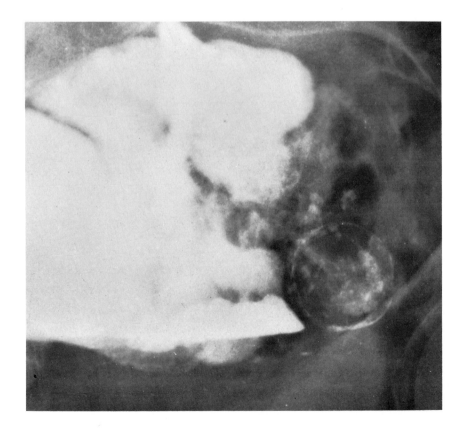

Figure 16-9 Lipoma. Same case as in Figure 16-8. There has been a slight change in the appearance of the lesion, which now appears circular. This change in shape is frequently seen with a lipoma and is due to the softness of the lesion.

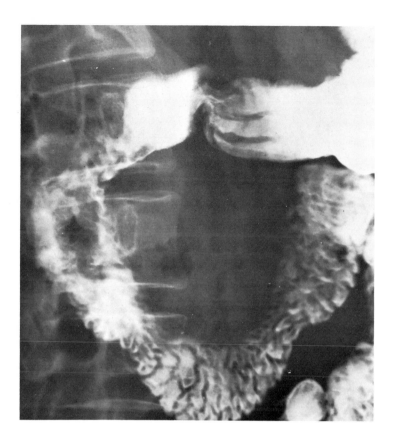

Figure 16-10 *Lipoma*. A short pedicle is seen attached to the tumor. It is impossible to make an exact diagnosis in this case.

Figure 16-11 *Lipoma* with intussusception.

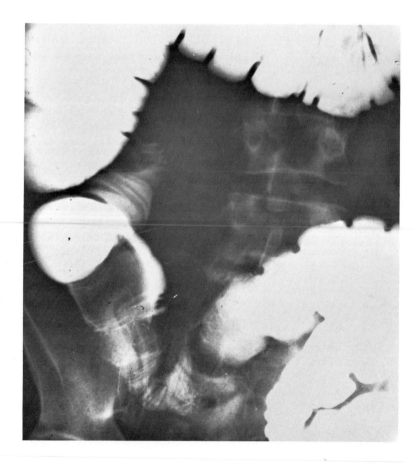

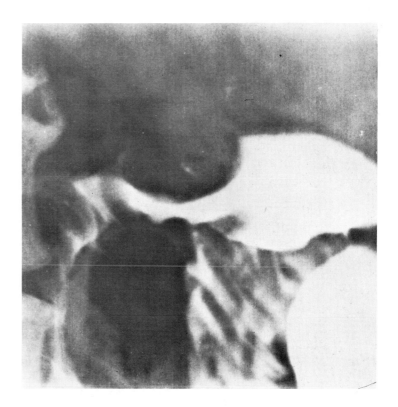

Figure 16-12 Lipoma within duodenal bulb. A tiny ulceration is noted in the central portion of this sharply demarcated submucosal tumor.

bowel. They can vary considerably in size and are sometimes huge. The tumors are intraluminal (Fig. 16-13), intramural (Figs. 16-14, 16-15), extramural, or both intraluminal and extramural. Leiomyomas are most often single but can be multiple. Bleeding is common and often severe. As the tumor grows, it tends to undergo central necrosis and replacement with vascular tissue and blood-filled cavities which perforate into the bowel wall and cause intestinal bleeding. Because of their varying size and location, a multiplicity of roentgen alterations may be seen. When intraluminal, they mimic adenomas and lipomas, and may be sessile or pedunculated and intussuscept. When intramural or extramural, varying degrees of compression of the bowel contour are produced (Figs. 16-16 to 16-18). Intussusception is common (Figs. 16-19 and 16-20).

Fibromas usually behave in a manner similar to leiomyomas. These tumors may produce intussusception, filling defects (Fig. 16-21), extrinsic compression by the tumor mass, kinking, volvulus, or ulceration.

Neurofibromas, which are interesting variants of fibromas, can be associated with generalized neurofibromatosis (Von Recklinghausen's disease).[6]

Hemangiomas are less frequent than any of the above tumors. They are unique in that they occur more frequently in the small bowel than in the remainder of the intestinal tract. Hemangiomas are cavernous, blood-filled, endothelially lined spaces, masses of capillaries, or mixtures of the two. Their roentgen appearance is that of diffuse expansive involvement of a fairly long segment of bowel, with nodular defects that are easily compressed (Fig. 16-22). Phleboliths within these lesions are common (Fig. 16-23). They have a tendency to change in size and shape. A rare example of an hemangioma is the Rendu-Osler-Weber syndrome, which is characterized by repeated hemorrhage, telangiectasia of the mucosa of the nasal and oral cavities, and a familial

(Text continued on page 313.)

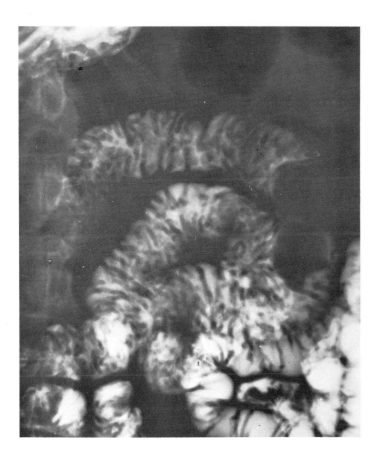

Figure 16-13 Leiomyoma. There is a dumb-bell-shaped intraluminal tumor in the proximal jejunum.

Figure 16-14 Leiomyoma. A sharply demarcated submucosal (intramural) filling defect is noted in the proximal jejunum.

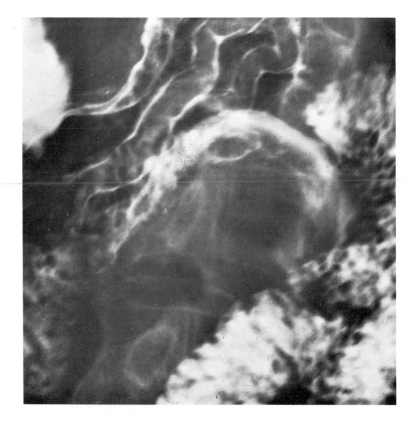

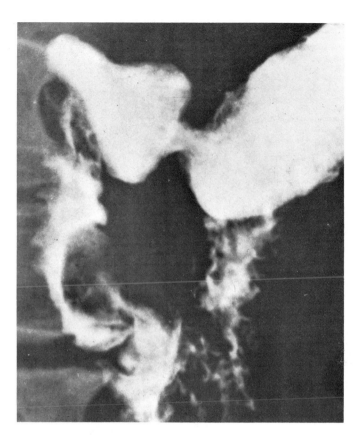

Figure 16-15 Leiomyoma. There is a sharply demarcated submucosal (intramural) filling defect in the second portion of the duodenum.

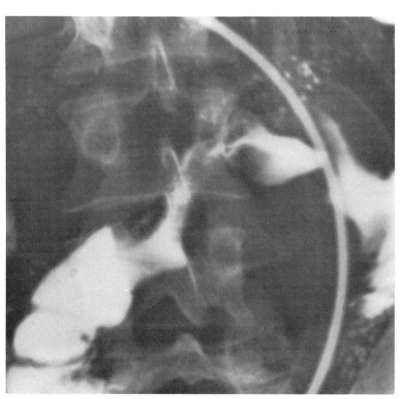

Figure 16-16 Leiomyoma. Multiple intraluminal and intramural defects are associated with extrinsic compression of a segment of ileum. A lobulated leiomyoma was resected. The roentgen appearance is unusual and the diagnosis difficult.

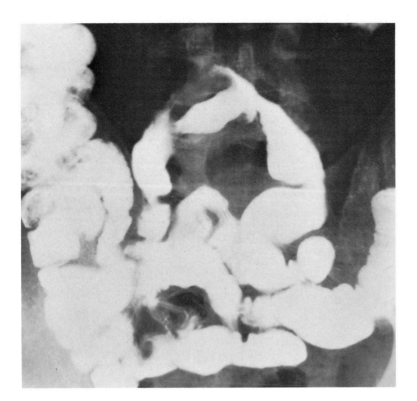

Figure 16-17 Leiomyoma. There is a sharply demarcated tumor compressing a segment of ileum. The tumor is primarily extramural. The appearance of the compressed segment could be confused with that of an ulcer.

Figure 16-18 Leiomyoma. There is a conical area of narrowing in the proximal ileum produced by compression secondary to an extramural tumor. This type of narrowing secondary to a benign tumor is unusual.

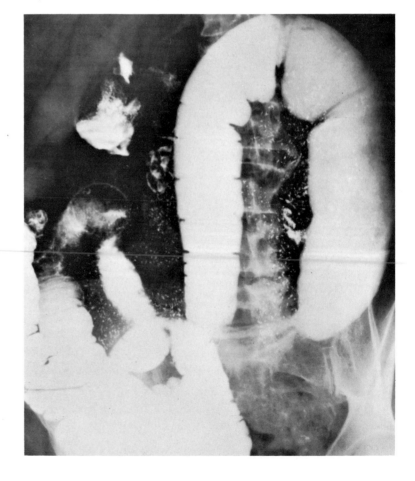

occurrence. Recognition of this lesion on x-ray is difficult. On occasion there may be a reticulated, foamlike appearance, which disappears readily on compression.

Lymphangiomas are rare tumors which involve the small bowel and produce multiple intraluminal and intramural filling defects (Fig. 16-24). They can be large and displace the small intestine. It is impossible to differentiate these lesions from many of the other lesions described previously.

Exotic pathologic entities may present as tumors involving the wall of the small bowel (Fig. 16-25A and B). They produce no distinctive roentgen features that are different from the main categories listed above.

Heterotopic pancreatic tissue may be seen any place in the intestinal tract but is most often found in the vicinity of the stomach and duodenal loop. These lesions are usually small and produce an intramural or intraluminal filling defect, which may have a central dimpling due to a depression at the apex of the tumor. They are innocuous lesions of little clinical significance.

Hyperplasia of Brunner's glands almost always occurs in the first portion of the duodenum. Lesions may be multiple or may present as a single large polypoid defect (Fig. 16-26).

When *endometriosis* involves the small bowel it is impossible to make a preoperative diagnosis, for there are no distinguishing characteristics.

It is obvious that benign tumors of the small bowel are most readily found when they are large enough to produce filling defects or when they intussuscept or ulcerate. Radiologists frequently comment on the overlapping loops of bowel which hinder the detection of these tumors. The overlapping loops are probably less of a problem than has been thought. It is not difficult, especially with compression, to visualize the entire small bowel and to see each loop separately from the others.

PEUTZ-JEGHERS SYNDROME

The association of intestinal polyposis with pigmentation of the skin and mucous membranes has been called the Peutz-Jeghers syndrome.[7] Initially described in 1921, the syndrome appears to be a hereditable disease transmitted as a mendelian dominant characteristic. The pigment, which is melanin, usually involves the lips and mouth in round or irregular spots, and at times involves the face and extremities.

The polyps of this syndrome may be present in the stomach, small bowel, and colon but are most frequent in the small bowel, where they produce symptoms by intussusception or bleeding (Fig. 16-27). Initially thought to be adenomas, the polyps have proved to be hamartomas and are not neoplasms.[8] Although in general the polyps of this syndrome appear to be entirely benign, several reports have appeared[9, 10] of gastrointestinal carcinoma in association with Peutz-Jeghers disease, suggesting that in the proximal gut the disease may have a malignant potential as yet not well defined. There have been no convincing reports of malignant changes in the polyps located in the mesenteric small bowel.

Roentgenologically the hamartomas are usually so small that recognition is difficult. When they are of sufficient size, roentgen characteristics typical of any adenomatous polyp are seen. Hamartomas may be pedunculated or sessile,

(Text continued on page 323.)

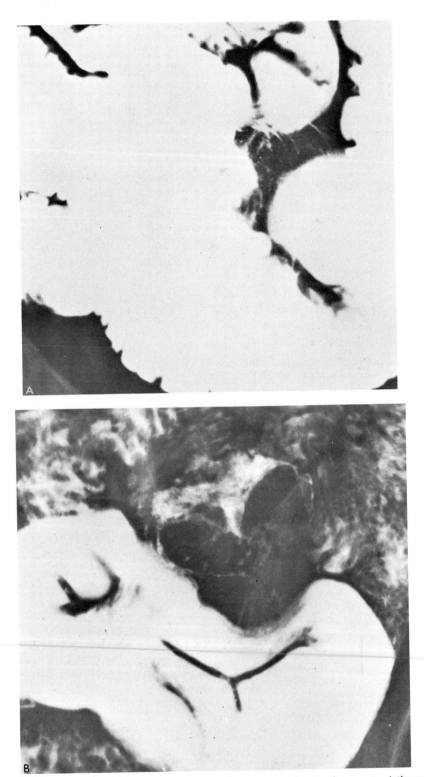

Figure 16-19 *Leiomyoma.* A, Early stage of intussusception in the proximal ileum. Note the thin, separated mucosal folds due to an early intussusception.

B, Later stage of intussusception of this tumor.

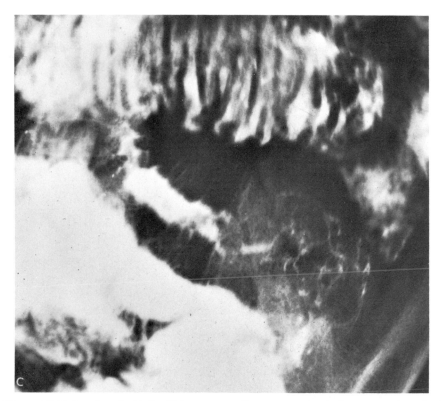

Figure 16-19 Continued   C, A still later stage of intussusception in the same patient. At this time the mucosal pattern is thickened and distorted as a result of edema induced by recurrent intussusception. It would be difficult to make a diagnosis of intussusception due to a benign tumor unless other films were available.

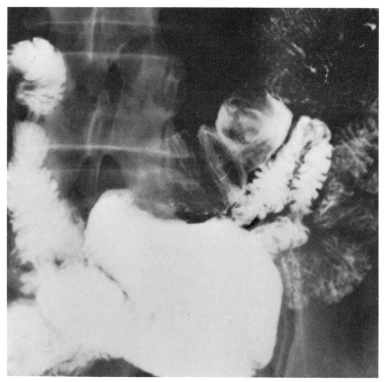

Figure 16-20   Leiomyoma. Intussusception is noted.

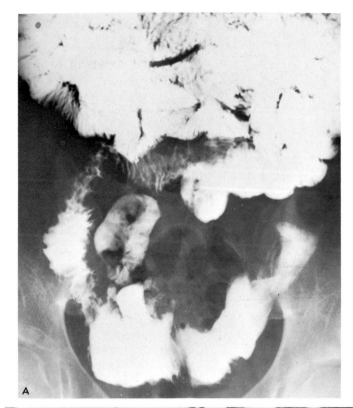

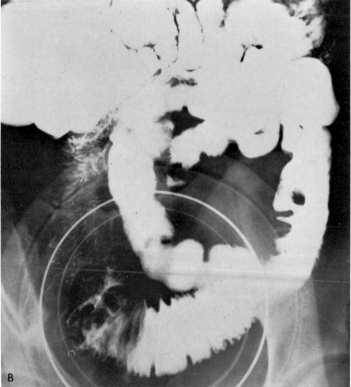

Figure 16-21 *Neurofibroma. A,* The mid-ileum for a distance of one foot reveals slight dilatation associated with moderate irregularity of the contours. In some areas there are submucosal defects. The mucosa appears to be slightly effaced.

B, The same patient one month later; minimal intussusception associated with slight dilatation of the mid-ileum is noted.

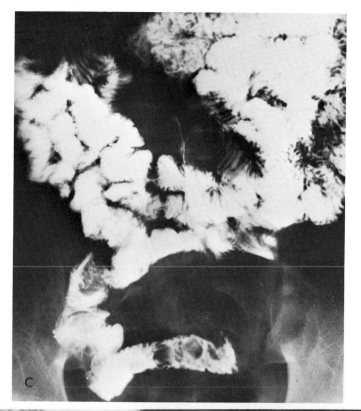

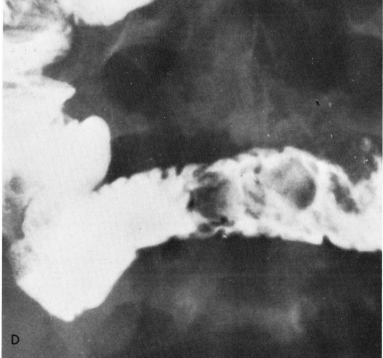

Figure 16-21 Continued C, Same patient three months later. Striking demonstration of multiple intraluminal and intramural filling defects.

D, Magnified view of *C.*

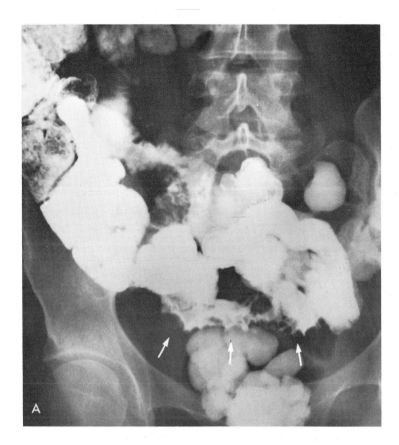

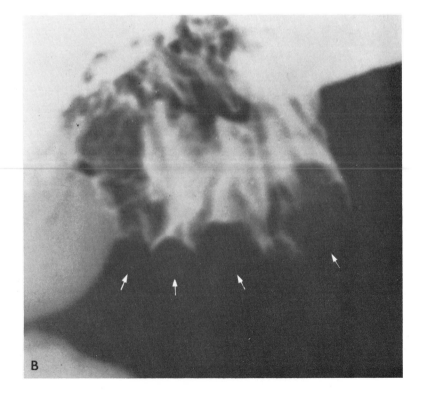

Figure 16-22 Hemangioma. A, Multiple, slightly irregular nodular filling defects are seen along the contour of the mid-ileum. These defects changed in size during compression.

Figure 16-22 B, Magnified view.

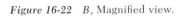

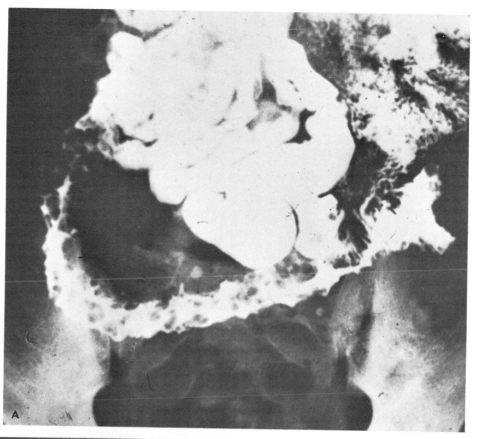

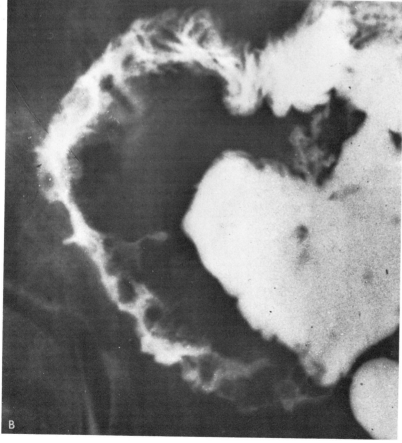

Figure 16-23   Hemangioma. A, Multiple submucosal and intraluminal defects are seen in the ileum. These are associated with many phleboliths, frequently seen in hemangiomas.

B, *Hemangioma.* There are multiple intraluminal and submucosal filling defects. On the preliminary film only an occasional phlebolith was seen.

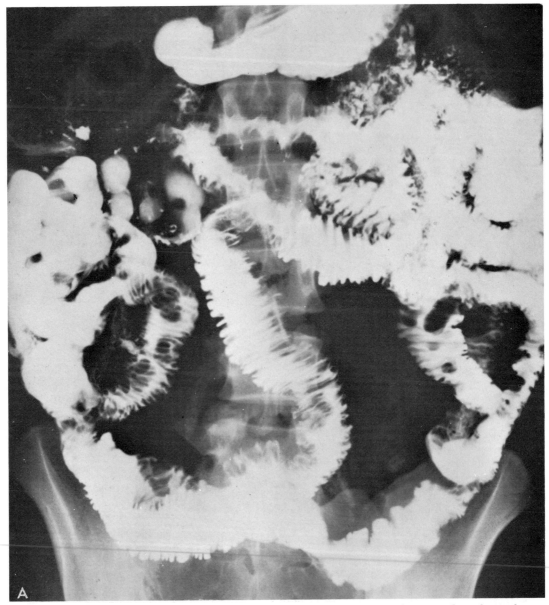

Figure 16-24 Lymphangioma. A, There are multiple small, sharply demarcated intraluminal and intramural filling defects. (Courtesy of Dr. Samuel Miller, Wilmington, Delaware.)

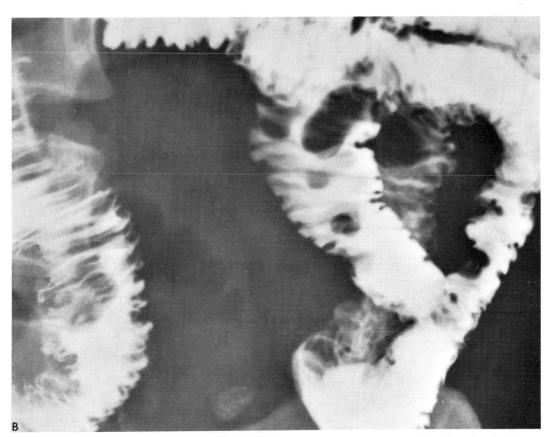

Figure 16-24 Continued   B, Film of the same patient as in Fig. 16-24A. Note the sharp borders of the lesions.

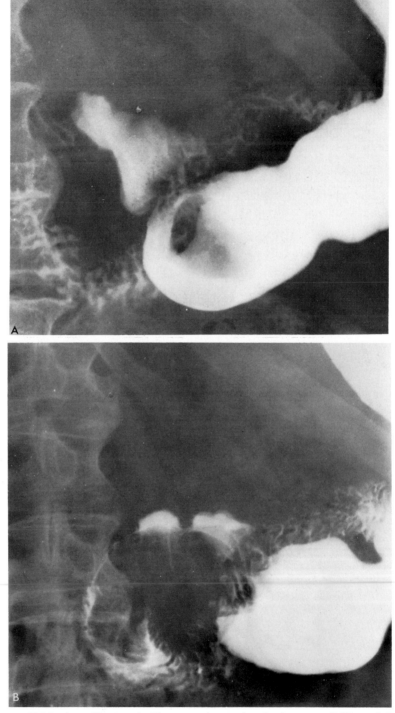

Figure 16-25 *Angiofibroma.* A, There is a large, sharply demarcated filling defect in the antrum of the stomach.

B, *Angiofibroma.* The lesion has intussuscepted into the second portion of the duodenum (gastroduodenal intussusception).

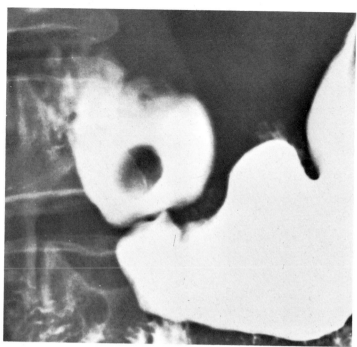

Figure 16-26 Adenoma of Brunner's glands. There is a small, sharply demarcated filling defect in the midportion of the duodenal bulb. Carcinoid tumors, single or multiple, can give a similar appearance, both in the duodenal bulb and the stomach.

or they may intussuscept (Figs. 16-28 and 16-29). They may be associated with lesions of the stomach and colon. It could be remembered that other syndromes are associated with multiple polyps of the small bowel, such as the rare cases of familial polyposis involving the entire intestinal tract, and the entity known as Canada-Cronkhite syndrome.[11] This disease is a hyperplasia of the mucosa which presents as polyposis associated with alopecia and onychia.

DUPLICATION CYSTS

Duplications may be seen at any level in the intestinal tract. Most commonly they are recognized when they become cystic and behave as submucosal tumors (Fig. 16-30). They can be intraluminal, intramural, or subserosal. When they are in any of these locations, differential diagnosis from benign tumors is difficult. If they are large and cystic in appearance, the diagnosis, especially in the region of the duodenum and distal ileum, may be suggested. Occasionally a large sinus tract parallel to the wall of the gut is noted and suggests a duplication.

MECKEL'S DIVERTICULUM

Meckel's diverticula are located along the antimesenteric border of the ileum, usually within 12 inches of the ileocecal valve but sometimes more distant. Heterotopic gastric and pancreatic tissue may occur within the diverticulum, and the gastric mucosa may be responsible for ulceration with hemor-

(Text continued on page 328.)

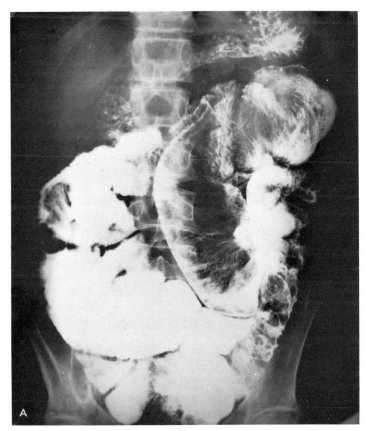

Figure 16-27 *Peutz-Jeghers Disease.* A, There is a long segment of intussusception with dilatation and obstruction produced by multiple polyps of the proximal small bowel.

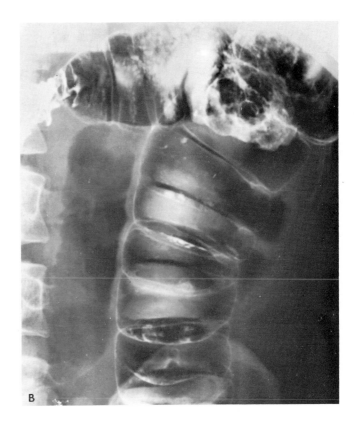

Figure 16-27 Continued *B*, Same case. There is an irregular polypoid filling defect in the splenic flexure of the colon.

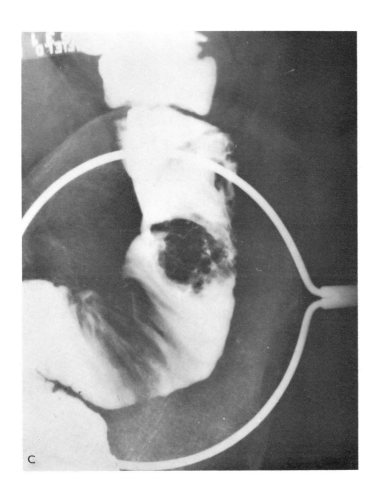

Figure 16-27 C, Same case. An irregular, large filling defect is seen in the sigmoid.

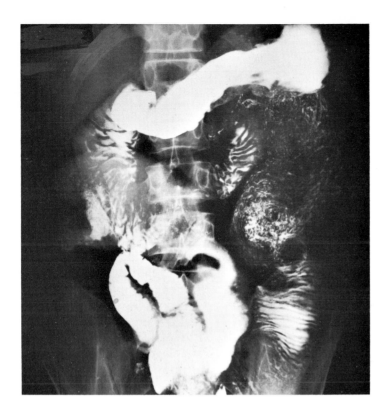

Figure 16-28 Peutz-Jeghers Disease. There are multiple areas of dilatation and intussusception due to multiple small polyps of the small bowel.

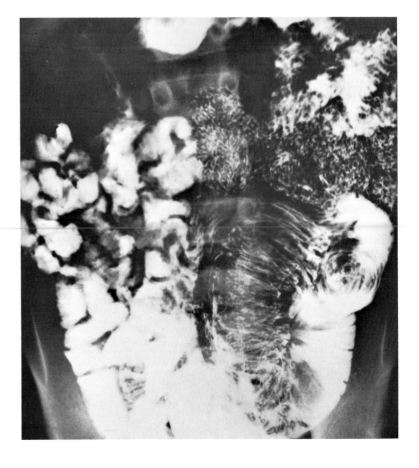

Figure 16-29 Peutz-Jeghers Disease. Intussusception produced by multiple polyps of the small bowel.

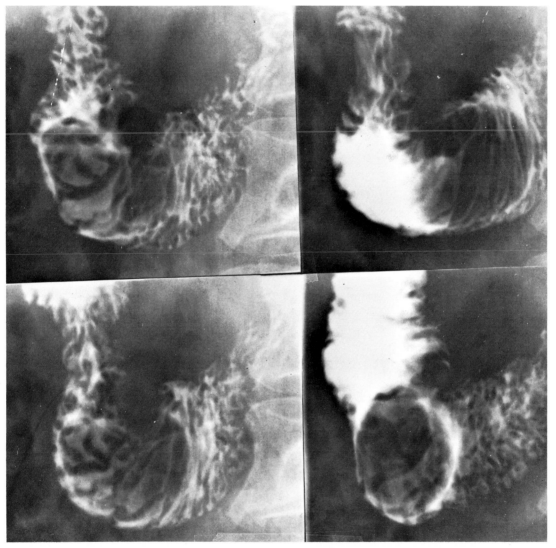

Figure 16-30 Duplication cyst. There is a sharply demarcated filling defect in the second portion of the duodenum. The lesion appears to conform to the bowel lumen. Differential diagnosis from a lipoma is impossible. (Courtesy of Dr. Mary F. Keohane, Yale University School of Medicine.)

rhage or perforation. The diverticulum may become inflamed and mimic appendicitis. We have seen the following roentgen configurations with Meckel's diverticula:

1. They may rarely be visualized by chance on a small bowel examination or a barium enema with reflux into the terminal ileum.

2. They not uncommonly produce intussusception (Figs. 16-31 and 16-32).

3. They can become huge, presenting as large, cystlike structures and can be located anyplace in the abdominal cavity, frequently with a fluid level and containing large amounts of mucoid secretions (Fig. 16-33).

4. When a diverticulum attains a large size, the pedicle may become elongated, twist, and produce a chronic intestinal obstruction. It should be remembered that a duplication cyst may also cause the findings described above (Fig. 16-34). Enteroliths may form within the diverticulum (Fig. 16-35).

SARCOMAS

Small bowel sarcomas, except for lymphosarcoma, are rare tumors, difficult to classify precisely by histologic criteria. Although any of the nonepithelial elements of the bowel wall could give rise to a sarcoma, most of the reported tumors have been leiomyosarcomas, fibrosarcomas, or neurofibrosarcomas.

Unlike lymphosarcoma, with its predilection for the ileum, the other sarcomas appear to occur about equally in all areas of the small bowel. Symptoms of sarcoma, which usually are insidious in onset, include abdominal pain,

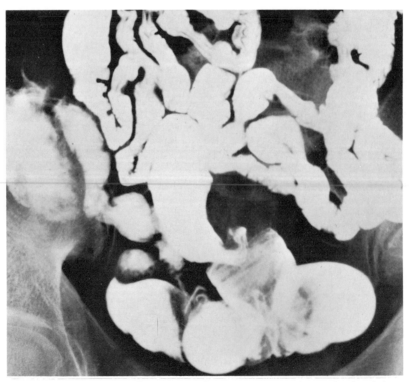

Figure 16-31 *Meckel's diverticulum* producing intussusception in the distal ileum.

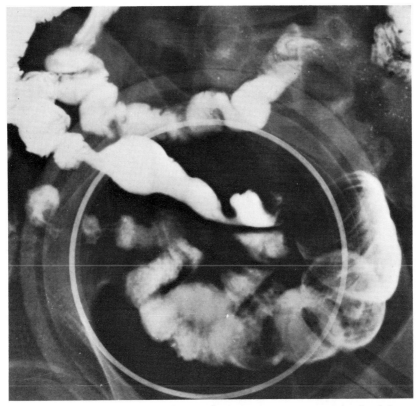

Figure 16-32 *Meckel's diverticulum* producing intussusception in the distal ileum.

Figure 16-33 *Meckel's diverticulum.* There is a tremendous biloculated saclike structure extending into the pelvis, with no intestinal obstruction. This appearance can also be seen with duplication cysts. (Courtesy of Dr. Harvey Peck, New York.)

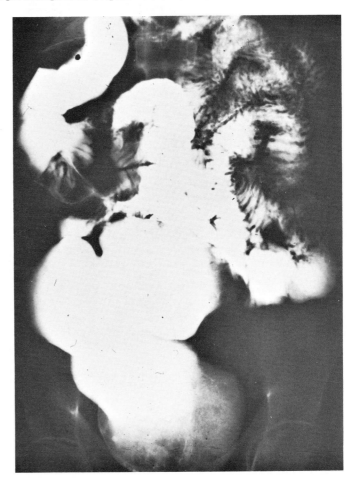

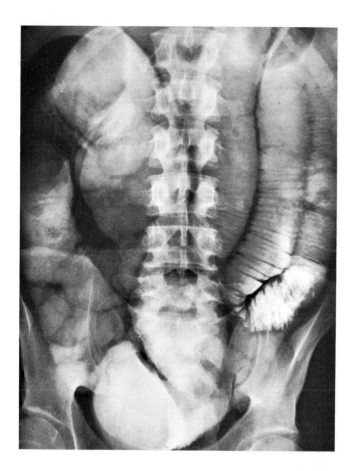

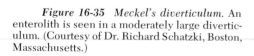

Figure 16-34 Meckel's diverticulum. A large amorphous sac is seen in the pelvis. This is a Meckel's diverticulum which has twisted the bowel and produced marked chronic obstruction.

Figure 16-35 Meckel's diverticulum. An enterolith is seen in a moderately large diverticulum. (Courtesy of Dr. Richard Schatzki, Boston, Massachusetts.)

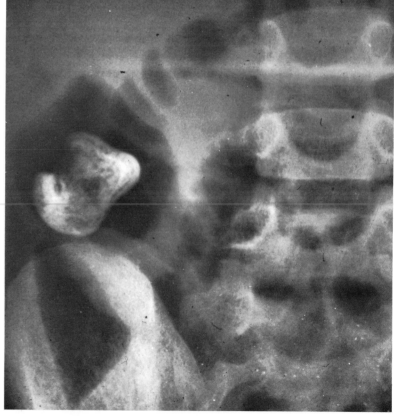

sometimes nausea and vomiting, weight loss, anemia, and change in bowel habits. At times the first finding is the presence of an abdominal mass. Occasionally the clinical presentation may be acute, with intestinal perforation, hemorrhage, or obstruction.

Leiomyosarcoma, the most common tumor in this group, usually occurs as a single lesion but may be multiple. Histologic distinction between benign leiomyoma and leiomyosarcoma may be very difficult, and at times the differentiation can be made with clinical certainty only by following the patient's course. Leiomyosarcomas are usually large, bulky, irregular polypoid lesions which may be intraluminal or extramural (Figs. 16-36 and 16-37). They tend to ulcerate and to undergo extensive central necrosis. Therefore, gastrointestinal bleeding is common (Figs. 16-38 to 16-40). Localized collections of air with irregular margins that do not conform to the usual configuration of the normal intestinal tract may be evident (Fig. 16-41). These changes are the result of excavation of the necrotic tumor which has communicated with the intestinal lumen. Perforation into the peritoneal cavity occurs. Large soft tissue masses are frequently seen. On occasion they grow to huge size and are attached to the bowel wall by a small pedicle which may twist and produce kinking and volvulus and a characteristic V-shaped configuration (Fig. 16-42). Ulceration within the tumor is easily recognized, and sometimes these ulcerations form deep pits, cavities, and fistulous tracts. The tumors not infrequently become detached from the intestinal wall and present as mesenteric masses (Fig. 16-41).

(Text continued on page 339.)

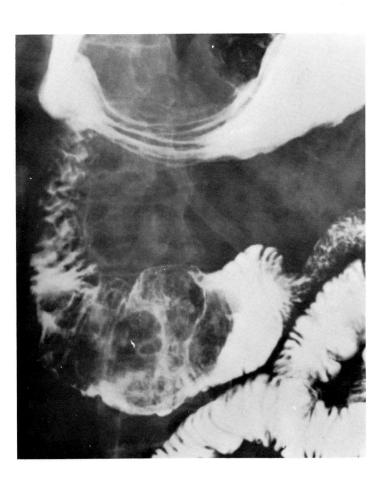

Figure 16-36 Leiomyosarcoma. There is a large, irregular filling defect dilating the third portion of the duodenum. This type of lesion is usually due to a sarcoma but occasionally may be seen in metastatic tumors.

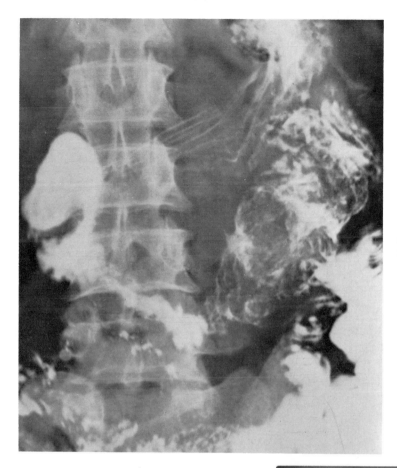

Figure 16-37 Leiomyosarcoma. A large, irregular filling defect which dilates the bowel lumen is noted immediately distal to the ligament of Treitz.

Figure 16-38 Leiomyosarcoma. There is a huge, irregular area of ulceration within a large mass in the distal jejunum. A single large mass with an irregular central ulceration usually proves to be a connective tissue sarcoma, such as a leiomyosarcoma; multiple masses suggest lymphosarcoma. Rarely is it due to a metastatic lesion.

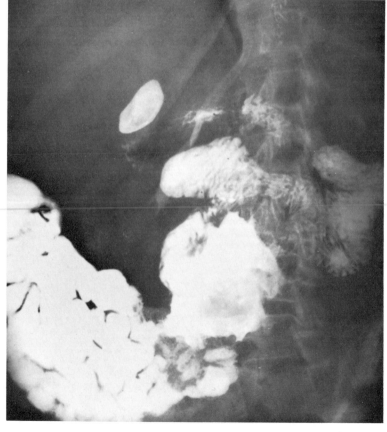

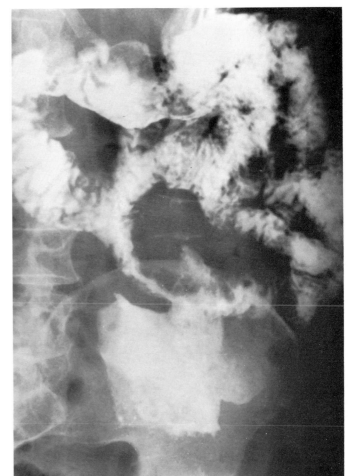

Figure 16-39 Leiomyosarcoma. A large irregular area of ulceration within a mass is noted in the distal jejunum.

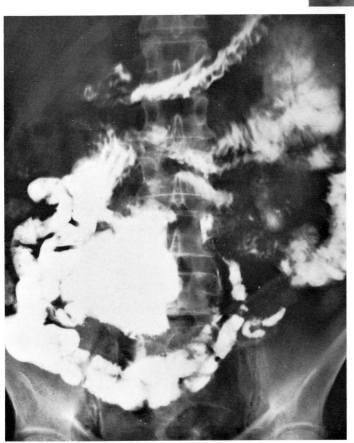

Figure 16-40 Leiomyosarcoma. A large irregular area of ulceration within a mass is seen in the proximal ileum.

333

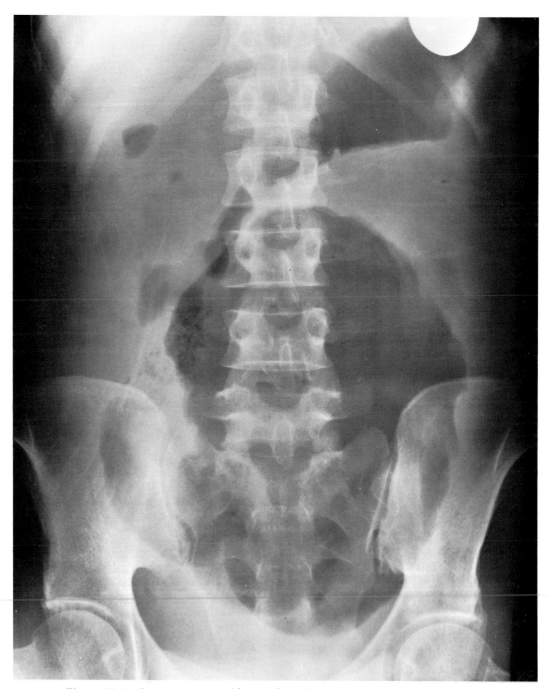

Figure 16-41 *Leiomyosarcoma* of low-grade malignancy. There is an enormous collection of air with irregular contours extending from the pelvis to the second lumbar vertebra.

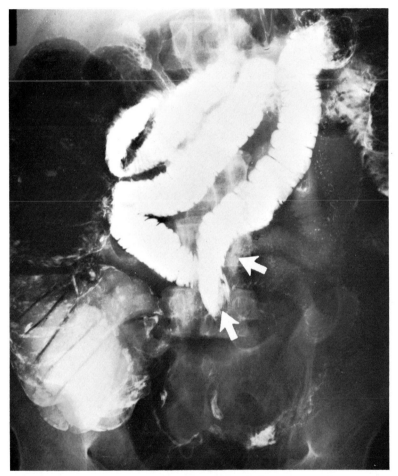

Figure 16-42 *Leiomyosarcoma.* There is intestinal obstruction with torsion and twisting of the small bowel, producing a V-shaped configuration. The small bowel loops are displaced from the pelvis and there is some extrinsic pressure.

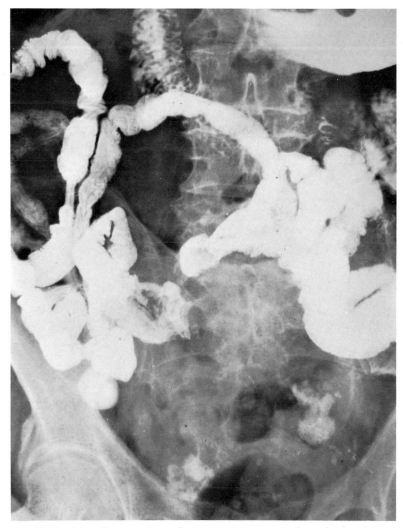

Figure 16-43 Neurofibrosarcoma. A large tumor is seen in the pelvis with irregular, mottled, amorphous calcifications. This may be mistaken for calcified fibroids. The small bowel has a peculiar triangular configuration on the right side, which is due to twisting and torsion of the small bowel by the large extramural tumor. The tumor which was removed was large, nodular, hemorrhagic and cystic, and arose from the outer aspect of the small bowel. At the sites of attachment of the tumor there was a dimple-like out-pouching of the mucosa, forming a small pseudodiverticulum in the depths of which a small ulcer was present.

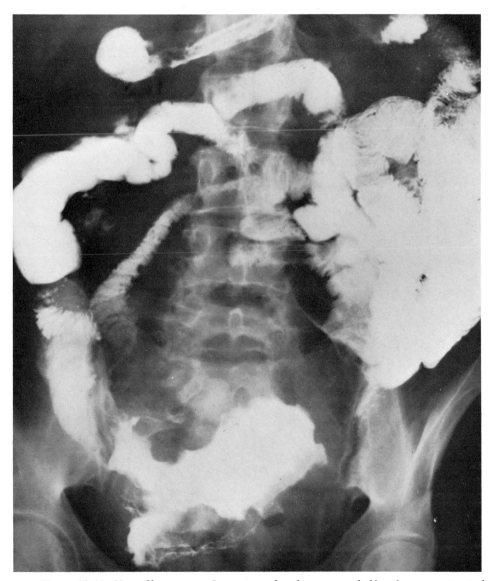

Figure 16-44 *Neurofibrosarcoma.* Large, irregular ulcer surrounded by a huge mass is noted. The fact that the lesion is single favors the diagnosis of connective tissue sarcoma rather than lymphosarcoma.

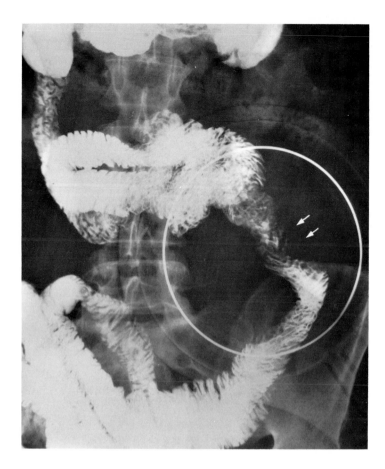

Figure 16-45 *Leiomyosarcoma.* The original tumor was removed several years ago and was called a cellular myoma. This is a recurrence producing extrinsic pressure on the distal jejunum. This demonstrates the difficulties in the differential diagnosis of benign connective tissue tumors and their malignant counterparts.

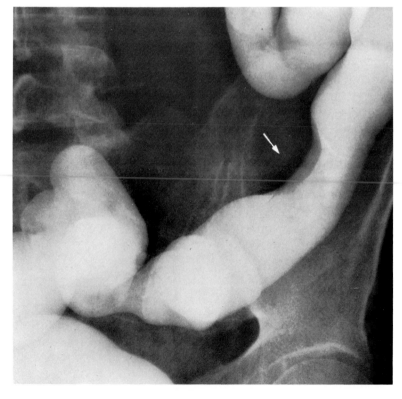

Figure 16-46 *Leiomyosarcoma.* Same case as in Figure 16-45. Recurrent tumor is producing extrinsic pressure on the sigmoid.

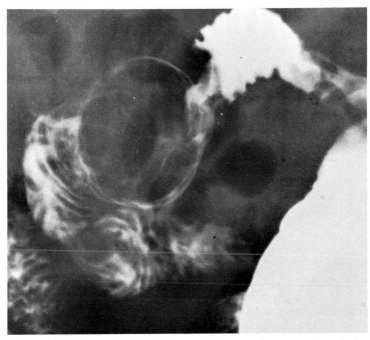

Figure 16-47 Metastatic hypernephroma. There is a large, circular, fairly sharply demarcated filling defect in the second portion of the duodenum. It mimics a benign tumor in this region. In most cases the tumor is irregular, extends from the posterior aspect, and its malignant nature is readily recognized.

Any benign tumor may have its malignant counterpart. Most have the same general appearance as leiomyosarcomas (Figs. 16-43 to 16-46).

Kaposi's sarcoma produces characteristic lesions of the skin which are manifested by an ulcerated hemorrhagic dermatitis. The entire intestinal tract may be involved by multiple reddish or bluish-red nodules which intrude into the lumen of the gut. They are sometimes intramural and extramural in loca-

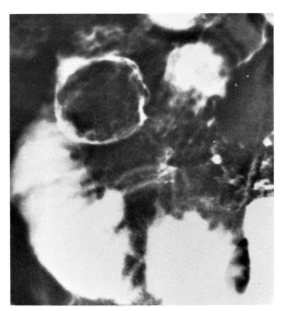

Figure 16-48 Metastatic melanoma. Multiple intraluminal defects produced intussusception. Only one of these is shown here. The appearance suggests a benign lesion.

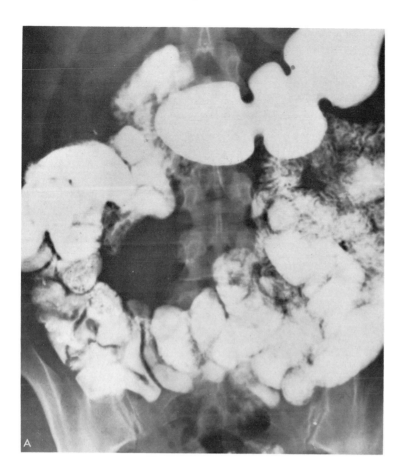

Figure 16-49   *A, Fibrosarcoma* of the mesentery.

Figure 16-49   *B*, Same patient. The mobility of this tumor is demonstrated.

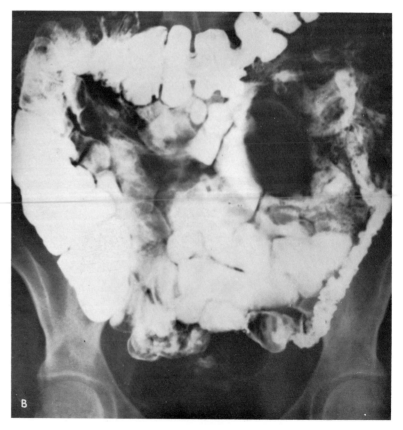

tion. They probably arise in the submucosa, and gastrointestinal bleeding is frequent. Opinions differ as to the exact nature of the disease but most authorities consider it as a vascular neoplasm with a low malignant potential. The lesions resemble lymphosarcoma and may produce central ulceration.

Metastatic hypernephroma, primarily a cellular tumor with little desmoplastic reaction, spreads to the intestinal tract and produces lesions which may mimic benign or malignant submucosal tumors (Fig. 16-47).

Metastatic melanoma (Fig. 16-48) and lymphosarcoma may on occasion mimic small bowel tumors, but usually they maintain their own roentgen characteristics (Fig. 16-49).

References

1. Calman, K. C.: Why are small bowel tumors rare? An experimental model. *Gut*, 15:552-554, 1974.
2. Jones, C. M.: Digestive Tract Pain: Diagnosis and treatment: Experimental observations. New York, The Macmillan Co., 1938.
3. River, L., Silverstein, J., and Tope, J. W.: Benign neoplasms of the small intestine; a critical comprehensive review with reports of 20 new cases. *Int. Abstr. Surg.*, 102:1, 1956.
4. Good, C. A.: Tumors of the small intestine. *Amer. J. Roentgen.*, 89:685, 1963.
5. Darling, R. C., and Welch, C. E.: Tumors of the small intestine. *New Eng. J. Med.*, 260:397-408, 1959.
6. Marshak, R. A., Freund, S., and Maklansky, D.: Neurofibromatosis of the small bowel. *Amer. J. Dig. Dis.*, 8:478-483, 1963.
7. Bartholomew, L. G., Dahlen, D. C., and Waugh, J. M.: Intestinal polyposis associated with mucocutaneous melanin pigmentation (Peutz-Jeghers syndrome). *Gastroenterology*, 32:434-451, 1957.
8. Weller, R. O., and McColl, I.: Electron microscope appearances of juvenile and Peutz-Jeghers polyps. *Gut*, 7:265-270, 1966.
9. Payson, B. A., and Moumgis, B.: Metastasizing carcinoma of the stomach in Peutz-Jeghers syndrome. *Ann. Surg.*, 165:145-151, 1967.
10. Reid, J. D.: Intestinal carcinoma in the Peutz-Jeghers Syndrome. *J. Am. Med. Assn.* 229:833-834, 1974.
11. Orimo, H., Fujita, T., Yoshikawa, M., Takamoto, T., Matsuo, Y., and Nakao, K.: Gastrointestinal polyposis with protein-losing enteropathy, abnormal skin pigmentation, and loss of hair and nails (Cronkhite-Canada Syndrome). *Am. J. Med.*, 47:445-449, 1969.

17

Carcinoid Tumors and the Carcinoid Syndrome

The carcinoid tumor has aroused a degree of interest among physicians well out of proportion to its incidence. The reason lies not only in the capacity of the tumor to become a relatively slow-growing malignancy, but in its ability to form and store serotonin, a hormone associated with a variety of clinical manifestations, as well as a still-undetermined number of potent vasoactive amines.

Carcinoid tumors are found throughout the gastrointestinal tract except for the esophagus, but they are most common in the appendix and in the small bowel. Identical tumors have been reported to arise from the mucosa of the respiratory tract and from the pancreas.

In the intestine the cell of origin is the Kulchitsky or argentaffin cell, one of the types of cells lining the crypts of Lieberkühn. Characteristic of this cell is the presence of cytoplasmic granules that are capable of reducing ammoniacal silver nitrate.

As a rule, carcinoid tumors of the intestine are small submucosal nodules or even simply focal areas of submucosal thickening.[1] Generally the tumors are firm, well circumscribed, and yellow-tan in color. Frequently they are multiple. The overlying mucosa is intact, and mucosal ulceration is uncommon. Muscle hypertrophy may be marked in the involved area, and because fibrosis is common there is a tendency for kinking and partial small bowel obstruction to occur. As the tumor grows, fibrosis in and about the mass becomes prominent. The tumor spreads slowly by infiltration through the bowel wall into the muscularis and serosa, to the mesenteric nodes and to distant sites of metastasis by both lymphatic and venous channels. Encroachment on the lumen of the bowel is unusual, and when this occurs it is usually due to fibrosis and kinking rather than to growth of tumor itself. Deep ulceration of the mucosa is uncommon, but the tumors may bleed from superficial erosions.

Histologically, carcinoid tumors are of two types. Classically, the tumor consists of solid nests of uniform small cells. Occasionally, however, the cells are arranged in a trabecular pattern; this uncommon type is more likely to be found in tumors arising in stomach, rectum, or bronchus than in those arising in the small bowel.

Despite the rather benign histologic appearance of the tumors, most pathologists believe that carcinoids, except those in the appendix, are potentially malignant. The tumors grow slowly, however, and patients with widespread metastases may live for many years.

In a careful survey of the literature, Sanders and Axtell[2] reported 2500 cases of gastrointestinal carcinoid and added 77 cases of their own. The greatest incidence of carcinoid tumor was in the appendix (1140 cases), and only 33 of these showed metastases. Sixty-four carcinoids were duodenal, and three-fourths of these were symptomatic, with duodenal obstruction, common bile duct obstruction, or an associated duodenal ulcer. There were 841 patients with carcinoids of the jejunum or ileum; the incidence in the ileum was eight times greater than in the jejunum. About one-third of the patients with jejunal and ileal carcinoids harbored metastases, but most of these were asymptomatic and were found at autopsy or as incidental tumors at laparotomy. The presence of metastasis in small bowel carcinoid was found to be correlated with symptoms (either carcinoid syndrome or partial small bowel obstruction) and with the size of the small bowel tumor (lesions larger than 1 cm. tended to have metastases).

Recommended treatment of small bowel carcinoid is wide resection. The prognosis is generally favorable, even with metastases.

CARCINOID SYNDROME

The carcinoid syndrome reflects the clinical manifestations of serotonin, and other compounds secreted by carcinoid tumor, upon the cardiovascular and respiratory systems and the gastrointestinal tract. The biologically active serotonin, transported in the blood by the platelets, is derived metabolically from the amino acid tryptophane. The initial step is hydroxylation to 5-hydroxytryptophane, which occasionally can itself be biologically active when released into the blood by some carcinoid tumors. As a rule, however, the compound undergoes decarboxylation by the argentaffin cells to form 5-hydroxytryptamine, or serotonin. In its subsequent metabolic pathway, serotonin undergoes oxidative deamination by the enzyme monoamine oxidase to 5-hydroxyindoleacetic acid, which is excreted in the urine. Monoamine oxidase is present in the gastrointestinal mucosa, lung, liver, brain, and kidney.

The most distinctive feature of the carcinoid syndrome is the flush, which varies in color from cyanotic to bright red and involves predominantly the head and neck. Usually the flush lasts only a few minutes but it may be recurrent and may be persistent. The flush has been observed to be triggered by palpation of the tumor, by exertion, or by emotional upsets, and it tends to become more frequent and intense as the disease progresses. In the past, the flush has been generally attributed to release of serotonin into the systemic circulation, but it has rarely been possible to document a rise in circulating serotonin during the flush; recent studies[3, 4] indicate that kallikrein, released by the tumor with consequent formation of bradykinin in the blood, is more likely a responsible agent. Yet other vasoactive substances may be involved in some patients.

Chronic diarrhea and intestinal colic are characteristic of carcinoid syndrome, effects reasonably attributable to the response of smooth muscle and intrinsic nerve fibers to serotonin. Malabsorption syndrome may develop in association with the diarrhea.[5]

Wheezing and asthmatic attacks occur in some patients, probably reflecting the bronchoconstriction of serotonin or bradykinin. Valvular heart disease, usually involving tricuspid or pulmonic valves, leads to right-sided heart failure. Pathologically there is dense, fibrous subendocardial thickening. It has been postulated that endocardial disease is an effect of circulating serotonin and that the left side of the heart tends to be spared in intestinal carcinoid because serotonin is destroyed in the lung by the monoamine oxidase present there. Bradykinin may also play a role in initiating an endocardial inflammation leading to fibrosis.

Liver metastases are invariably present in patients with the carcinoid syndrome when the tumor arises in the intestine. In the absence of hepatic metastases, the serotonin released by the tumor can be inactivated by liver monoamine oxidase and does not reach the general circulation.

Diagnosis of carcinoid syndrome is made by the clinical features and by the finding of elevated levels of 5-hydroxyindoleacetic acid in the urine. Normal excretion of the compound is 2 to 10 mg. a day. Urinary outputs of 50 to 1000 mg. a day have been reported in a carcinoid syndrome, and most patients excrete more than 100 mg. a day.

Treatment of carcinoid syndrome is resection of both primary and metastatic tumor whenever possible, an approach made feasible by the slow growth

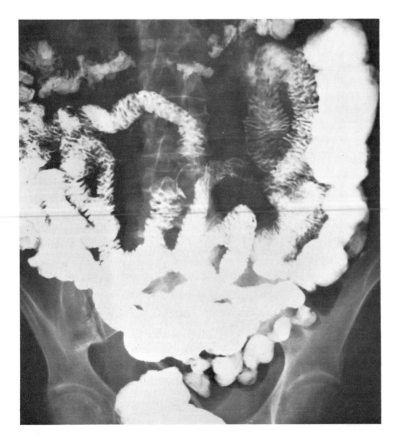

Figure 17-1 A, Carcinoid of the small bowel. There is a submucosal defect measuring 2 cm. in diameter in the distal jejunum. The adjacent folds both proximally and distally are thickened and distorted. Slight separation of the loops of bowel is noted.

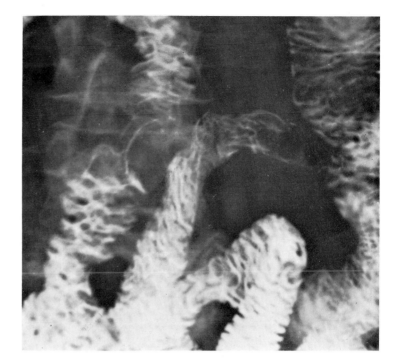

Figure 17-1 Continued *B*, Same case as in Figure 17-1A. Magnified.

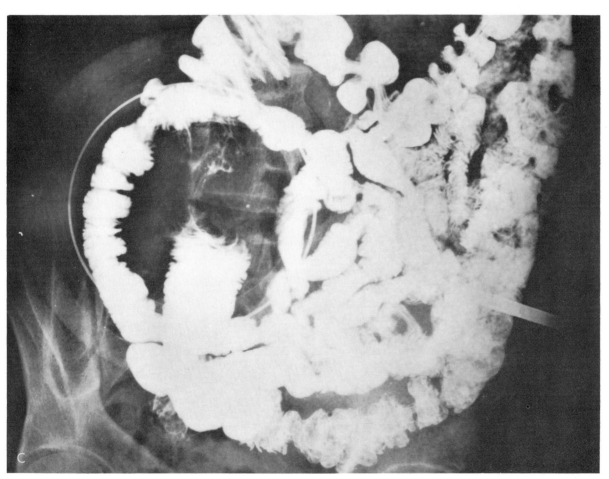

Figure 17-1 *C, Carcinoid of the small bowel.* There is a 3 cm. submucosal nodule in the distal ileum, with moderate obstruction.

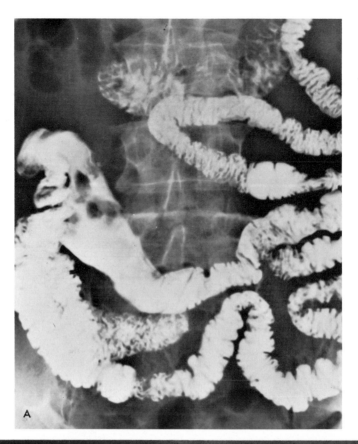

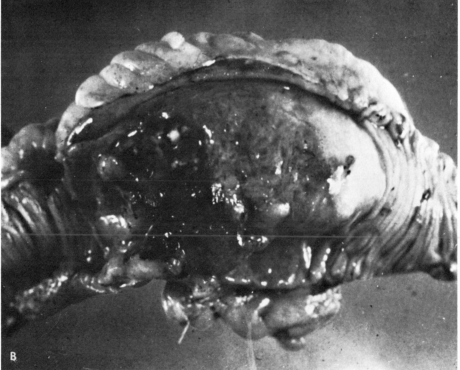

Figure 17-2 A, Carcinoid of the small bowel. A segment of proximal ileum is dilated and contains multiple irregular nodular filling defects. (Courtesy of Dr. Irving Bluth, Brooklyn, New York).

B, Same case as in A. Excised specimen demonstrating the polypoid lesion, dilatation of the bowel, and the multiple nodular excrescences.

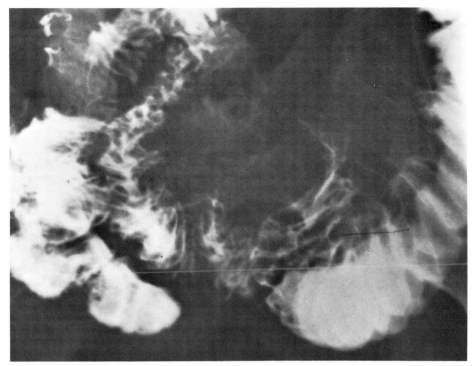

Figure 17-3 *Carcinoid of the small bowel.* The distal ileum is angulated, moderately rigid, and narrowed. The folds are thickened and stretched. Submucosal defects are identified on the superior surface of the involved segment of ileum.

of the tumor. Drug treatment utilizing antiserotonin compounds has not been generally effective, but parachlorophenylalanine, an inhibitor of serotonin synthesis, lessens the gastrointestinal symptoms of some patients with the carcinoid syndrome, and methysergide and cyproheptadine, serotonin antagonists, are sometimes effective as well.[3, 6]

Roentgen Findings

Although carcinoids are the most common tumors in the small intestine, they are infrequently diagnosed on roentgen examination.[7] This is due to several factors. Most carcinoids are tiny and therefore are not seen. When they become sufficiently large, carcinoids produce such a variety of roentgen findings that it is difficult to define a characteristic pattern. Despite this difficulty, certain roentgen alterations are noted which aid in their detection.

The primary mucosal lesion grows submucosally, producing an intramural or intraluminal defect that is indistinguishable from submucosal tumors (Figs. 17-1A, 17-1B and 17-1C). These lesions can be multiple and are either confluent or widely separated. When confluent, the nodules may produce large filling defects, and in some cases aneurysmal dilatation of the bowel is noted (Fig. 17-2). When the tumors are widely separated they can produce local stenosis and alternating areas of constriction and dilatation.

More commonly, because of the associated desmoplastic reaction, angulation, kinking of the bowel wall, partial intestinal obstruction, and stretching and rigidity of the folds are noted. These alterations can be seen with or

(Text continued on page 356.)

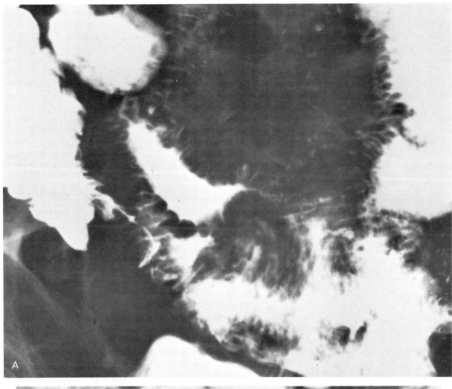

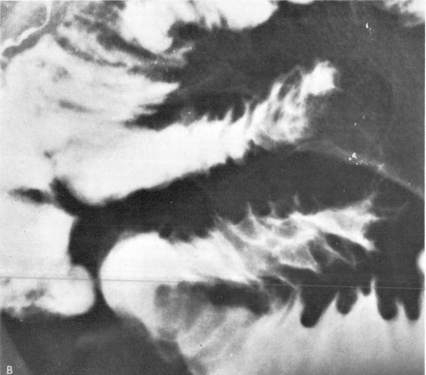

Figure 17-4 Carcinoid of the small bowel. A, The distal ileum is involved. There is narrowing and rigidity, with multiple submucosal nodules, angulation of the bowel, stretching of the folds, and partial obstruction. (Courtesy of Dr. I. Weinfeld, Miami, Florida.)

B, Same case as in *A.* The short segment of narrowing in an arcuate fashion is again identified. This is secondary to submucosal involvement. The folds proximally and distally are fixed, thickened, distorted, and stretched.

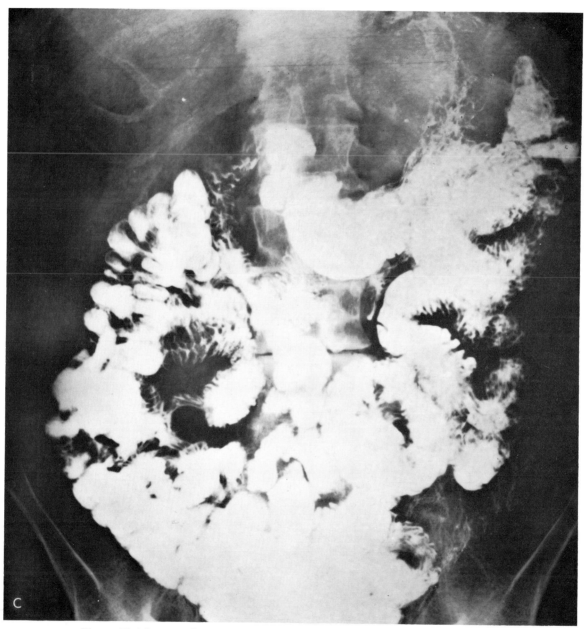

Figure 17-4 Continued *C, Carcinoid of the small bowel.* There is a small mass in the right lower quadrant, with pleating of the folds and a submucosal nodule. No obstruction is seen.

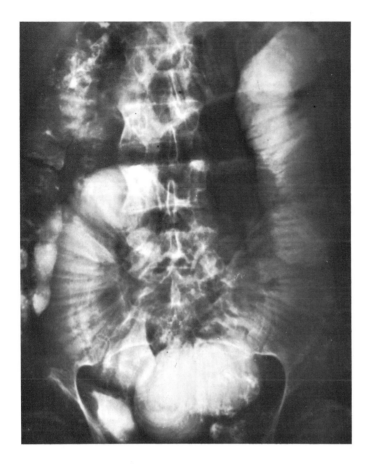

Figure 17-5 Carcinoid of the small bowel. Considerable small bowel obstruction secondary to a carcindoid tumor is seen. The actual tumor is not visualized.

Figure 17-6 Carcinoid of the small bowel. Complete obstruction to the retrograde flow of barium due to an encircling carcinoid of the ileum. Only the distal inch of ileum is seen protruding from the barium filled cecum as a sausage-like structure.

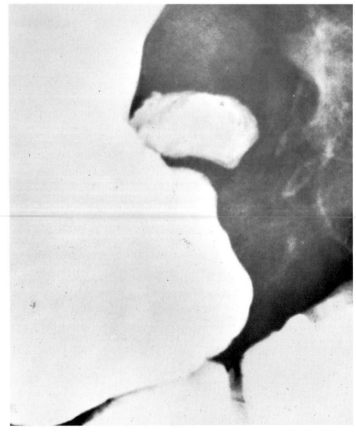

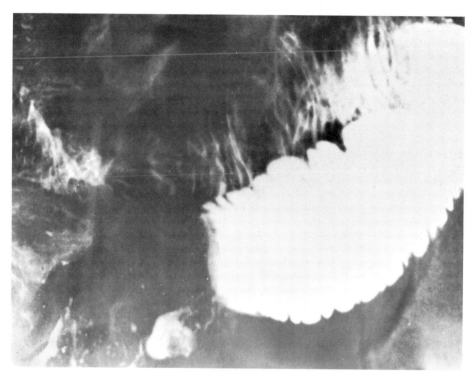

Figure 17-7 *Carcinoid of the small bowel.* There is marked obstruction due to a large ulcerating lesion. The edges of the obstructed segment are everted, suggesting that the tumor is eccentric and extending into the lumen from the outside. It is impossible to differentiate this lesion from metastatic carcinoma.

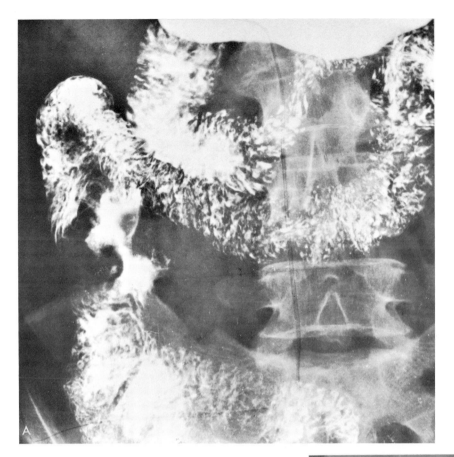

Figure 17-8 A Carcinoid of the small bowel. An ulcerating tumor with minimal obstruction is noted. The appearance simulates a lymphoma.

Figure 17-8 B, Carcinoid tumor. Same case as Figure 17-8A. Intussusception of the tumor is noted.

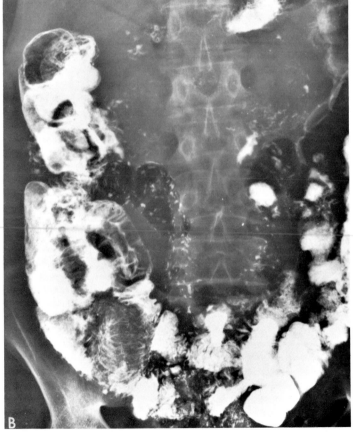

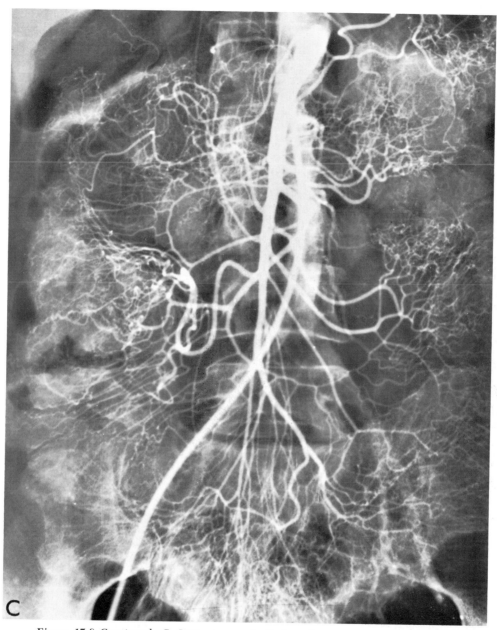

Figure 17-8 Continued C, Same case as in B. Superior mesenteric artery injection. The tumor is vascular.

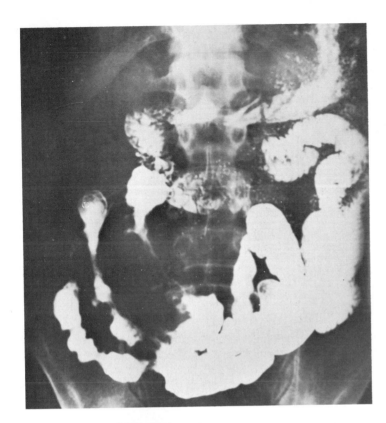

Figure 17-9 A, *Carcinoid tumor simulating regional enteritis.* There is marked narrowing and rigidity of the involved loops of bowel with separation of the loops. This is due not only to the thickened mesentery but also to the thickened submucosa. (Courtesy of Dr. I. Bluth, Brooklyn, New York.)

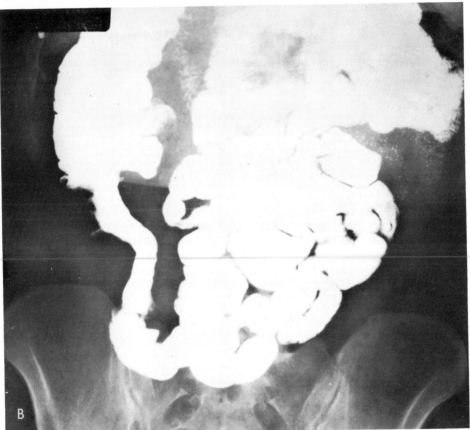

Figure 17-9 B, *Carcinoid of the small bowel.* The distal 5 inches of ileum are narrowed and rigid, with smooth contours. Tiny projections are identified extending from the margins of the distal ileum. The mucosa appears effaced. The cecal cap is obliterated. These roentgen alterations suggest that the cecum and terminal ileum are encased in a mass. At laparotomy, a carcinoid tumor mass was found to be producing these findings.

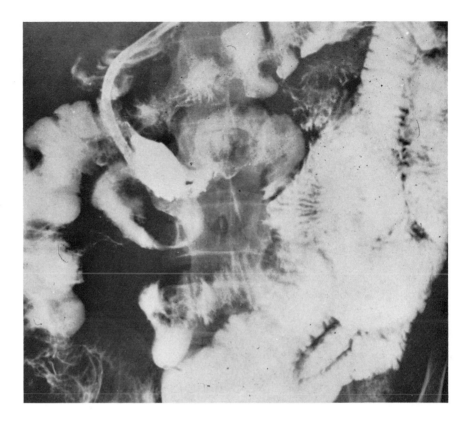

Figure 17-10 *Carcinoid tumor.* Several segments of small bowel are involved. The one adjacent to the colon on the right side demonstrates narrowing, rigidity, and effacement of the mucosa. The findings are those usually associated with infarction. The loops of small bowel inferior to this segment reveal fixation and stretching of the folds. Slight obstruction is noted.

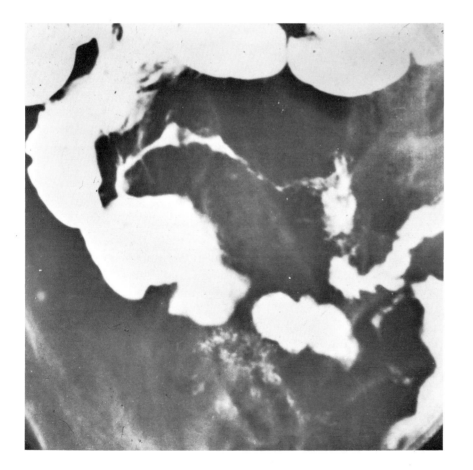

Figure 17-11 *Carcinoid of the small bowel.* There is considerable narrowing of the terminal ileum with irregularity of the contour. This patient had severe diarrhea and rapid motility of the barium through the small bowel. Multiple metastases to the liver were demonstrated by angiography.

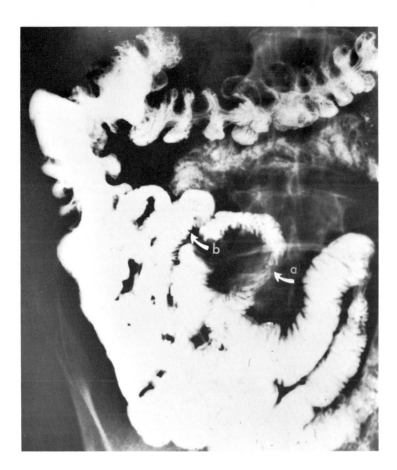

Figure 17-12   Carcinoid of the small bowel. There are 2 short segments of narrowing with stretching and irregularities of the folds.

without single or multiple submucosal tumors.[8, 9] The findings are so similar to metastatic carcinoma that whenever the latter lesion is suspected one should also consider the possibility of a carcinoid (Figs. 17-3 and 17-4). In some cases the tumor nodule completely encircles the bowel, producing varying degrees of obstruction (Fig. 17-5), mimicking either a primary carcinoma or a metastatic lesion (Fig. 17-6). Despite the fact that bleeding occurs, deep ulcerations are uncommon (Figs. 17-7 and 17-8).

The resemblance of carcinoid tumors and regional enteritis has been noted.[10] Because of the marked smooth muscle hypertrophy, long areas of stenosis are seen with separation of the loops of bowel. Cases have been observed for years under the erroneous diagnosis of regional enteritis (Fig. 17-9). The lack of mucosal changes, however, may suggest to the radiologist that the lesion is not regional enteritis.

Small bowel infarction is also seen in association with carcinoids.[11] Several factors have been implicated, including vascular compromise produced by metastatic nodes at the root of the mesentery, angulation of the bowel due to fibrosis, and adhesions (Fig. 17-10).

Rapid motility through the small bowel is a feature associated with carcinoid syndrome and when this phenomenon is observed the diagnosis should be considered (Figs. 17-11 and 17-12).

References

1. Teitelbaum, S. L.: The carcinoid. A collective review. *Amer. J. Surg.*, 123:564-572, 1972.
2. Sanders, R. J. and Axtell, H. K.: Carcinoids of the gastrointestinal tract. *Surg. Gynec. Obstet.*, 119:369-380, 1964.
3. Leading article: Taking stock of the carcinoid flush. *Lancet*, 2:711-712, 1973.
4. Ureles, A. L.: Diagnosis and treatment of malignant carcinoid syndrome. *J.A.M.A.*, 229:1346-1348, 1974.
5. Kowlessar, O. D., Law, D. H., and Sleisenger, M. H.: Malabsorption syndrome associated with metastatic carcinoid tumor. *Am. J. Med.*, 27:673-677, 1959.
6. Engelman, K., Lovenberg, W., and Sjoerdsma, A.: Inhibition of serotonin synthesis by para-chlorophenylalanine in patients with the carcinoid syndrome. *New Eng. J. Med.*, 277:1103-1108, 1967.
7. Moertel, C. G., Sauer, W. G., Dockerty, M. B., and Baggenstoss, A. H.: Life history of the carcinoid tumor of the small intestine. *Cancer*, 14:901-912, 1961.
8. Miller, E. R. and Herrmann, W. W.: Argentaffin tumors of the small bowel: roentgen sign of malignant change. *Radiology*, 39:214-220, 1942.
9. Wilson, J. W. and Waugh, J. M.: Metastasizing carcinoid of the ileum simulating metastasis from a carcinoma of the rectosigmoid. *Canad. Med. Ass. J.*, 59:268-271, 1948.
10. Stark, S., Bluth, I., and Rubenstein, S.: Carcinoid tumor of the ileum resembling regional enteritis clinically and roentgenologically. *Gastroenterology*, 40:813-817, 1961.
11. Ritchie, A. C.: Carcinoid tumors. *Med. Clin. N. Amer.*, 44:465-474, 1960.

18

Primary and Metastatic Carcinoma of the Small Bowel

PRIMARY CARCINOMA

Adenocarcinoma of the duodenum or small bowel is a rare lesion. Within the duodenum, carcinoma may present clinically with ulceration and bleeding, obstruction, perforation, or jaundice. The usual classification[1] divides carcinoma of the duodenum into suprapapillary, peripapillary, and infrapapillary neoplasms. The predominant clinical manifestations depend upon the location within the duodenum. Lesions superior to the papilla tend to cause obstruction and bleeding; periampullary lesions cause obstructive jaundice; and tumors below the ampulla cause ulceration, bleeding and obstruction. Carcinoma of the papilla of Vater is a distinct entity and has a characteristic roentgen appearance. Primary carcinoma elsewhere in the duodenum is rare and may be difficult to distinguish from metastatic disease or extension from the pancreas.

In the mesenteric small bowel, primary adenocarcinoma occurs more frequently in the jejunum than in the ileum.[2] The most common clinical features are abdominal pain and evidence of intermittent bowel obstruction. Such obstruction may occur by growth of an annular constricting lesion, by intussusception of a polypoid mass, or by progressive encroachment on the lumen by tumor. Bleeding is common, as either occult blood loss or massive hemorrhage. Occasionally free perforation of the tumor mass occurs.

It is often difficult for the pathologist to determine whether a duodenal or small bowel adenocarcinoma is a primary or a metastatic lesion and therefore data on incidence from different institutions are difficult to compare. Because the area of the ligament of Treitz is a common site of metastatic carcinoma, lesions here carry a high suspicion of being metastatic, rather than primary tumors.

Roentgen Features

Peripapillary carcinomas are usually polypoid and ulcerated, and are immediately adjacent to the papilla of Vater. Obstruction is not a conspicuous feature. The roentgen features of carcinoma of the remainder of the duodenum (Figs. 18-1*A* to 18-1*D*) and the small bowel (Figs. 18-2 to 18-12) are similar to those seen in the colon or esophagus. There is usually a constricting lesion of varying length, associated with an eccentric and irregular channel and with overhanging edges. The mucosa in the region of the lesion is ulcerated, and partial obstruction is common. It is unusual to find a carcinoma of the small bowel limited to one wall, as seen in the colon. In some cases the lesion is huge and polypoid in configuration, and may or may not be associated with intussusception.

Carcinoma of the small bowel has been seen with sprue and with regional enteritis. In both conditions the neoplasm is difficult to recognize because roentgen changes in the underlying disease obscure the characteristic features of the tumor, unless it is large.

METASTATIC CARCINOMA OF THE SMALL BOWEL

Metastatic carcinoma of the small bowel and its mesentery, although a common finding at necropsy, may pass unrecognized roentgenologically.[3-7] A study of these patients reveals a multiplicity of roentgen changes which, while they are not pathognomonic, are highly suggestive. The presence of abdominal carcinomatosis may be obvious clinically, and small bowel examination demonstrates findings indicative of multiple large metastatic masses. Difficulties arise, however, when a primary site is not known or when the disease is less advanced. In such instances, only a single lesion may be discovered, or there may be no constant morphologic alterations in the small bowel but rather functional motor changes or ascites.

The most frequent sites of origin of metastatic disease to the small bowel are the ovary, pancreas, stomach, colon, breast, lung, and uterus. Patients usually present with symptoms indicative of intestinal obstruction, such as pain and increasing abdominal girth, or weight loss. Gastrointestinal bleeding may occasionally be the first manifestation of metastatic disease. Abdominal examination will usually reveal distention, intra-abdominal masses, or ascites.

Pathologically, the metastatic lesion may originate in the wall of the bowel, beneath the serosa, or in the mesentery. A submucosal lesion may develop a pseudopedicle and present as an intestinal polyp, and may cause intussusception and bleeding. More commonly, mesenteric or serosal deposits extend secondarily into the wall of the bowel, producing angulation, fixation, and flattening of the contour of the bowel wall. With continued growth, the tumor may extend through the bowel wall and present as an intraluminal sessile mass, with or without ulceration. In other instances, the appearance of an intraluminal mass may be simulated by invagination of the wall and tumor toward the lumen. Intestinal obstruction is caused by a combination of encroachment on the lumen, local fixation, and deformity, as well as angulation and twisting of the bowel. For descriptive purposes, these metastatic lesions related to the small intestine may be arbitrarily divided into three groups,

(Text continued on page 368.)

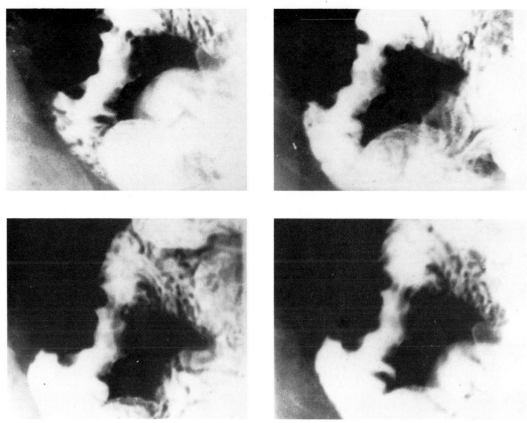

Figure 18-1   A, Carcinoma of the duodenum. There is a constricting lesion involving the second portion of the duodenum with eccentric lumen and overhanging edges. The findings are typical of a primary carcinoma of the second portion of the duodenum. This patient is alive and well 8 years after resection of the tumor.

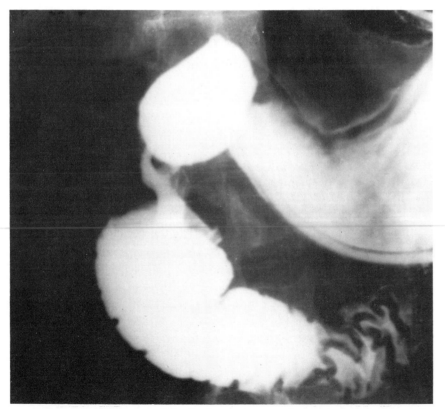

Figure 18-1   B, Carcinoma of the duodenum. An irregular constricting lesion involves the proximal half of the second portion of the duodenum. Both prestenotic and post-stenotic dilatation are noted.

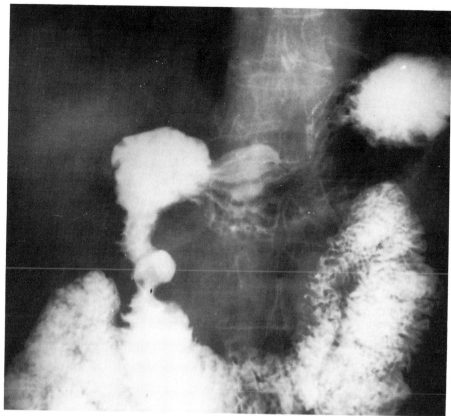

Figure 18-1 Continued C, Carcinoma of the duodenum. There is an irregular constricting lesion involving the second portion of the duodenum. An ulcer crater is seen on the medial aspect of the mid-portion of the lesion. Although the ulcer itself appears benign, in association with the irregular channel a diagnosis of carcinoma should be made. The absence of overhanging margins suggests a component of extension and therefore the possibility that the lesion represents a carcinoma of the pancreas involving the duodenum should also be considered.

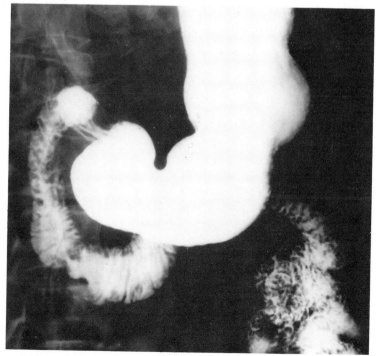

Figure 18-1 D, Carcinoma of the duodenum. A short constricting lesion with overhanging edges is seen in the distal descending duodenum. The mucosa is ulcerated.

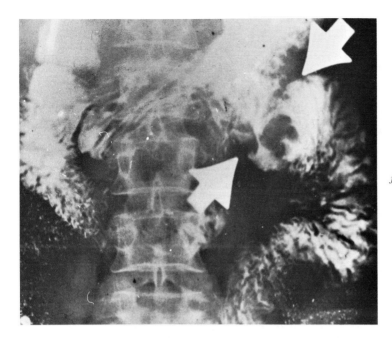

Figure 18-2 Small primary carcinoma of the jejunum which produced intermittent obstruction.

Figure 18-3 Primary carcinoma of the jejunum. There is a short constricting lesion in the proximal jejunum with overhanging edges, eccentric lumen, and ulceration of the mucosa. Slight obstruction is noted.

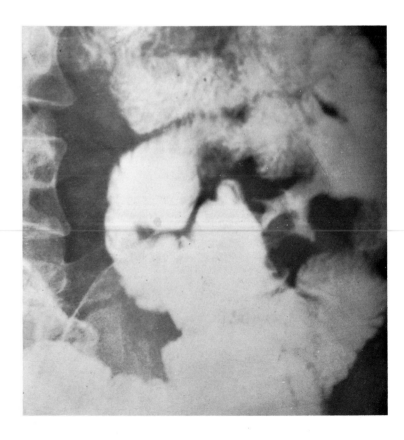

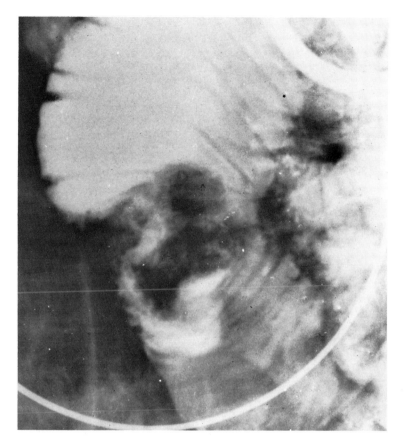

Figure 18-4 *Primary carcinoma of the jejunum.* Similar changes to those of Figure 18-3, except there is more proximal obstruction.

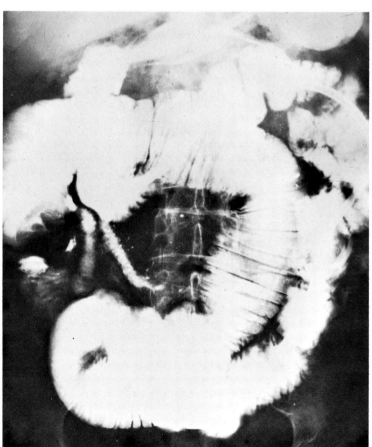

Figure 18-5 *Primary carcinoma of the jejunum.* Considerable obstruction proximal to an annular carcinoma in mid-jejunum.

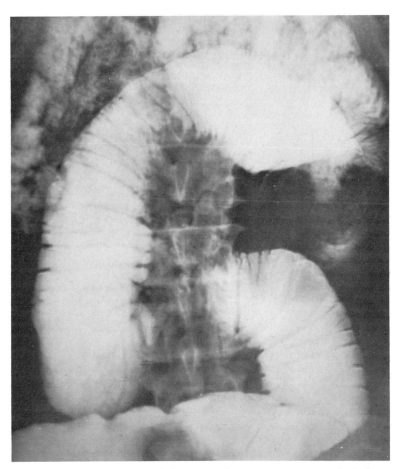

Figure 18-6 *Primary carcinoma of the proximal jejunum* causing marked obstruction.

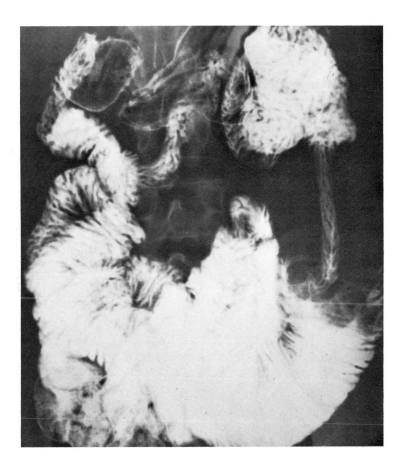

Figure 18-7 A, Polypoid carcinoma of the jejunum causing intussusception.

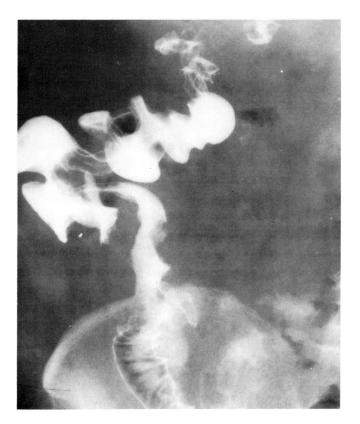

Figure 18-7 B, Primary carcinoma of the ileum. The distal 4 inches of ileum proximal to the ileocecal valve is involved. There is moderate rigidity and narrowing, with multiple nodular defects, especially along the mesial aspect. At the proximal edge of the lesion slight overhanging edges are seen. Minimal obstruction is identified. Lymphosarcoma and carcinoid were considered in the differential diagnosis. At laparotomy a primary carcinoma of the ileum was found.

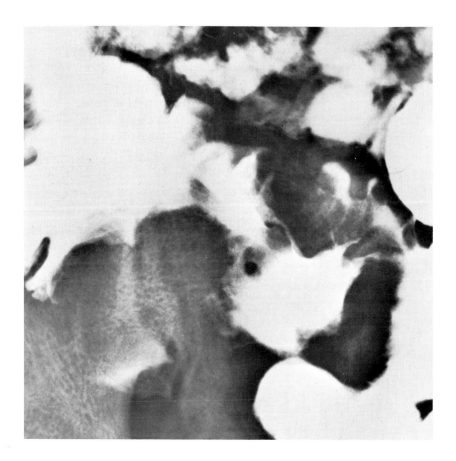

Figure 18-8   Carcinoma of the cecum with extension into the terminal ileum. Whenever a carcinoma is seen in the terminal ileum the possibility that it arises in the cecum should be considered. The characteristic findings of cecal carcinoma permit distinction from lymphosarcoma but sometimes, especially where there is no obstruction, this differentiation is impossible. In this patient the multiple irregular polypoid lesions exclude an inflammatory process.

Figure 18-9   Primary or metastatic carcinoma of the small bowel at the ligament of Treitz. There is a long, irregular, ulcerated neoplasm without proximal obstruction. The length of the lesion, the location, and the lack of obstruction all favor a metastatic lesion but the pathologist could not determine whether this was primary or metastatic carcinoma.

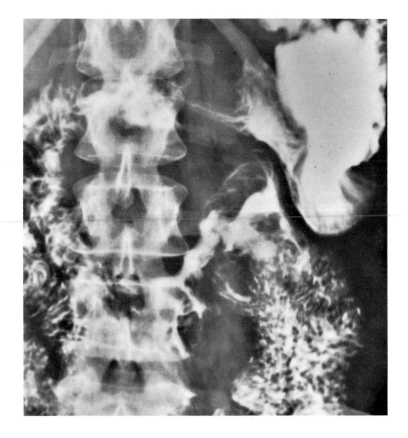

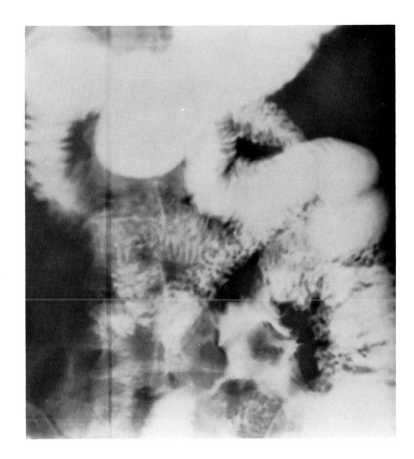

Figure 18-10 *Primary or metastatic carcinoma.* A large irregular ulcer is noted in the proximal jejunum without obstruction. The pathologist could not determine whether this lesion was primary or metastatic carcinoma.

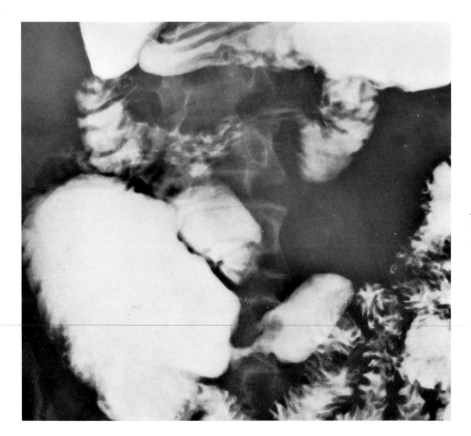

Figure 18-11 *Carcinoma of the jejunum in a blind loop.* This patient had an enteroenteric anastomosis several years before; the reason for the procedure is not known.

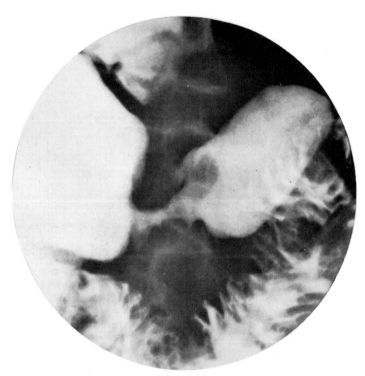

Figure 18-12 Same case as in Figure 18-11, magnified view.

depending on the predominant type of roentgen change. There is obviously considerable overlap of these groups.

Roentgen Classification

Group 1. Single or multiple metastatic lesions involving primarily the wall of the small bowel.

Group 2. Metastatic lesions involving primarily the mesentery, with or without involvement of the adjacent wall of the bowel.

Group 3. Multiple metastatic nodules involving both the small bowel and the mesentery. Ascites is particularly common in this group.

Group 1

The earliest finding in Group 1 is that of a discrete, intramural, extra-mucosal tumor, which produces a contour defect similar to that produced by any other submucosal tumor (Fig. 18-13). Continued growth of the lesion may cause marked and irregular narrowing of the lumen and partial obstruction (Fig. 18-14). Most of the growth may occur intraluminally with the production of a false pedicle and an intraluminal polypoid defect, simulating an adenomatous polyp (Fig. 18-15). A metastatic lesion originating in the wall of the bowel may also, as it grows, extend into the mesentery and present as a so-called "endoexo-centeric mass." When necrosis of the tumor is extensive, irregular ulceration similar to a primary carcinoma may be seen (Fig. 18-16).

(Text continued on page 373.)

Figure 18-13 A, Metastatic carcinoma from body of uterus. There is a localized, 3 cm., slightly irregular submucosal nodule in the fourth portion of the duodenum (arrows). There is no mucosal ulceration or proximal dilatation. The defect does not have the exquisite sharpness usually associated with benign intramural tumors. This type of nodular defect can also be seen as a result of direct extension from a carcinoma of the body of the pancreas.

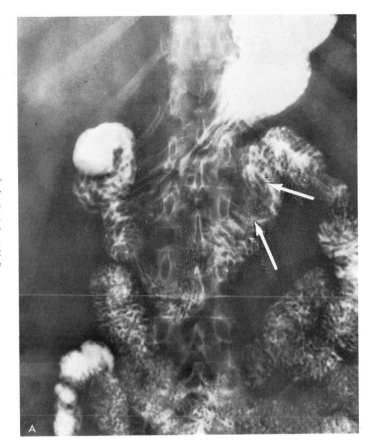

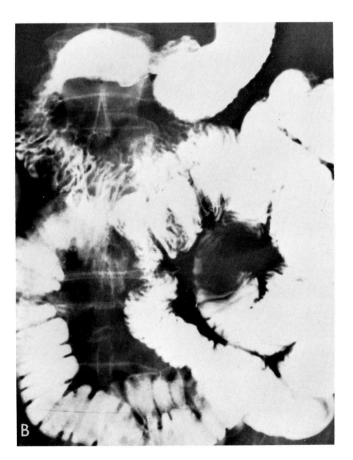

Figure 18-13 B, Metastatic carcinoma from the ovary. A solitary, submucosal lesion is present in the jejunum. The margins of the mass are not exquisitely sharp. Despite this, however, differentiation from a benign submucosal tumor is difficult.

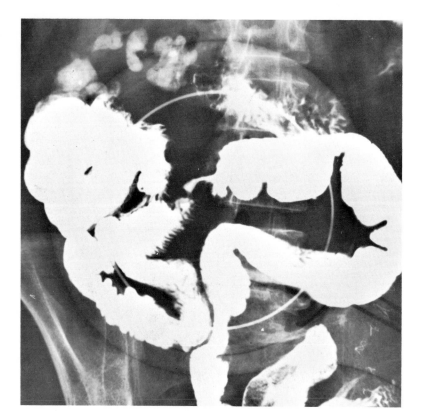

Figure 18-14 Metastatic carcinoma from the colon. There is a short, annular, constricting lesion with an eccentric lumen, and slight proximal dilatation. The margins terminate abruptly without overhanging edges. Slight nodularity of the superior wall of the narrowed segment is also evident. There is no extrinsic component.

Figure 18-15 Metastatic carcinoma from the kidney. There is a single polypoid intraluminal mass in the proximal jejunum (arrows) associated with a slightly eccentric lumen and minimal intussusception. A single small metastatic nodule such as this is difficult to differentiate from a submucosal tumor or intraluminal polyp.

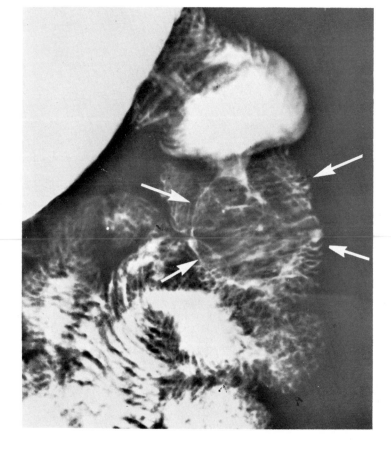

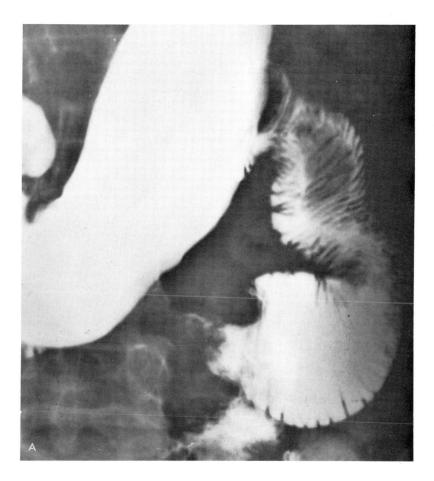

Figure 18-16 A, Metastatic adeno-carcinoma, primary unknown. There is an irregularly constricting lesion in the proximal jejunum showing mucosal ulceration and an eccentric lumen. Dilatation proximally produces an apparent overhanging edge.

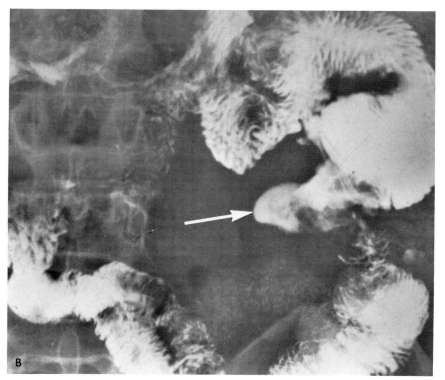

Figure 18-16 B, The same patient one hour later. The irregular ulceration is now more obvious. In addition, angulation and fixation at the tumor site are demonstrated (arrow). Despite the narrowing and dilatation, barium passes readily into the distal bowel.

(Illustration continued on following page.)

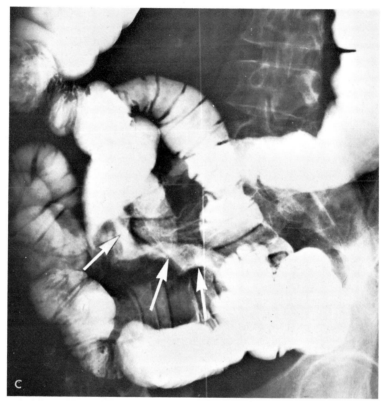

Figure 18-16 Continued   C, Metastatic carcinoma from the colon. There is a large, irregular ulceration (upper left arrow) within a lobulated endoexoenteric mass (lower arrows) in the ileum proximal to the ileotransverse colostomy. There is only minimal obstruction. This appearance is also seen with other submucosal tumors such as lymphosarcoma.

Group 2

In Group 2, the metastatic mass arises in the mesentery rather than in the wall of the bowel. In the initial stage, single or multiple areas of smooth indentation upon the loops of small bowel are seen (Fig. 18-17A). At this stage, the small bowel loops are normally distensible. The appearance is not pathognomonic of metastatic disease, since it is also seen with other retroperitoneal masses. When the mass infiltrates the bowel wall the indentation may become irregular, and fixation of the segment of bowel occurs, associated with obvious evidence of extrinsic pressure along the mesenteric border (Fig. 18-17B). The involved part of the bowel is then flattened or convex toward the lumen. As the mass continues to grow, the appearance is that of segments of small bowel wrapped around a mesenteric mass without evidence of mucosal ulceration or intraluminal polypoid masses (Fig. 18-17C and D). Obstruction in this group is usually associated with angulation and fixation of the intestinal loops. This is in contrast to lymphoma where compression of the bowel loops occurs but usually without fixation, angulation, or intimate adherence to the bowel wall.

(Text continued on page 376.)

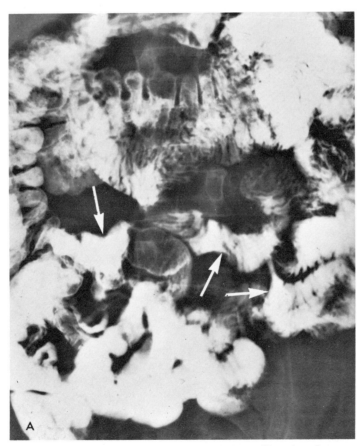

Figure 18-17 A, *Metastatic carcinoma* from retroperitoneal lymph nodes, primary unknown. Metastatic nodules produce separation of the loops of bowel with evidence of extrinsic pressure (arrows).

(Illustration continued on following page.)

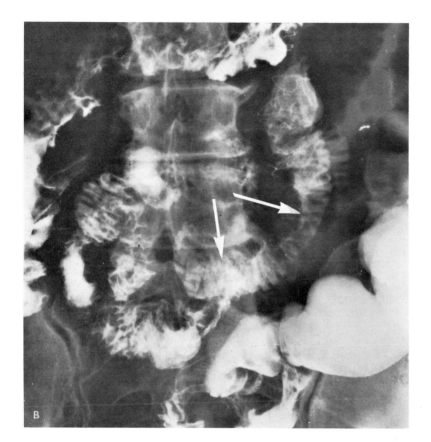

Figure 18-17 Continued B, Metastatic carcinoma, primary unknown. Fixation of the loop with invasion of the mesenteric aspect (arrows) is demonstrated.

Figure 18-17 C, Metastatic carcinoma from the lungs. Fixation and infiltration of several loops of bowel around a mesenteric mass are seen. At this time partial intestinal obstruction is evident.

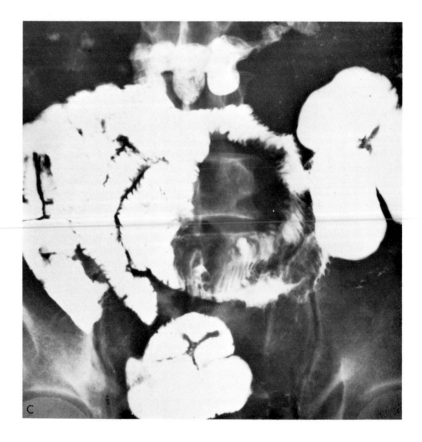

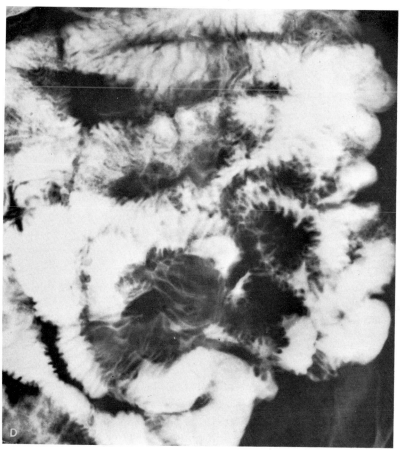

Figure 18-17 *Continued D, Metastatic carcinoma.* Fixation and infiltration of the mid-intestinal loops.

These four cases show the varying degrees of involvement of the bowel wall by large mesenteric masses.

Group 3

In Group 3, multiple implants produce changes not only in the wall of the bowel but also in the mesentery. This results in multiple areas of eccentric or concentric constriction with intervening segments of dilatation. The folds in the narrowed segments are distorted and not destroyed (Fig. 18-18A). The metastatic process in the mesentery produces shortening, rigidity, and thickening of this structure. As a result of the shortening of the mesentery, the small intestine appears short. Shortening of the mesentery is also associated with a peculiar crowding of the valvulae conniventes, which may be referred to as "pleating" or "shirring." This roentgen appearance is similar to that noted in small intestinal intubation (Fig. 18-18B and C).

The small bowel at the ligament of Treitz presents a rather special problem because both metastatic lesions and extension into the bowel from carcinoma of the pancreas are frequent in this area (Fig. 18-19A and B). Since the bowel in the region of the ligament of Treitz may be obscured by the overlying stomach, a supine or lateral decubitus projection may provide better visualization (Fig. 18-19B). Often the first suspicion of the presence of a tumor in this area arises from the presence of dilatation of the proximal portion of the duodenum. Distortion, fixation, and stretching of the folds, irregular ulcerations, and obstruction are features which should suggest an infiltrating neoplasm in the region of the ligament of Treitz.

As a result of extensive involvement of the mesentery and bowel wall, there may be ascites. Ascites can be recognized by bulging flanks and the central position of the small intestinal loops. On occasion a peculiar appearance of the valvulae conniventes, a "herringbone" configuration, is seen (Fig. 18-20A). This pattern is presumably due to trapped air distributed throughout the bowel, producing an air contrast study. This is best seen with partial intestinal obstruction and is more commonly noted with metastatic lesions, but not in ascites or diseases of other etiologies.

Because of the marked mesenteric involvement, there is fixation and drawing together of the bowel loops with central location of the loops, which remain fixed despite changes in position of the patient (Fig. 18-20B and C). Occasionally, the eccentric clumping and fixation of loops by carcinomatosis produce a pseudointernal hernia configuration (Fig. 18-21A).

Plain roentgenograms of the abdomen may be diagnostic of carcinomatosis. These show segments of irregularly contoured, dilated loops of small bowel scattered in different portions of the abdomen. If this appearance is associated with bulging of the flanks and central location of the bowel, the presence of metastatic carcinoma is likely (Fig. 18-21B). Fixed soft intrusions on the gas column of dilated loops may also be seen. An occasional finding is the presence of multiple small, psammoma-like calcifications. These are tiny, 1 to 2 mm. in diameter, and so faint that they may be overlooked (Fig. 18-22). On occasion, the calcific densities in metastatic tumors may be large and irregular, and may superficially resemble calcified mesenteric lymph nodes or uterine fibroids. Metastatic calcifications, however, tend to be less confluent and less dense in contrast to those seen in fibroids and lymph nodes, where these are lumpy, confluent, and sharply defined. Peritonitis with ascites resulting from an inflammatory process such as tuberculosis may produce some of the findings described.

(*Text continued on page 385.*)

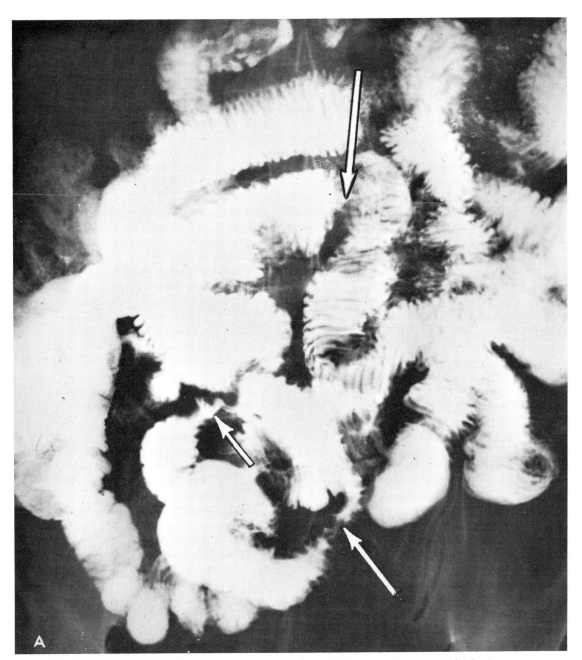

Figure 18-18 A, Metastatic carcinoma, primary unknown. There are multiple short segments of irregular narrowing where the mucosal folds are distorted, blunted, and fixed (arrows). The intervening bowel segments are slightly dilated due to obstruction. There is no discrete mass, nor is there mucosal ulceration. The bowel appears short, presumably from mesenteric infiltration, and its central location suggests ascites.

(Illustration continued on following page.)

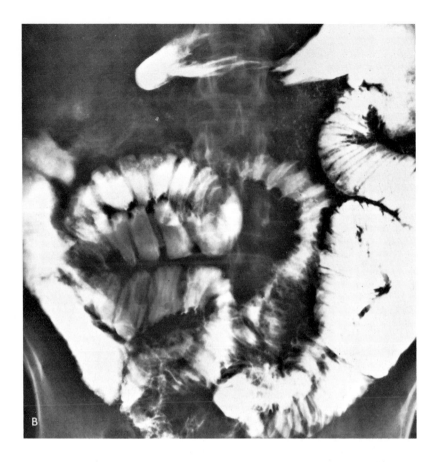

Figure 18-18 B, Metastatic carcinoma from the ovary. There is partial intestinal obstruction secondary to multiple irregular narrowed segments of ileum. The dilated bowel on the left side of the abdomen is due to obstruction. On the right, the loop is not only dilated but fixed, and the valvulae are separated. This is due to both obstruction and adjacent mesenteric involvement. The long narrowed segment in the midabdomen shows irregular indentations due to mural infiltration and is separated from adjacent loops because of the mesenteric mass.

Figure 18-18 C, Metastatic carcinoma from the ovary. Advanced cases of metastatic disease demonstrating multiple areas of alternating narrowing and dilatation with fixation, angulation of the bowel loops, shortening, and ascites.

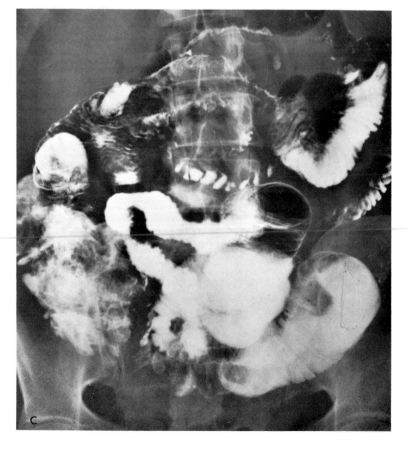

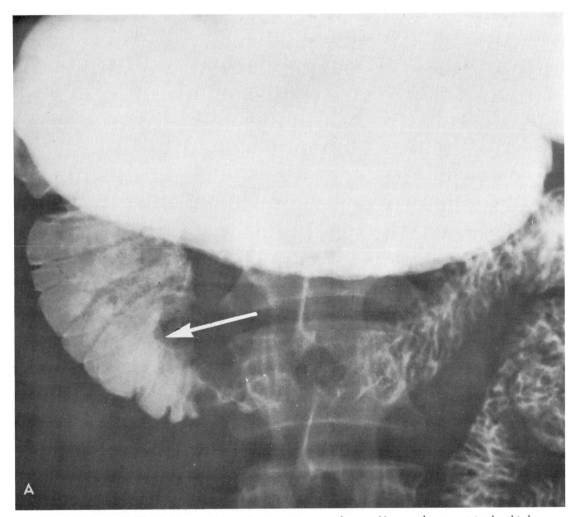

Figure 18-19 *A, Metastatic carcinoma, primary unknown.* Narrowed segment in the third portion of the duodenum (arrow) with thickened nodular folds and obstruction. It is impossible to distinguish invasion by carcinoma of the pancreas from metastatic implants in this region.

(Illustration continued on following page.)

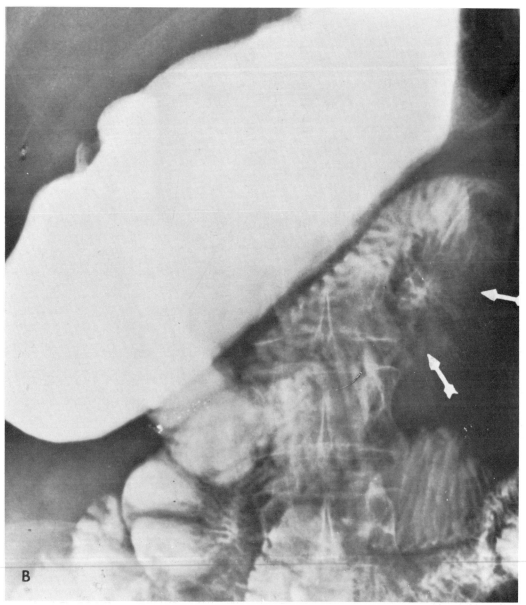

Figure 18-19 *Continued* **B,** *Metastatic carcinoma from the cervix.* There is an obstructing lesion at the ligament of Treitz, which is best visualized in the lateral decubitus position (arrows).

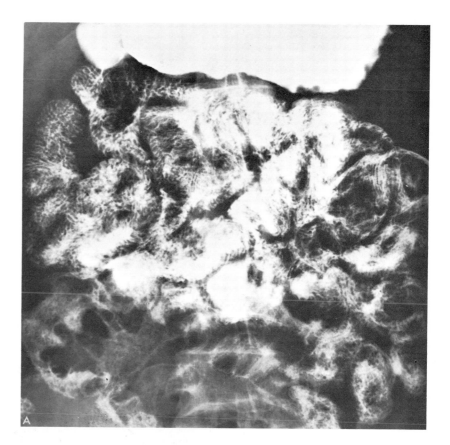

Figure 18-20 Metastatic carcinoma from fundus of stomach. A, The central location of the small intestine with bulging flanks is due to ascites. The normal feathery appearance of the mucosal folds is enhanced by trapped intraluminal air.

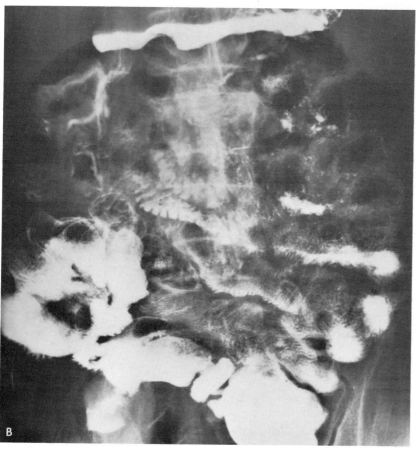

Figure 18-20 B, An erect roentgenogram of the same patient shows no change in the position of the small intestine. This is presumably due to a combination of fixation of the bowel and the mesentery, and ascites.

(Illustration continued on following page.)

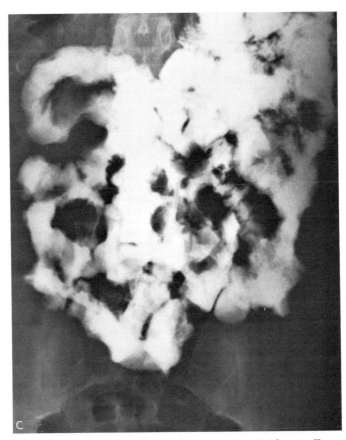

Figure 18-20 Continued   C, Metastatic carcinoma, primary unknown. Erect study. There are multiple small, sharply demarcated pressure defects on the loops of small bowel. The mucosa is intact. The ascites was minimal and the fixed location of the loops was due to extrinsic carcinomatosis. (Courtesy of H. Johnson, M.D., Riverside Hospital, Jacksonville, Florida.)

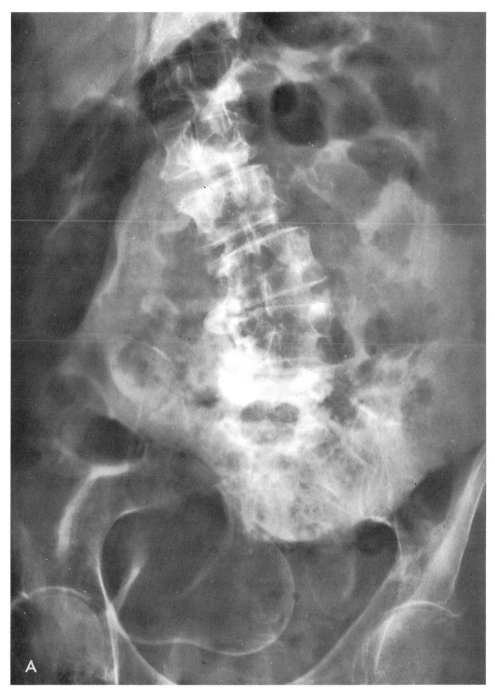

Figure 18-21 *A, Abdominal carcinomatosis, primary unknown.* The large central irregular mass is due to matted, fixed mesentery and small bowel infiltrated by metastatic carcinoma. Free intraperitoneal air outlines the cecum and accentuates the mass which simulates an internal hernia.

(Illustration continued on following page.)

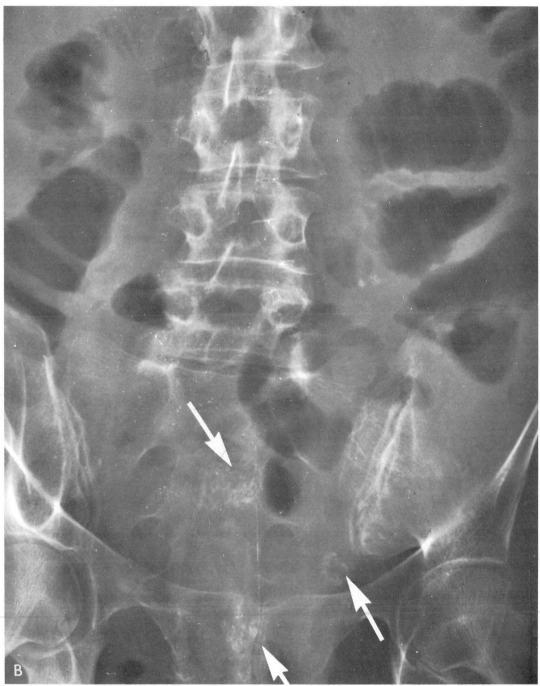

Figure 18-21 Continued *B, Metastatic carcinoma from the appendix.* Multiple dilated small bowel segments, some of which have irregular contours and a conical appearance, are scattered in the abdomen. This is due to trapped air secondary to multiple partial obstructions. The calcifications are within metastases and are larger than psammoma bodies (arrows).

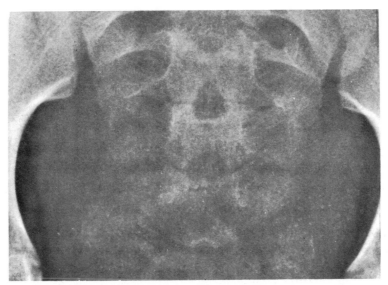

Figure 18-22 Multiple punctate psammoma-like calcifications are seen in the pelvis of an 11 year old child. Diagnosis: Undifferentiated carcinoma, probably arising in teratoma of ovary.

Differential Diagnosis

When a metastatic lesion presents as a solitary defect, differentiation from a primary tumor may not be possible. However, the classic appearance of a primary carcinoma with a short segment of stenosis and symmetric overhanging edges is uncommon in a metastatic process. The ulcerations in metastatic tumors, when present, are usually larger and more irregular, and the bowel is frequently angulated and fixed at the site of the tumor. Intestinal obstruction, although present in both, is usually more marked in primary carcinoma. A metastatic process presenting as a single constricting lesion must also be distinguished from inflammatory lesions, a stricture secondary to infarction, and a lymphoma, specifically Hodgkin's disease. Irregularity of the contour and eccentricity of the process are features not ordinarily found in segmental infarction, where the walls are more often tapering and conical. In regional enteritis, single short segments of involvement are rare, and the inflammatory nature of the process will usually be evident by characteristic mucosal changes. In lymphosarcoma, there is often local dilatation of the bowel lumen despite the infiltrating nature of the tumor process. Hodgkin's disease, on the other hand, may produce narrowing and irregularity of the contour, as seen in metastatic or primary carcinoma. When a large mass is present, obviously displacing adjacent small bowel, both lymphoma and metastatic disease must be considered. Angulation and fixation as well as direct involvement of the bowel by retroperitoneal lymphosarcoma is not common, and lymphoma of this type is rarely associated with any significant degree of obstruction.

The chief problem in differential diagnosis in the region of the ligament of Treitz is direct extension from a carcinoma of the pancreas. In most of these instances, the possibility of metastatic disease will arise only when a previous primary neoplasm has been evident.

Metastatic carcinoma which has caused shortening of the mesentery and

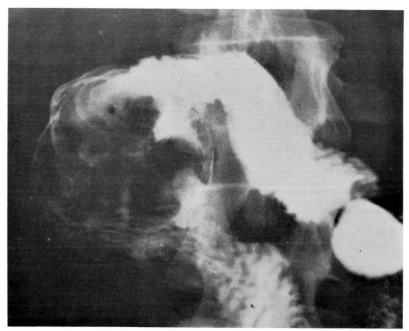

Figure 18-23 Metastatic hypernephroma to second portion of duodenum, producing a large, bulky, irregular mass.

multiple areas of narrowing and intervening dilatation may result in a superficial resemblance to granulomatous ileojejunitis. Absence of involvement of the terminal ileum suggests metastatic disease. Moreover, in metastatic carcinoma confined to the wall of the bowel or the adjacent mesentery, the mucosal folds, although distorted and angulated, are still present, and diffuse ulceration and a cobblestone pattern are not evident. Sinus tracts and fistulas are uncommon in metastatic carcinoma.

Hypernephromas on occasion metastasize by direct extension to the adjacent small bowel. Since the original lesion is primarily cellular, with little desmoplastic reaction, the metastases have a similar cellular appearance, producing a large, bulky, irregular mass. This is most often seen in the second portion of the duodenum (Fig. 18-23), but may also be observed in the small bowel or colon.

References

1. Eaton, Jr., S. B. and Ferrucci, Jr., J. T.: Radiology of the Pancreas and Duodenum. Philadelphia, W. B. Saunders Co., 1973. p. 299.
2. Good, C. A.: Tumors of the small intestine. *Am. J. Roentgen.*, 89:685-705, 1963.
3. DeCastro, C. A., Dockerty, M. B., and Mayo, C. W.: Metastatic tumors of small intestines. *Surg. Gynec. Obstet.*, 105:159-165, 1957.
4. Graham, W. P., III, and Goldman, L.: Gastrointestinal metastases from carcinoma of breast. *Ann. Surg.*, 159:477-480, 1964.
5. Legré, J., Padovani, J., Salamon, G., and Clement, J. P.: Tumeur métastatique du grêle. *J. Radiol. Electrol.*, 44:126-127, 1963.
6. Tillotson, P. M., and Douglas, G. R.: Metastatic tumor of small intestine: three cases presenting unusual clinical and roentgenographic findings. *Am. J. Roentgenol.*, 88:702-706, 1962.
7. Willis, R. A. The Spread of Tumours in the Human Body. Second edition. Butterworth & Co., Ltd., London, 1952.

19

Patterns of Spread of Malignancy to the Small Bowel

by MORTON A. MEYERS, M.D.

The spread of neoplasms within the peritoneal cavity occurs by intraperitoneal seeding, embolic metastases, direct invasion, and lymphatic extension.[1,2] Recent insights and basic correlation with the pathogenesis of the intra-abdominal spread of malignancies have established that the *pattern* of involvement as well as the individual effects of secondary malignancies of the bowel often present characteristic roentgen features.[1,3,4,6] These reflect the mode of dissemination and thereby indicate the primary site. Distinction between the major pathways of spread is of critical practical importance: (*1*) It correlates the roentgen changes closely with the pathogenesis and provides a rational system for radiologic analysis. (*2*) Since it is not rare for a malignant neoplasm to be manifested initially by its gastrointestinal metastasis or extension,[6] recognition of the *type* of secondary involvement can aid in the search for the primary lesion. Confronted with a lesion of the bowel which he can identify as secondary in nature, the clinical radiologist is then in a crucial position—by recognizing the particular mode of dissemination—to determine the further investigation in the search for the primary lesion. (*3*) If there is a known primary tumor and gastrointestinal symptoms develop, particular radiologic attention can be directed to the most likely secondary sites in the abdomen for that type of lesion. (*4*) Identification of the type of secondary involvement of bowel can help in planning treatment. Awareness that involvement of a portion of the alimentary tract is secondary to invasion from an adjacent primary tumor allows for adequate preoperative preparation for wider surgical excision. Localized embolic metastases are subject to segmental resection.[6,7] Radiotherapy and chemotherapy may be reserved for disseminated metastases or implants.

INTRAPERITONEAL SEEDING

It has been generally assumed that transcoelomic spread is random or, at least, a function of serosal implantation in the immediate area of a primary neoplasm. Recent observations, however, have shown that the deposition and growth of secondarily seeded neoplasms in the abdomen are dependent upon the natural flow of ascites within the peritoneal recesses.[3] In breaking through into the peritoneal cavity, a primary neoplasm or even its intra-abdominal lymph node metastases can shed cells into the ascitic fluid induced. The degree of ascites need not be great for the transportation and deposition of malignant cells. Investigative fluoroscopic and roentgen observations following the intra-peritoneal instillation of positive contrast medium clearly and consistently demonstrate that intraperitoneal fluid, rather than being static, continually follows a circulation through the abdomen.[3, 8, 9] These dynamic pathways of distribution and sequential spread are dependent particularly on mesenteric reflections and peritoneal recesses, as well as on the forces of gravity and negative subdiaphragmatic pressure.

The peritoneal cavity is subdivided by peritoneal reflections and mesenteric attachments into several compartments and recesses (Fig. 19-1A).

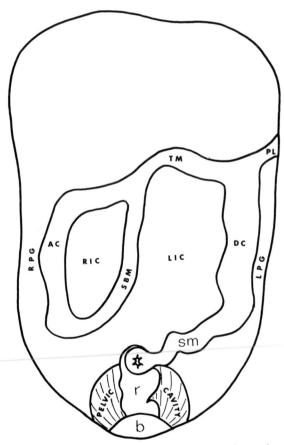

Figure 19–1 A, Posterior peritoneal reflections and intra-abdominal spaces. TM = transverse mesocolon; PL = phrenicocolic ligament; SMB = small bowel mesentery; AC = attachment of ascending colon; DC = attachment of descending colon; SM = sigmoid mesocolon; r = rectum; b = urinary bladder; RIC = right infracolic space; LIC = left infracolic space; RPG = right paracolic gutter; LPG = left paracolic gutter. (From Meyers, M. A.: Distribution of intra-abdominal malignant seeding: Dependency on dynamics of flow of ascitic fluid. *The American Journal of Roentgenology, Radium Therapy and Nuclear Medicine.* Reproduced with permission.)

These are anatomically continuous, either directly or indirectly. The major barrier dividing the abdominal cavity is the *transverse mesocolon*. Below this, the obliquely oriented *small bowel mesentery* divides the inframesocolic space into two compartments of unequal size: the *right* and *left infracolic spaces.* Its main axis, nevertheless, is directed toward the right lower quadrant in relation to the terminal ileum and cecum. The right infracolic space terminates at their junction. The left infracolic space is anatomically open to the pelvis to the right of the midline; toward the left, it is restricted from continuity with the pelvis cavity by the sigmoid mesocolon. The *right* and *left paracolic gutters* are lateral to the attachments of the peritoneal reflections of the ascending and descending colon. They represent potential communications between the lower abdomen and pelvis below, with the supramesocolic area above. On the left, however, the phrenicocolic ligament[10] partially separates the paracolic gutter from the perisplenic (left subphrenic) space. The *pelvis* is the most dependent portion of the peritoneal cavity in either the supine or erect position. Its compartments include the midline cul-de-sac or *pouch of Douglas* (rectovaginal pouch in the female and rectovesical pouch in the male) and the *lateral paravesical recesses.*

The transverse mesocolon, small bowel mesentery, sigmoid mesocolon, and the peritoneal attachments of the ascending and descending colon serve as

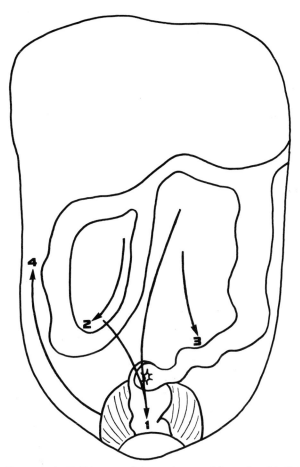

Figure 19–1 Continued B, Diagram of the pathways of flow of ascitic fluid and the four predominant sites. (From Meyers, M. A.: Distribution of intra-abdominal malignant seeding: Dependency on dynamics of flow of ascitic fluid. *The American Journal of Roentgenology, Radium Therapy and Nuclear Medicine.* Reproduced with permission.)

watersheds directing the flow of ascites (Fig. 19-1*B*). The force of gravity operates to pool peritoneal fluid in dependent peritoneal recesses. Fluid in the inframesocolic compartments preferentially seeks the pelvic cavity. From the left infracolic space, flow is directed along the right side of the rectum. Some fluid is temporarily arrested along the superior plane of the sigmoid mesocolon but gradually channels into the pelvis. From the right infracolic space, spread occurs along the small bowel mesentery. It is not until a pool is formed at the apex, at the termination of the ileum with the cecum, that some begins to overflow into the pelvis. From this point the fluid ascends both paracolic gutters. Passage up the shallower left one is slow and weak, and cephalad extension is limited by the phrenicocolic ligament. The major flow from the pelvis is up the right paracolic gutter. This recess serves also as the main communication from the upper to the lower abdominal compartments.

Four predominant sites are therefore clearly identified for the preferential, repeated, or arrested flow of ascitic fluid: (*1*) the pelvic cavity, particularly the pouch of Douglas; (*2*) the right lower quadrant at the termination of the small bowel mesentery; (*3*) the superior aspect of the sigmoid mesocolon; and (*4*) the right paracolic gutter. These pathways are illustrated in Figure 19–1*B*. Analysis of a series of proved cases from The New York Hospital and Memorial Hospital for Cancer and Allied Diseases has shown that the sites of lodgement and growth of intraperitoneal seeded metastases clearly follow the pathways of flow of ascitic fluid.[3] In males, the primary carcinoma most commonly arises in the gastrointestinal tract (stomach, colon, pancreas) and in females, in the genital system (ovary).[11, 12] Stasis or pooling of ascitic fluid favors the processes of deposition, fixation, and growth of seeded malignant cells. The seeded deposits coalesce and are then fixed to the serosal surfaces by fibrinous adhesions which quickly become organized.[13]

Seeding in the pouch of Douglas is the most common and is identifiable in 56 per cent of those cases with involvement of the peritoneal cavity at single or multiple sites. On barium enema study, the process results in a characteristic pattern of fixed parallel folds or a nodular indentation upon the anterior aspect of the rectosigmoid junction.[1, 3] These changes reflect the coalescence of deposits with a dense fibrous reaction which may be clinically palpable as the classic Blumer's shelf.[14]

The root of the small bowel mesentery extends from the left side of the second lumbar vertebra near the duodenojejunal junction downward to the right, across the aorta and inferior vena cava, to the cecocolic junction near the right sacroiliac joint, a distance of only 15 cm. From the root, a series of mesenteric ruffles support the small bowel loops (Fig. 19–2). It is these fan-like mesenteric extensions which contribute to the characteristic undulating nature and position of the coils of small bowel, which averages 15 to 20 feet in length. A series of peritoneal recesses is thus formed extending along the right side of the ruffled small bowel mesentery obliquely toward the right lower quadrant of the abdomen. It has been shown that these also serve to pool collections of ascitic fluid.[1, 3, 4] Spread here occurs in a series of cascades or rivulets from one mesenteric ruffle to the next, directed along the axis of the small bowel mesentery toward the right lower quadrant in relation to distal ileal loops and the cecum (Fig. 19–3). It is here, within the lower recesses of the small bowel mesentery, that the most consistent pool of fluid forms before overflow into the pelvis occurs.

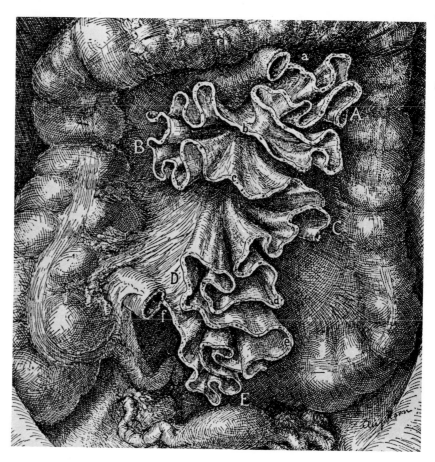

Figure 19–2 The small bowel mesentery, illustrating its ruffled nature. A series of peritoneal recesses is formed along its right side. (From Kelly, H. A.: Appendicitis and other Diseases of the Vermiform Appendix. J. B. Lippincott Co., Philadelphia, 1909. Reproduced with permission.)

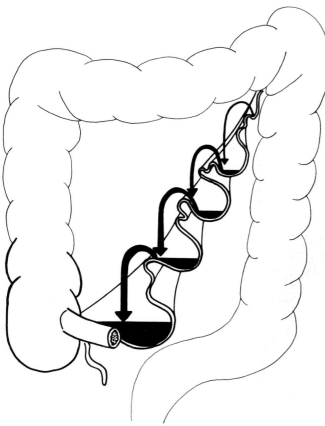

Figure 19–3 The flow of ascites forms a series of pools within the recesses of the small bowel mesentery. The most consistent drainage is to its lower end, in relation to distal ileal loops and the cecum. (From Meyers, M. A.: Malignant seeding along small bowel mesentery: roentgen features. *The American Journal of Roentgenology, Radium Therapy and Nuclear Medicine.* Reproduced with permission.)

Seeded deposits lodging within the lower recesses of the small bowel mesentery in the right infracolic space are clinically identifiable in over 40 per cent of cases by their displacement of distal ileal loops, perhaps with pressure effects also upon the medial contour of the cecum and ascending colon.

Symmetric growth within multiple adjacent mesenteric recesses results in discrete separation of ileal loops in the right lower quadrant. Angulated tethering of the mucosal folds indicates an associated desmoplastic response. Significantly, these and any serosal masses are therefore identifiable on the concave (mesenteric) borders.[4] The narrowed loops may be aligned in a parallel configuration which we describe as "palisading" (Fig. 19–4). The axis of the serosal masses as well as of the affected intestinal loops conforms to the axis of the small bowel mesentery. As the seeded growths become somewhat larger, they may displace the bowel loops in a gently arcuate manner (Fig. 19–5). The striking symmetry of size, mass displacement from the mesenteric border of the loops and orientation to the concave mesenteric borders in the right lower quadrant characterize the process (Fig. 19–6).

If the desmoplastic response to the seeded metastases is severe, marked fixation and angulation of ileal loops in the right lower quadrant result (Figs. 19–7 and 19–8). The most extreme fibrous reaction has been encountered in metastatic seeding from pancreatic carcinoma and mucin-producing gastric carcinoma. Serosal mass displacement may remain evident. The points of acute angulation tend to conform to the axis of the mesentery. Despite the narrowing and sharp course, obstruction may not be conspicuous.

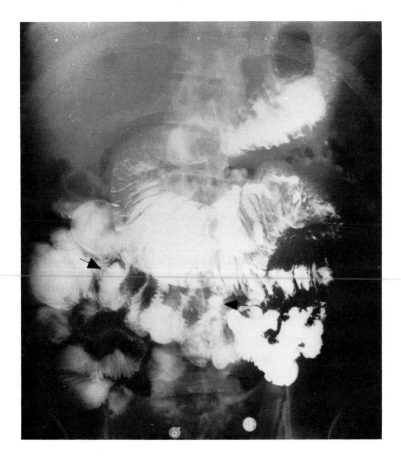

Figure 19–4 Seeded gastric carcinoma along lower small bowel mesentery. There is palisaded separation of ileal loops in the right lower quadrant (arrows). Mucosal folds are mildly tethered. (Sites of obstruction are also present proximally.) (From Meyers, M. A.: Malignant seeding along small bowel mesentery: roentgen features. *The American Journal of Roentgenology, Radium Therapy and Nuclear Medicine.* Reproduced with permission.)

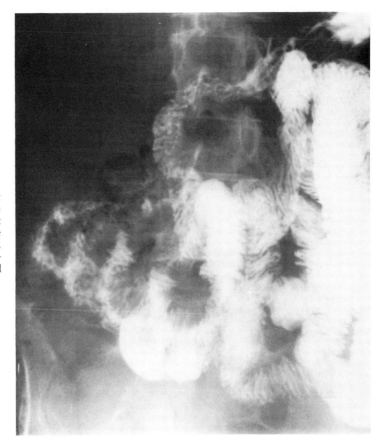

Figure 19–5 *Seeded ovarian carcinoma along lower small bowel mesentery.* There is striking scalloped displacement of multiple ileal loops in the right lower quadrant, following the axis of the mesenteric recesses. The mucosal folds are mildly tethered. (Meyers, M. A., and McSweeney, J.: Secondary neoplasms of the bowel. From *Radiology.* Reproduced with permission.)

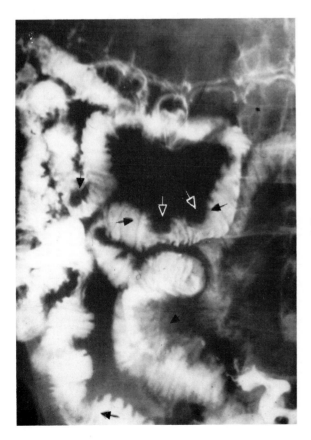

Figure 19–6 *Seeded gastric carcinoma along lower small bowel mesentery.* Multiple extrinsic, serosal masses (arrows) are localized to the mesenteric sides of ileal loops in the right lower quadrant.

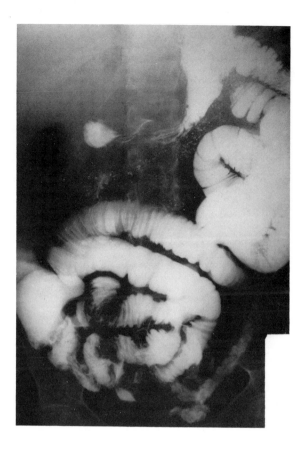

Figure 19-7 *Seeded ovarian carcinoma along lower small bowel mesentery.* Nodular serosal masses on the mesenteric borders of distal ileal loops are associated with fibrotic narrowing and angulation. These produce some proximal obstruction.

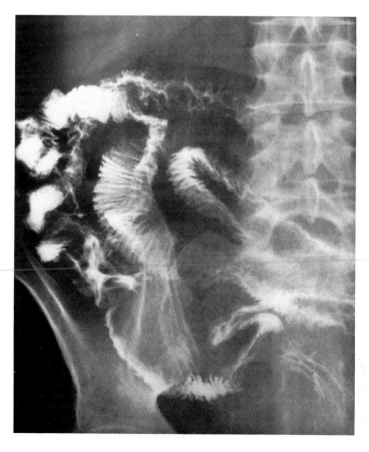

Figure 19-8 *Seeded pancreatic carcinoma along lower small bowel mesentery.* Mass separation and striking angulation of fixed ileal loops in right lower quadrant from extensive desmoplastic reaction. (From Meyers, M. A.: Malignant seeding along small bowel mesentery: roentgen features. *The American Journal of Roentgenology, Radium Therapy and Nuclear Medicine.* Reproduced with permission.)

If no significant fibrous reaction is elicited as the metastases increase in size, gross extrinsic mass displacement may be shown (Fig. 19–9). The mesenteric masses, however, tend to be multiple and they maintain their relationship to the lower small bowel mesentery. They displace ileal loops predominantly inferiorly and medially and may exert pressure upon the ascending colon medially and the proximal transverse colon inferiorly.

Since the small bowel mesentery most commonly inserts at the cecocolic junction, the effects of seeded metastases upon the cecum are shown typically upon its medial and inferior contours.[4] The level of involvement is thus usually below the ileocecal valve in the caput of the cecum. The extrinsic mass indenting the cecum may be smooth or lobulated (Fig. 19–10), of variable size, and at times may encircle the cecum. The mass changes upon the cecum are not, in themselves, specific for seeded metastases and may simulate appendiceal abnormalities, other mesenteric masses, or even primary lesions of the cecum. However, they are almost invariably accompanied by the more characteristic changes involving distal small bowel loops. If first discovered by a barium enema study, these can be identified by reflux into the terminal ileum or in a subsequent small bowel series. The association of findings may occasionally closely simulate granulomatous ileocolitis[15] (Fig. 19–11). The small bowel alterations are usually not difficult to distinguish from other common disease states. The lack of inflammatory features such as spasm, ulcerations, and sinus tracts and the characteristic spectrum of changes help in the differential diagnosis from regional enteritis, tuberculosis, amebiasis, and peritoneal adhesions.

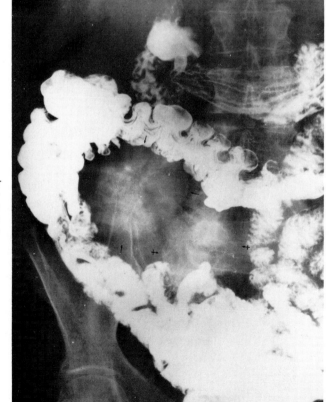

Figure 19–9 *Seeded ovarian carcinoma along lower small bowel mesentery.* Two masses with psammomatous calcifications (arrows) in the right lower quadrant displace ileal loops and press upon the ascending and transverse colon. (From Meyers, M. A., and McSweeney, J.: Secondary neoplasms of the bowel. *Radiology.* Reproduced with permission.)

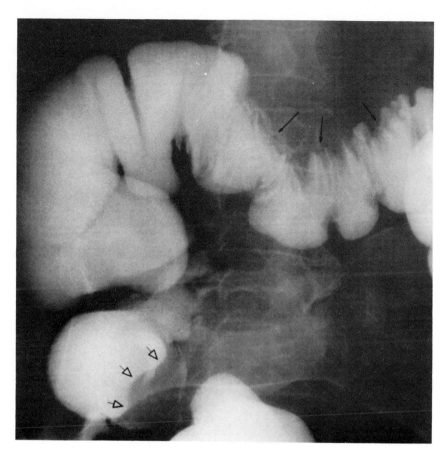

Figure 19–10 Carcinoma of the gallbladder. Seeding in the right lower quadrant results in a mass eccentrically indenting the medial contour of the cecum (open arrows). There is also direct invasion of the transverse colon (black arrows). (From Meyers, M. A.: Malignant seeding along small bowel mesentery: roentgen features. *The American Journal of Roentgenology, Radium Therapy and Nuclear Medicine.* Reproduced with permission.)

When the seeded metastases are diffuse throughout the small bowel (Fig. 19–12), the changes secondary to the desmoplastic process may resemble carcinoid or radiation enteritis. Fixed angulation and alternating areas of narrowing and dilatation are accompanied by serosal masses identifiable on the mesenteric borders and conspicuous tethering of mucosal folds.

Lodgement and growth of deposits arrested along the barrier of the sigmoid mesocolon in the left lower quadrant result in irregular, nodular changes characteristically localized to the superior border of the sigmoid colon. The associated desmoplastic reaction causes tethering of the mucosal folds. This localization occurs in over 20 per cent of cases of metastatic seeding.[3]

Flow of ascitic fluid from the pelvis is preferentially upward within the right paracolic gutter. Egress from the pelvis upward is not a function simply of overflow. Fluid surmounts the sacral promontory and flank muscles to extend upward, whether the patient is horizontal or erect. In addition to the anatomic pathways and action of gravity, variations in intraperitoneal pressure also determine the distribution of peritoneal fluid. The hydrostatic pressure of the contents of the abdominal cavity together with the flexibility of a portion of the abdominal walls determine, for the most part, the pressure within the abdominal cavity. The intraperitoneal pressure in the upper abdomen is subatmospheric and decreases further during inspiration. This negative subdiaphragmatic pressure and its relation to breathing are maintained in the horizontal or erect position. This is explained by the outward movement of the ribs during inspiration,

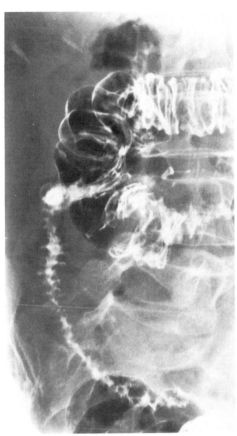

Figure 19–11 Seeded pancreatic carcinoma along lower small bowel mesentery. Barium enema with air-contrast studies demonstrate changes involving the cecum and terminal ileum closely simulating granulomatous ileocolitis. (From Meyers, M. A., Oliphant, M., Teixidor, H., and Weiser, P.: Metastatic carcinoma simulating inflammatory colitis. *The American Journal of Roentgenology, Radium Therapy and Nuclear Medicine.* Reproduced with permission.)

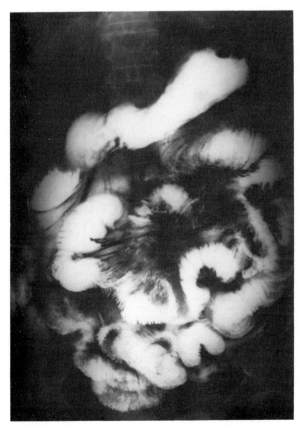

Figure 19–12 Diffuse seeded metastases from gastric carcinoma along small bowel mesentery. Serosal masses are present predominantly on the mesenteric borders of small bowel loops, including the ileum in the right lower quadrant. The mucosal folds are tethered, and there are angulations and alternating constrictions of loops. These changes are consequent to the fibrotic reaction.

which enlarges the space in the upper abdomen more than it is decreased by the descent of the diaphragm. Deposition and growth in this peritoneal process, particularly its inferior portion, are shown by mass changes lateral and posterior to the cecum and proximal ascending colon. Tethering of mucosal folds or angulated fixation of a small bowel loop in this area may occur as a consequence of an associated fibrous reaction. This localization occurs in 18 per cent of cases.[3]

Multiple sites of seeded deposition are somewhat more common than a solitary focus. Seeding in other disparate sites may be related to adhesions, perhaps resulting from previous abdominal operations.

EMBOLIC METASTASES

The commonest primary neoplasms which embolize to bowel include melanoma and tumors of breast and lung. The presenting picture is usually one of incomplete obstruction or bleeding, often occurring several years after treatment of the original neoplasm. At times, the symptoms of the bowel metastases may be the first clinical manifestation of an occult primary malignancy.[6, 7, 16, 17] Partial or complete obstruction is the result of the bulk of the metastatic mass, accompanied by either angulation of the bowel from a fibrotic response or intussusception. The appearance of a hematogenous metastasis to bowel is dependent upon the characteristics of the lesion.[1] These include both the degree of vascularity in relation to the rate of growth and the desmoplastic capabilities.

Metastatic melanoma is by far the commonest of these tumors to be clinically encountered, and it may be taken as a prototype. The hematogenous deposition is usually in the submucosal layer, and growth typically results in intramural masses with a bulky polypoid extension into the lumen.[6, 7] There is no significant desmoplastic response. Central ulceration is especially common as the metastasis outgrows its blood supply, producing a "bull's eye" or "target" lesion (Fig. 19–13). Characteristically, the borders of the filling defect are well defined and the ulcer is quite large in proportion to the metastatic mass. Rarely, the central collection is not necessarily secondary to necrotic ulceration but may reflect an epithelialized umbilication on the intraluminal surface of the metastasis.[18] However, linear fissures over the surface of the mass radiating distinctly to the central collection invariably indicate ulceration. This produces what we have designated as a "spoke-wheel" pattern.[1]

Dissemination may be single but is more commonly multiple. While the lesions of metastatic melanoma may involve any portion of the alimentary tract, they tend to be more numerous and more frequent in the small bowel. When multiple, they may be either widespread or confined to a segment of intestine (Fig. 19–14). This reflects their mode and periodicity of vascular distribution.[1] Diffuse metastases are often of different sizes, indicating periodic embolic showers. At times, the secondary deposits are present within the field of a specific arterial distribution when, typically, the nodules are of approximately the same size (Fig. 19–14). A further observation which is very useful in identifying such submucosal masses as embolic metastases relates to their specific sites on the bowel wall.[1] When the lesion is localized to one wall of the bowel, a distinct predilection is shown for the antimesenteric border. In the small intestine this is readily identifiable as the convex margin of the loop, since the

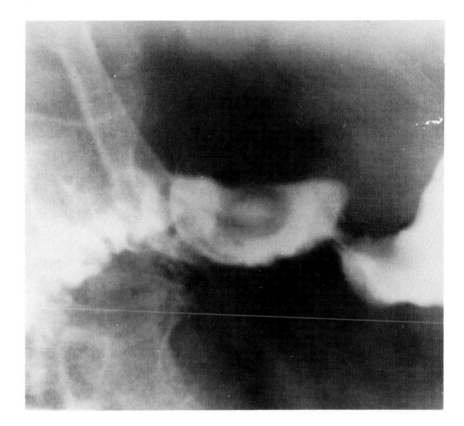

Figure 19–13 Metastatic melanoma to duodenal bulb. A, A filling defect with sharply demarcated borders contains a proportionately large ulcer crater. These features are helpful in identifying this lesion as a submucosal nodule with secondary central ulceration, in contrast to a benign peptic ulcer with surrounding edema, the borders of which usually fade away gradually.

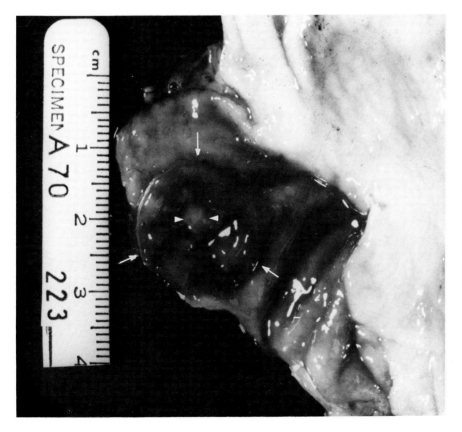

Figure 19–13 B, Gross specimen demonstrates prominent submucosal mass (arrows) with central ulceration (arrowheads). Pathologically, this type of hematogenous metastasis is described as a "buttercup" lesion. (From Meyers, M.A., and McSweeney, J.: Secondary neoplasms of the bowel. *Radiology.* Reproduced with permission.)

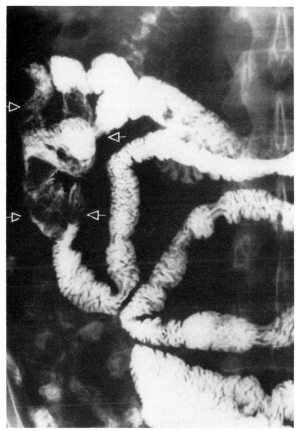

***Figure 19–14* *Metastatic melanoma to small bowel*.** Multiple submucosal masses of approximately equal sizes confined to one segment of small bowel indicate embolic metastases within a discrete arterial distribution.

mesentery supports the concave surface. These findings are apparently related to the entrance of the intestinal vessels on the mesenteric border and their intramural ramifications toward the antimesenteric side. They are in agreement with Coman's experimental work revealing that strictly mechanical and circulatory factors can account for the distribution of some secondary tumors.[19]

Breast metastases to the gastrointestinal tract result in a different pattern. Autopsy series record an incidence of breast metastases to the gastrointestinal tract as high as 16.4 per cent.[16] Attention has been focused on the frequency of the stomach and duodenum as metastatic sites in patients with breast carcinoma being treated with adrenal steroids.[20] The need for surgical intervention for an abdominal complication of the metastasis, often many years after a mastectomy, is not uncommon.[16, 17] The type that gives rise to gastrointestinal metastases and symptoms most commonly is the poorly differentiated breast cancer that grows in rows of small anaplastic cells.[21] No significant desmoplastic response accompanies the highly cellular secondary deposits. While all layers of the bowel wall may be diffusely infiltrated, the majority of the embolic deposits reside in the submucosa,[17] where they are more readily subject to radiologic identification.

Breast metastases to the small bowel may result in single or, more commonly, multiple neoplastic strictures with alternating areas of narrowing and interval dilatations (Fig. 19–15). The stomach is also frequently involved, presenting a linitis plastica appearance.[1] Although no desmoplastic response is

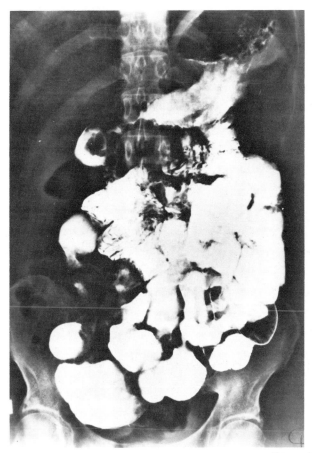

Figure 19–15 *Metastatic breast carcinoma to small bowel. Small bowel series.* There are multiple skip areas of strictures with intervening dilatation. Diffuse submucosal metastases are also present within the stomach, producing the rigid appearance of a linitis plastica. (From Meyers, M. A., Oliphant, M., Teixidor, H., and Weiser, P.: Metastatic carcinoma simulating inflammatory colitis. *The American Journal of Roentgenology, Radium Therapy and Nuclear Medicine.* Reproduced with permission.)

elicited by breast metastases, the highly cellular submucosal deposits may narrow and deform the lumen, resulting in a scirrhous appearance. With small bowel involvement, evidence of hematogenous spread to the colon is also commonly present. The associated spread to the large intestine may be easily mistaken for primary inflammatory processes such as granulomatous ileocolitis both clinically and radiologically.[15] Diarrhea may be a conspicuous clinical presentation, occasionally of several years' duration, and perhaps associated with some blood and mucus. Deep biopsy and cytologic analysis of any ascitic fluid may be confirmatory.

Metastases to the bowel from carcinoma of the lung frequently result in large mesenteric masses, with infiltration of the bowel wall and fixation and angulation of the bowel and its mucosal folds (Fig. 19–16). In such cases, the findings are indistinguishable from those in widespread intra-abdominal metastases from other sources. Occasionally, extensive ulceration supervenes (Fig. 19–17), or the lesions may show as discrete submucosal masses, perhaps with central "bull's eye" ulceration.

Hematogenous metastasis to bowel from a renal carcinoma is rare. In some cases, Batson's vertebral venous plexus is a possible route. It typically presents as a solitary, bulky intramural lesion.[22]

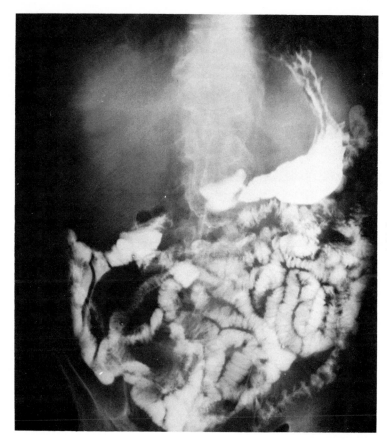

Figure 19–16 *Metastatic lung carcinoma to small bowel.* Hematogenous spread results in large mesenteric masses displacing and fixing intestinal loops.

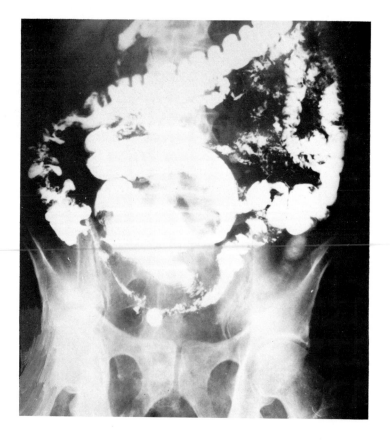

Figure 19–17 *Metastatic lung carcinoma to small bowel.* There is extensive ulceration of dilated fixed ileal loops associated with a large mesenteric mass.

DIRECT INVASION

Intrinsic involvement of the alimentary tract from an immediately contiguous neoplasm indicates a locally aggressive tumor which has usually broken through fascial planes. By virtue of their anatomic relationships, the small bowel loops are much less commonly involved by such direct extension than the colon. Since the second portion of the duodenum descends immediately anterior to the medial aspect of the right kidney, secondary invasion may result from underlying renal neoplasms. This may be seen in clinically occult hypernephromas or as recurrences many years after nephrectomy for malignancy. With growth, they tend to produce bulky intraluminal masses without significant obstruction since they generally elicit no desmoplastic response.[1, 22] Occasionally, however, we have found they may produce luminal narrowing with mucosal destruction simulating a primary carcinoma of the bowel (Fig. 19–18). Recognition of the usual site of involvement and identification of any extraluminal soft-tissue mass lead to the correct diagnosis.

Invasion may also occur from noncontiguous primary tumors by means of mesenteric reflections or direct lymphatic extension. The duodenum is most commonly involved by these processes. As the hepatic flexure of the colon crosses anterior to the descending duodenum, the two structures are in very close anatomic relationship, separated only by the short beginning of the transverse mesocolon[5] (Fig. 19–19). In this way, the paraduodenal area may be involved by direct spread from an infiltrating carcinoma of the hepatic flexure

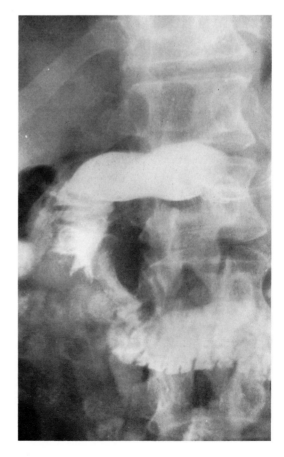

Figure 19–18 Direct invasion of the descending duodenum by right renal hypernephroma. Mucosal destruction simulates a primary neoplasm of the duodenum. (From Meyers, M. A., and McSweeney, J.: Secondary neoplasms of the bowel. *Radiology.* Reproduced with permission.)

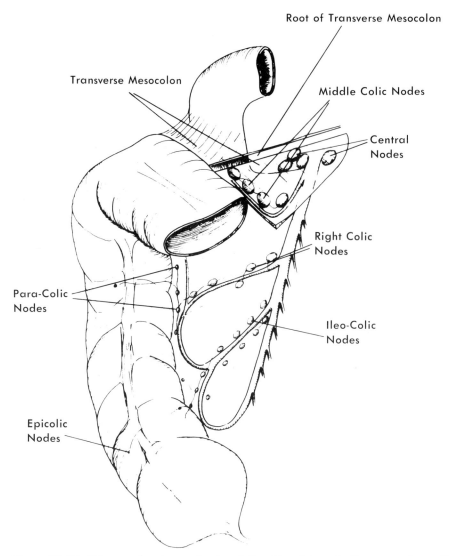

Figure 19–19 Diagram showing anatomic relationship of hepatic flexure to descending duodenum and the lymphatic drainage of the right colon. The central nodes are in relationship to the duodenum.

across the beginning reflection of the transverse mesocolon[5, 23] (Fig. 19–20). Carcinomas of the right colon are notoriously clinically occult and the palpation of an epigastric or right upper quadrant mass in such a patient may lead to initiation of radiologic investigation with an upper gastrointestinal series (Fig. 19–20). This may be very misleading unless the underlying anatomic relationships are kept in mind and a barium enema administered.

Direct lymphatic extension along the draining chain of lymph nodes may be occasionally identifiable by barium studies.[5, 24] By its relationship to the central lymph nodes draining the colon, the duodenum may reflect changes of lymph node spread from a remote carcinoma of the colon. The lymphatic vessels draining the colon parallel the arterial supply. Those draining the right side of the colon are located near the origin of the superior mesenteric artery, in close relationship to the superior border of the horizontal (third) portion of the duodenum (Fig. 19–19). Those draining the distal transverse and descending

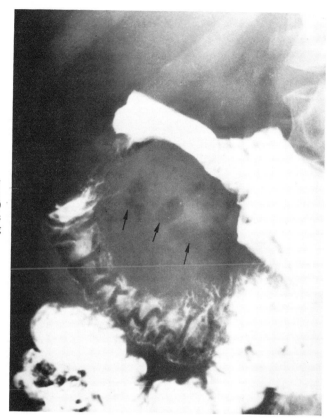

Figure 19–20 Extension of colonic carcinoma across the mesocolon to the paraduodenal area. A, Upper gastrointestinal series reveals numerous gas-containing abscess cavities (arrows) within a mass in the area of the head of the pancreas. There is edema and distortion of the mucosal folds of the descending duodenum.

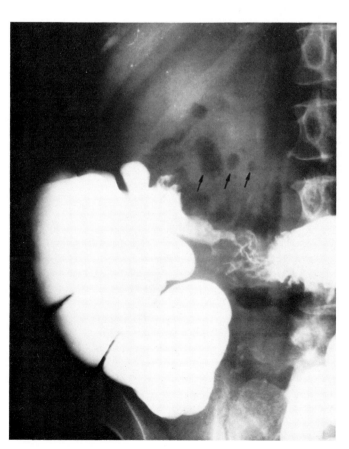

Figure 19–20 B, A subsequent barium enema study shows a primary infiltrating carcinoma of the anterior hepatic flexure with a pericolonic-paraduodenal abscess.

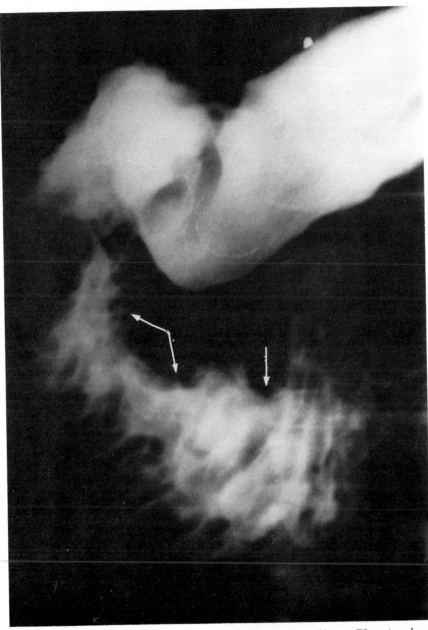

Figure 19-21 *Nodal spread from right colonic carcinoma.* Upper GI series documents metastases within the enlarged, draining lymph nodes by virtue of their extrinsic impressions upon the duodenum (arrows).

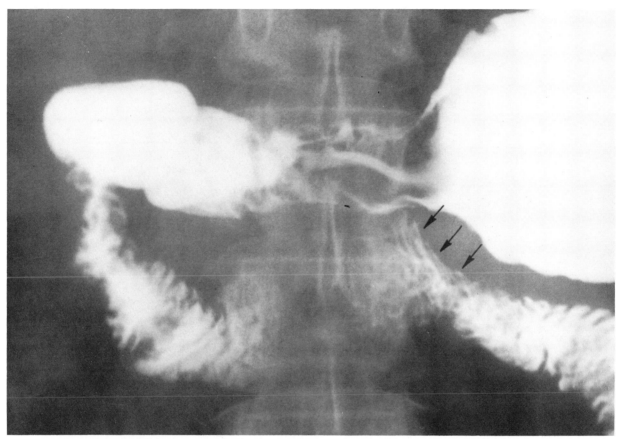

Figure 19–22 *Metastases within the draining central inferior mesenteric lymph nodes* from a carcinoma of the left colon. These are shown by the extrinsic pressure effect upon the lateral aspect of the duodenojejunal junction (arrows). (From Meyers, M. A., and Whalen, J. P.: Roentgen significance of the duodenocolic relationships: An anatomic approach. *The American Journal of Roentgenology, Radium Therapy and Nuclear Medicine.* Reproduced with permission.)

colon are partially located in the transverse mesocolon and near the ascending left colic branch of the inferior mesenteric artery which courses lateral to the ascending (fourth) portion of the duodenum. By roentgenologically recognizing changes of nodal impressions upon the superior contour of the third portion of the duodenum (Fig. 19–21), or upon the lateral aspect of the duodenojejunal junction (Fig. 19–22), it is possible to determine the extent of a colonic carcinoma preoperatively or the development of lymph node metastases postoperatively.[5, 24]

References

1. Meyers, M. A., and McSweeney, J.: Secondary neoplasms of the bowel. *Radiology,* 105:1–11, 1972.
2. Willis, R. A.: The Spread of Tumours in the Human Body. Second edition. Butterworth and Co. Ltd., London, 1952.
3. Meyers, M. A.: Distribution of intra-abdominal malignant seeding: dependency on dynamics of flow of ascitic fluid. *Amer. J. Roentgen.,* 119:198–206, 1973.
4. Meyers, M. A.: Malignant seeding along small bowel mesentery: roentgen features. *Amer. J. Roentgen.,* 123:67–73, 1975.
5. Meyers, M. A., and Whalen, J. P.: Roentgen significance of the duodenocolic relationships: An anatomic approach. *Amer. J. Roentgen.,* 117:263–274, 1973.
6. Farmer, R. G., and Hawk, W. A.: Metastatic tumors of the small bowel. *Gastroenterology,* 47:496–504, 1964.

7. De Castro, C. A., Dockerty, M. B., and Mayo, C. W.: Metastatic tumors of the small intestines. *Internat. Abstr. Surg.* 105:159–165, 1957. In *Surg. Gynec. Obstet.*, June, 1957.

8. Meyers, M. A.: The spread and localization of acute intraperitoneal effusions. *Radiology*, 95:547–554, 1970.

9. Meyers, M. A.: Peritoneography: Normal and pathologic anatomy. *Amer. J. Roentgen.*, 117: 353–365, 1973.

10. Meyers, M. A.: Roentgen significance of the phrenicocolic ligament. *Radiology*, 95:539–545, 1970.

11. Raiford, T. S.: Tumors of small intestine. *AMA Arch. Surg.*, 25:321–355, 1932.

12. Walther, H. E.: Krebsmetastasen. Benno Schwabe, Basel, 1948.

13. Sampson, J. A.: Implantation peritoneal carcinomatosis of ovarian origin. *Amer. J. Path.*, 7:423–443, 1931.

14. Blumer, G.: Rectal shelf: neglected rectal sign of value in diagnosis of obscure malignant and inflammatory disease within abdomen. *Albany M. Ann.*, 30:361, 1909.

15. Meyers, M. A., Oliphant, M., Teixidor, H., and Weiser, P.: Metastatic carcinoma simulating inflammatory colitis. *Amer. J. Roentgen.* 123:74–83, 1975.

16. Asch, M. J., Wiedel, P. D., and Habif, D. V.: Gastrointestinal metastases from carcinoma of the breast: autopsy study and 18 cases requiring operative intervention. *Arch. Surg.*, 96:840–843, 1968.

17. Graham, W. P. III: Gastrointestinal metastases from carcinoma of the breast. *Ann. Surg.*, 159: 477–480, 1964.

18. Pomerantz, H., and Margolin, H. N.: Metastases to the gastrointestinal tract from malignant melanoma. *Amer. J. Roentgen.*, 88:712–717, 1972.

19. Coman, D. R., De Long, R. P., and McCutcheon, M.: Studies on the mechanism of metastasis: the distribution of tumors in various organs in relation to the distribution of arterial emboli. *Cancer Res.*, 11:648–651, 1951.

20. Hartmann, W. H., and Sherlock, P.: Gastroduodenal metastases from carcinoma of the breast: an adrenal steroid-induced phenomenon. *Cancer*, 14:426–431, 1961.

21. Choi, S. H., Sheehan, F. R., and Pickren, J. W.: Metastatic involvement of the stomach by breast cancer. *Cancer*, 17:791–797, 1964.

22. Khilnani, M. T., and Wolf, B. S.: Late involvement of the alimentary tract by carcinoma of the kidney. *Amer. J. Dig. Dis.*, 5:529–540, 1960.

23. Treitel, H., Meyers, M. A., and Maza, V.: Changes in the duodenal loop secondary to carcinoma of the hepatic flexure of the colon. *Brit. J. Radiol.*, 43:209–213, 1970.

24. McCort, J. J.: Roentgenographic appearance of metastases to central lymph nodes of superior mesenteric artery in carcinoma of right colon. *Radiology*, 60:641–646, 1953.

20

Lymphosarcoma, Hodgkin's Disease, and Melanosarcoma

LYMPHOSARCOMA

Studies of lymphoid tumors in all areas of the body are complicated by differences in nomenclature used by authors, and studies in the small bowel are still further complicated by difficulties in determining whether a patient with a small bowel lymphoid tumor has a primary disease of the intestine or whether the bowel involvement is but one manifestation of a systemic disease. Despite these very real problems, useful clinical information about lymphoid tumors of the small bowel has become available, and the roentgen features have been delineated.

In this discussion, the term lymphosarcoma will be used to include the histologic entities of lymphosarcoma and reticulum cell sarcoma. Hodgkin's disease will be discussed in another section.

Pathology

It is difficult to determine, even in retrospect, whether a given case represents at the onset primary intestinal lymphosarcoma or systemic disease. Dawson, Cornes, and Morson[1] suggest that the following strict criteria be employed for classifying intestinal lymphosarcoma as primary: no peripheral lymphadenopathy, no adenopathy on chest x-ray, normal peripheral blood count and smear, and abdominal lesions confined to the intestine and regional nodes, with liver and spleen free of tumor. The distinction between primary and secondary involvement of the intestine has significant prognostic implications but is less important in considering the roentgenologic aspects of the disease in the bowel.

Within the small bowel, lymphosarcoma involves the terminal ileum most commonly, perhaps because lymphoid tissue is abundant there. In the

409

Memorial Hospital series[2] of 1269 cases of lymphosarcoma, small bowel involvement was found in 138 patients. Of these, 15 occurred in duodenum, 11 in jejunum, 33 in ileum, and 13 in the appendix. In 66 cases the site was either multiple or undetermined.

The tumor may arise in the lymphoid tissue of mucosa or submucosa. It tends to extend along the long axis of the bowel and may have its origin in multiple sites. This behavior is in contrast to that of carcinoma, which usually produces a single short segmental constricting lesion.

In the initial stages lymphosarcoma may appear as a discrete, thickened plaque with relatively intact overlying mucosa. Growth may be predominantly toward the lumen, causing no rigidity in the adjacent bowel wall. Exaggerated peristalsis induced by the intraluminal mass may cause intussusception with subsequent intestinal obstruction.

Lymphosarcoma may, however, extend intramurally, causing a diffuse thickening of the wall of the small intestine over a considerable distance. When this occurs in the submucosa the mucosal folds may be intact, or they may be smoothed out by the submucosal thickening. At times they may even appear coarsely thickened. When the infiltration is quite superficial, the overlying mucosa may be thrown up into many small polypoid projections. This diffusely infiltrating form is not associated with a single mass but occurs along the course of the involved bowel. Areas of greater and lesser involvement may be found, producing a grossly irregular and rigid appearance.

In contrast to this type of extension along the longitudinal axis of the bowel, growth may be predominantly outward. The mass is usually large in such cases and is both endo- and exointestinal in location. As the mass enlarges it destroys the intestinal wall and extends into the mesentery, infiltrating and destroying adjacent intestinal loops. Ulceration of the tumor occurs with the formation of many communicating channels within the tumor mass as well as into the adjoining bowel loops. Ulceration and necrosis within the tumor produce a large irregular excavation which communicates with several loops of bowel. When perforation occurs, therefore, it is rarely into the free peritoneal cavity but rather into the agglutinated mass of tumor, mesentery, and small intestine. Involvement of the mesentery and extension into the peritonum may cause ascites which at times is chylous.

Because lymphosarcoma is a medullary tumor it does not evoke a desmoplastic response. There is little tendency for scirrhous tissue to form or for stenosis to occur. Some narrowing of the bowel lumen may be observed because of extrinsic compression and marked thickening of the bowel wall, but stricture formation of sufficient severity to cause intestinal obstruction is rare. When stricture formation does occur it is usually associated with ulceration and secondary infection.

In some cases the infiltrated bowel wall reveals a remarkable local segmental dilatation, which has been called aneurysmal dilatation. The apparent atonicity has been explained as the result of infiltration of muscle layers by tumor and destruction of nerve plexuses in the bowel wall.[3]

On histologic examination, the nodal architecture in *lymphosarcoma* is replaced by diffuse masses of small round cells which resemble mature lymphocytes. Usually the capsule is infiltrated, but there is no proliferation of the reticulum. In *reticulum cell sarcoma* the predominant cell is less mature than in lymphosarcoma, and it has a larger nucleus. Reticulum is increased, and large, bizarre reticulum cells may be seen. Intermediate and coexistent forms are found within these arbitrary groups of lymphoid tumors, and pathologists will not always agree on a precise diagnosis. It is often difficult for pathologists to distinguish reticulum cell sarcoma from anaplastic carcinoma in biopsy material.

Clinical Features

The most common features of small bowel lymphosarcoma are abdominal pain, either dull or colicky, anorexia, weakness, malaise, weight loss, a palpable abdominal mass, and anemia. Because lymphosarcoma tends not to obstruct the lumen, the tumor may be very large and the disease process far advanced before the patient is seen by a physician. The reported complications of lymphosarcoma provide a list of almost all major abdominal catastrophes, including massive hemorrhage, perforation, intussusception, intestinal obstruction and intra-abdominal fistulas. Malabsorption syndrome has been occasionally reported[4] in patients with small bowel lymphosarcoma.

In the Memorial Hospital series, small bowel involvement was seen more commonly in children than in adults. Initial clinical involvement of the small bowel was found in 9 per cent of 69 children but only 1 per cent of 1200 adults studied. Eventual clinical small bowel disease was found in 19 per cent of the children and 4 per cent of the adults. Involvement of the small bowel at autopsy was found in 58 per cent of 26 children but only 29 per cent of 251 adults.

There is general agreement[1] that wide surgical excision of the intestinal lesion and adjacent lymph nodes is the treatment of choice. Most authorities feel that radiation therapy should be used in inoperable cases, in patients with regional lymph node involvement, and in patients in whom tumor is found at the resected end of the surgical specimen. Whether radiation therapy confers added benefit to patients in whom the bowel lesion can be completely removed is uncertain. Dawson, Cornes, and Morson[1] note that all the reported patients with a primary intestinal lesion who survived ten years after diagnosis had been treated by surgery or by combined surgery and radiation therapy; these authors were unable to demonstrate that radiation therapy significantly increased a patient's chance of survival.

Roentgen Features

We have classified the roentgenologic changes as follows:
1. Multiple nodular defects.
2. Infiltrating form.
3. Polypoid form (intussusception).
4. Endo-exoenteric form with excavation and fistula formation.

5. Predominantly invasive form of the mesentery with (a) large extra-luminal masses (single or multiple with extrinsic pressure upon the small intestine) and (b) production of the sprue pattern.

Multiple Nodular Defects (Figs. 20-1 to 20-9)

These appear as multiple intraluminal nodules or intramural defects of varying size which alter the mucosal pattern and produce an irregular, coarse scalloping of the bowel contour. Ulceration may be seen within the nodules because of central necrosis. The bowel lumen is of normal or increased caliber. These changes are more often found in the ileum and involve segments varying from one to several feet in length. The altered segments retain their pliability and are not fixed in position. This type may occur as the sole manifestation of this entity or may be associated with other intestinal changes. Not infrequently, when the terminal ileum is involved, the nodules extend into the cecum and ascending colon. In some cases the nodules are tiny and difficult to identify.

(*Text continued on page 419.*)

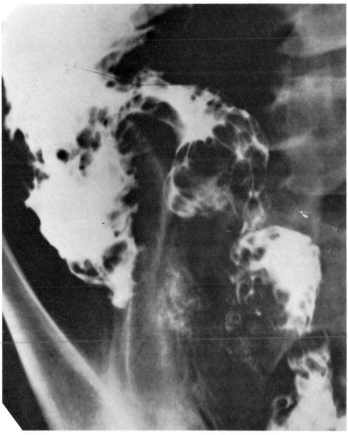

Figure 20–1   Lymphosarcoma. Multiple tumor nodules of varying size are present in the terminal ileum, cecum and ascending colon. The terminal ileum is slightly dilated. There is a superficial resemblance to nodular lymphoid hyperplasia, but the nodules are larger and asymmetrical.

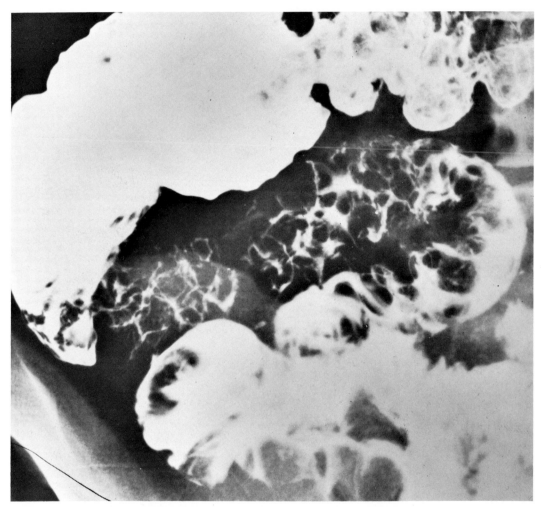

Figure 20-2 *Lymphosarcoma.* The mucosal pattern is replaced by numerous polypoid intramural and intraluminal defects which alter the caliber of the bowel lumen. There is no evidence of obstruction.

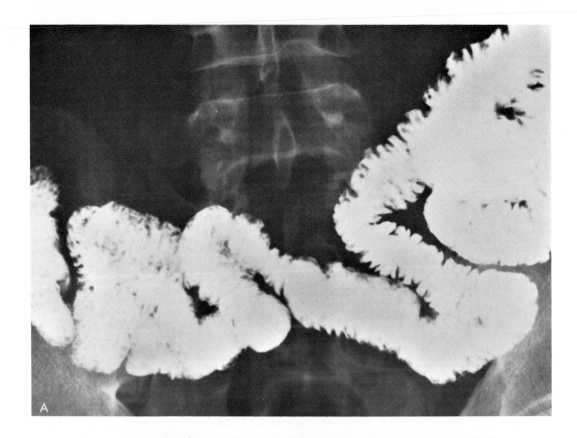

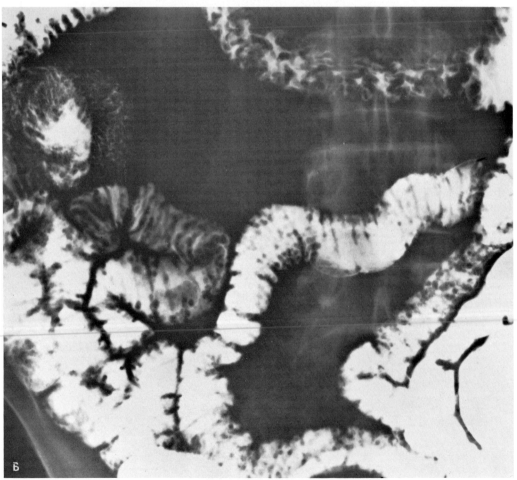

Figure 20–3 A and B See legend on opposite page.

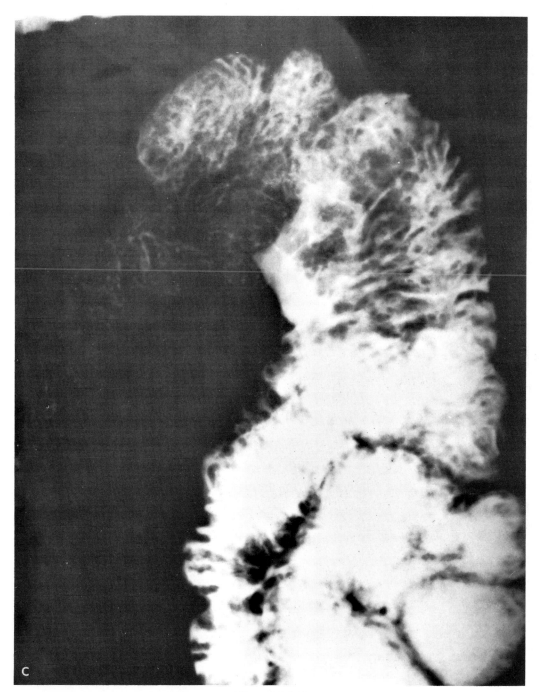

Figure 20–3 C

Figure 20–3 Lymphosarcoma. A, A barium mixture containing a poor suspending agent failed to reveal an abnormality. *B,* with use of a different barium mixture, numerous tiny circular filling defects are seen throughout the midportion of the small bowel. The appearance is consistent with a diagnosis of nodular lymphoid hyperplasia or lymphosarcoma.

C, Same patient, one year later. There is a segment of midjejunum, measuring 3 inches in length, in which the mucosa is ulcerated, thickened, and nodular in configuration. Some of the tiny defects previously described are again identified. At surgery, almost the entire small bowel as well as the mesentery was involved with lymphosarcoma. Extensive nodular lymphoid hyperplasia may be related to lymphosarcoma. (Courtesy of Dr. Roger Blahut, Burlingame, California.)

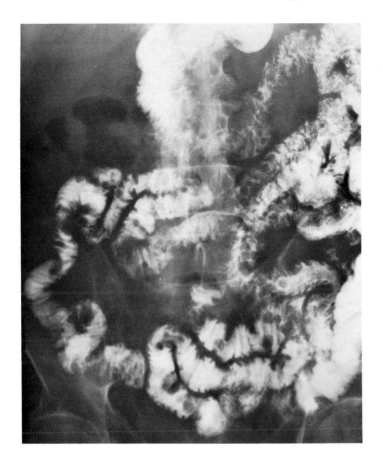

Figure 20–4 *Lymphosarcoma.* Numerous small polypoid intramural and intraluminal defects are distributed throughout the small bowel.

Figure 20–5 *Lymphosarcoma.* Multiple polypoid intraluminal and intramural defects are identified.

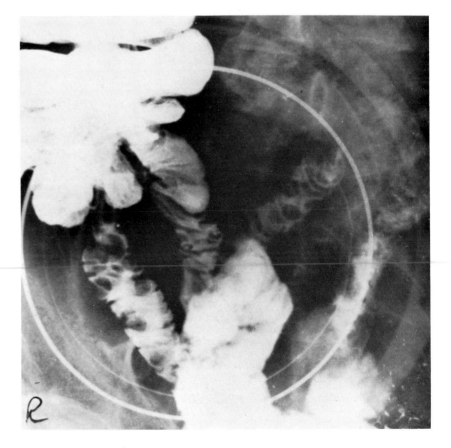

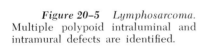

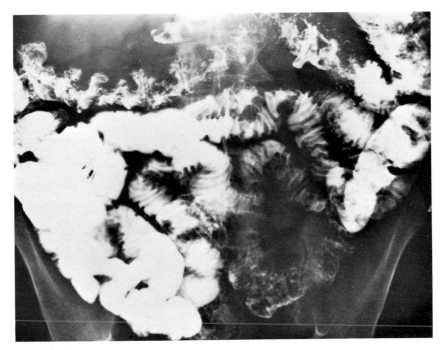

Figure 20–6 Lymphosarcoma. The polypoid and nodular defects are associated with tiny central ulcerations. Such specks of barium may also be seen in melanosarcoma and metastatic carcinoma.

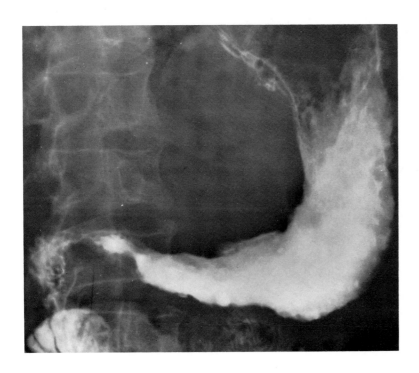

Figure 20–7 Same patient as in Figure 20–6. Similar polypoid defects associated with central ulceration are noted throughout the stomach.

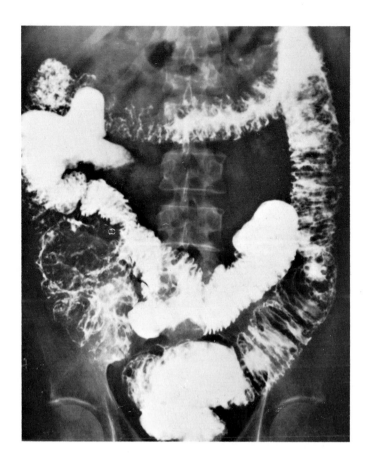

Figure 20–8 Lymphosarcoma. Multiple polypoid and nodular defects are identified throughout the colon and distal terminal ileum.

Figure 20–9 Lymphosarcoma. Multiple polypoid intraluminal defects are identified, especially in the sigmoid. This is a consistent pattern in lymphosarcoma. The entire intestine was involved in this case.

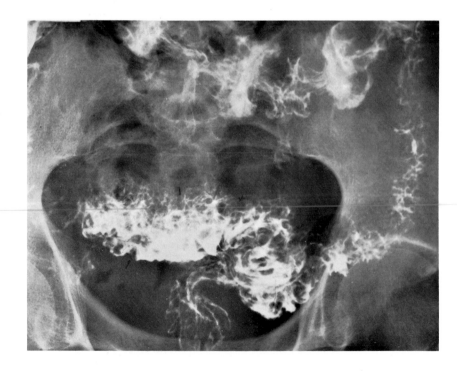

The Infiltrating Form (Figs. 20-10 to 20-16)

The bowel wall becomes diffusely infiltrated and thickened. The degree of thickening varies from area to area, producing irregular segments of narrowing and relative dilatation. The degree of narrowing is never as marked as that observed in cancer or inflammation. The mucosal folds may become flattened and effaced, or they may be thickened and thrown up into irregular nodular projections, producing coarse, irregular scalloping of the bowel contour with intraluminal filling defects of varying size. The mural thickening causes separation and straightening of the intestinal loops which stand out clearly from the closely approximated normal small intestine. The barium column may have a mottled appearance because of the increased secretions within the lumen of the affected segment. The infiltration may be limited to short segments, either single or multiple, which appear as short areas of eccentric narrowing of the bowel lumen with effacement or thickening of the mucosal

(*Text continued on page 423.*)

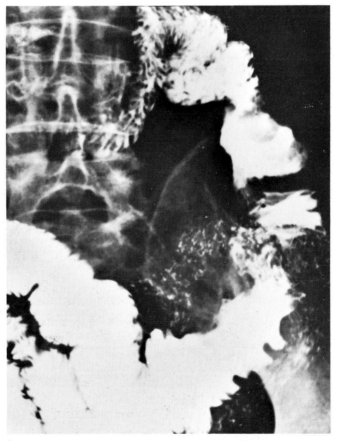

Figure 20–10 Lymphosarcoma. Infiltration of multiple short segments of jejunum is noted. In this case several areas are involved. The proximal areas of involvement show segmental areas of irregular dilatation of the bowel lumen, destroyed mucosal folds and a suggestion of an intramural mass. The other lesions, a few inches caudad, show flattening and rigidity of one wall and abnormal valvular markings on the contour of the opposite wall.

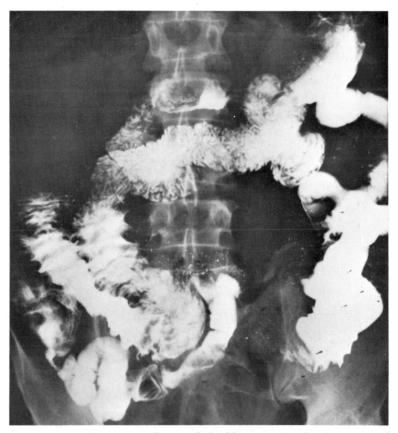

Figure 20-11 Lymphosarcoma. There is slight dilatation of the distal jejunum, which shows thickening and blunting of the folds with effacement in some areas. The contours are coarsely irregular. One short segment of narrowing is seen. The appearance simulates that of the nonstenotic phase of regional enteritis. Unlike regional enteritis, the contours are nodular due to tumor.

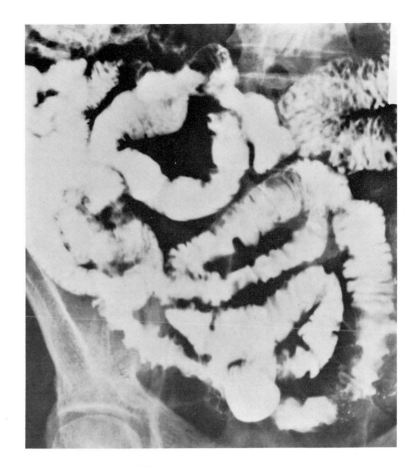

Figure 20–12 Lymphosarcoma. There is thickening and blunting of the folds, with some encroachment upon the bowel lumen but no obstruction. In some areas small tumor nodules can be identified along the contour of the bowel lumen. Again the nonstenotic phase of regional enteritis is simulated.

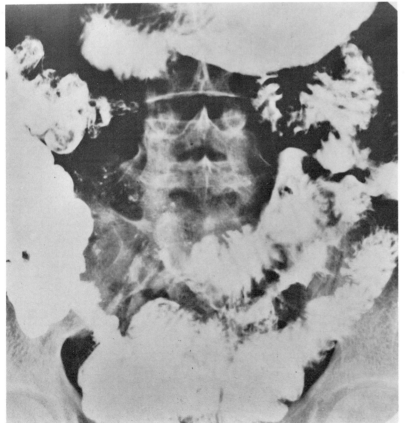

Figure 20–13 Lymphosarcoma. Irregular narrowing of a segment of small bowel mimicking regional enteritis. The narrowing in lymphosarcoma is due to encroachment of the lumen by tumor and is usually not associated with any significant proximal obstruction.

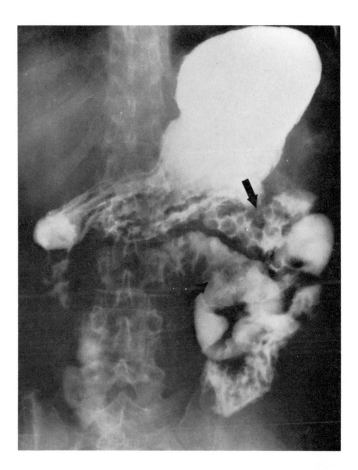

Figure 20–14 Lymphosarcoma. Diffuse infiltrating lymphosarcoma involving the entire small intestine. In the jejunum, multiple intramural and intraluminal tumor nodules (arrow) alter the bowel contour. This diagnosis was confirmed by small bowel biopsy.

Figure 20–15 Same case as in Figure 20–14. In the ileum, the bowel is dilated. The mucosal folds are thickened and blunted. Mural tumor nodules can still be identified (arrows).

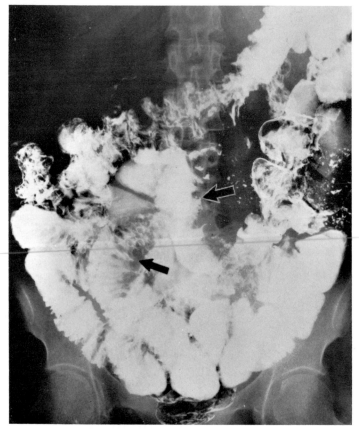

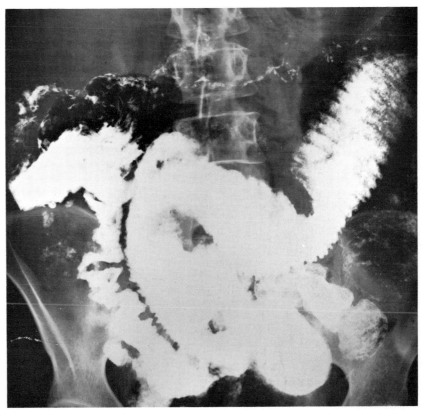

Figure 20–16 *Lymphosarcoma.* Diffuse infiltrating lymphosarcoma of the jejunum and ileum. In some segments the lumen is dilated with irregular or saw-toothed contours. Elsewhere the folds are thickened.

folds and evidence of tumor formation. As noted previously, lymphosarcoma is primarily a medullary tumor and produces no desmoplastic reaction. Because of this, marked rigidity of the involved segments is uncommon, and there is usually insufficient stenosis to produce dilatation of the small intestine proximally. Stricture formation, however, sufficient to cause intestinal obstruction, has been noted in association with ulceration and secondary infection. In several instances a discrete ulceration within a mass evoked mechanical intestinal obstruction by producing spasm or by completely encircling the lumen of the bowel (Fig. 20-17).

Another form of segmental infiltration of the bowel wall in lymphosarcoma is characterized by marked localized dilatation. This has been referred to as aneurysmal dilatation (Figs. 20-18 to 20-20). The increased thickness of the bowel wall is demonstrated by increased separation from adjacent loops. The barium tends to pool within the widened lumen, and no mucosal pattern can be seen. The contours of the dilated segment may be smooth, coarsely irregular, or show scalloping and nodularity due to intramural tumor formation. The adjacent mucosa may appear intact or thickened and nodular. In an unusual form of lymphosarcoma, diffuse thickening of the folds throughout the small bowel is seen with little evidence of nodularity or intraluminal defects (Fig. 20-21).

(Text continued on page 428.)

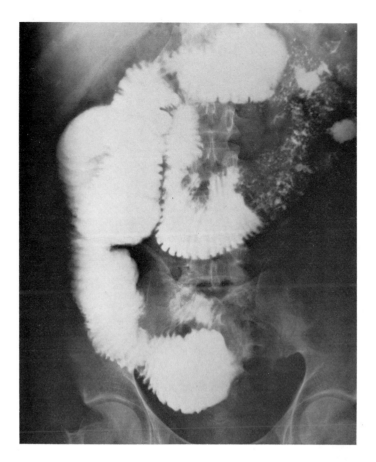

Figure 20–17 Lymphosarcoma. Unusual instance of obstruction, produced by kinking and spasm at the site of an ulcerated intraluminal lymphosarcoma. The lesion was flat and in itself did not compromise the bowel lumen.

Figure 20–18 Lymphosarcoma. Aneurysmal dilatation in diffuse infiltrating lymphosarcoma. Tumor nodules encroaching upon the bowel lumen can be identified. Other segments of small intestine as well as the duodenum are involved.

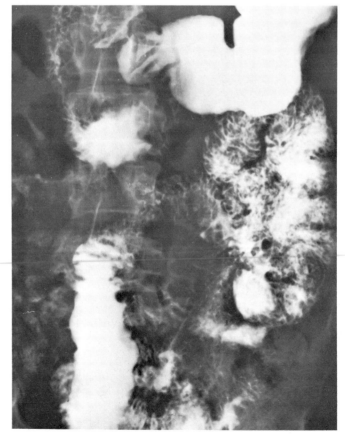

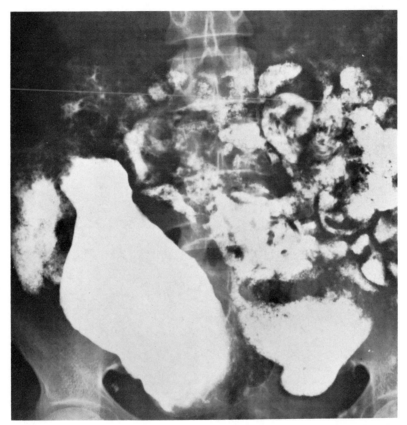

Figure 20–19 *Lymphosarcoma.* Marked aneurysmal dilatation in the ileum. The increased thickness of the bowel wall is indicated by the increased distance between the involved bowel and adjacent loops.

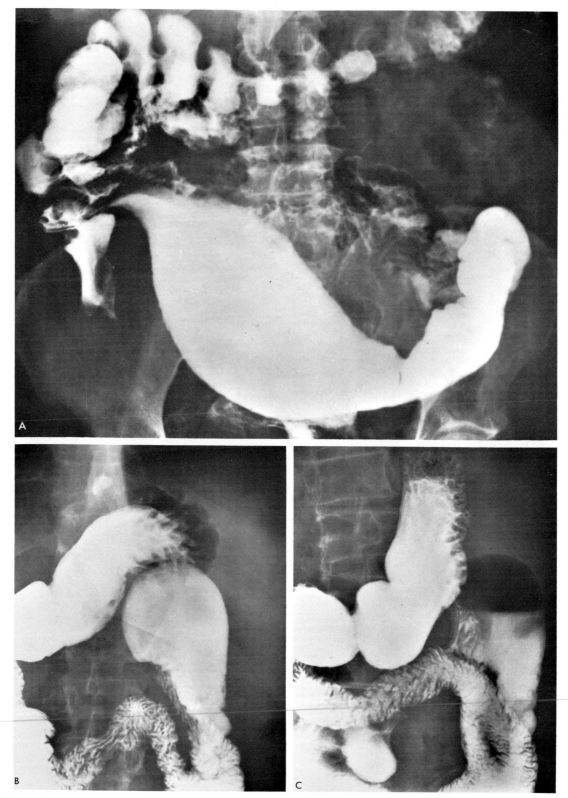

Figure 20-20 A, *Lymphosarcoma.* Tremendous dilatation of the terminal ileum due to lymphosarcoma. (Courtesy of Dr. Jerome Shapiro, Boston City Hospital, Massachusetts.)

B, *Lymphosarcoma.* There is a large saclike structure extending superiorly from the jejunum and mimicking a cyst. The right inferior wall is moderately irregular. The resected specimen revealed marked aneurysmal dilatation and a thickened wall.

C, Erect film of same patient shows a fluid level within the dilated segment.

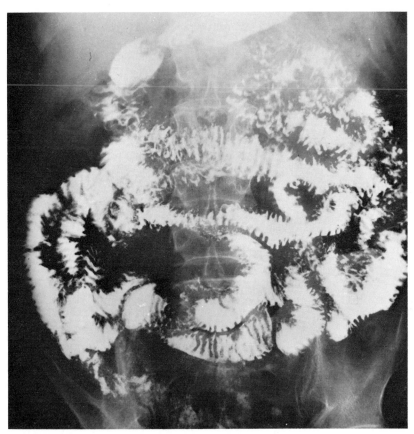

Figure 20–21 *Lymphosarcoma.* Diffuse thickening of the folds without nodularity. This is an unusual radiological appearance of lymphosarcoma.

The Polypoid Form (Figs. 20-22 to 20-25)

When the tumor has grown to a size sufficient to produce a discrete intraluminal mass and is without intramural extension, it may be drawn forward by peristalsis, forming a pseudopedicle, and may become the leadpoint of an intussusception. Unless there are other clues to the nature of the underlying lesion, the cause of the intussusception cannot be determined from the roentgenograms. At times the polypoid tumor presents predominantly as an intraluminal lesion without intussusception. This is especially true when the lesion is large and bulky.

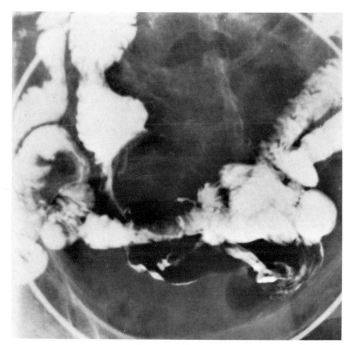

Figure 20–22   Lymphosarcoma. There is a single smooth submucosal defect in the distal jejunun. At surgery, this proved to be a lymphosarcoma. The surgeon could find no further evidence of any abnormality. Four years later, however, the patient had disseminated lymphosarcoma. A single lesion does occur in lymphosarcoma but is unusual.

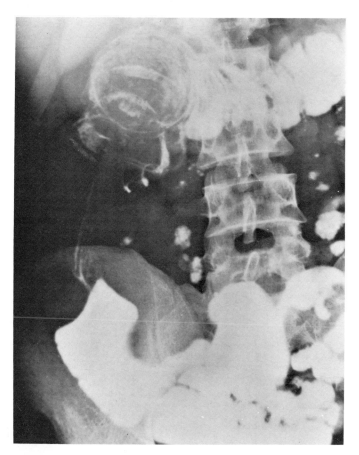

Figure 20–23 *Lymphosarcoma.* Polypoid lymphosarcoma of the terminal ileum, resulting in an ileocecal intussusception with minimal obstruction. The lesion is obscured by the intussusception.

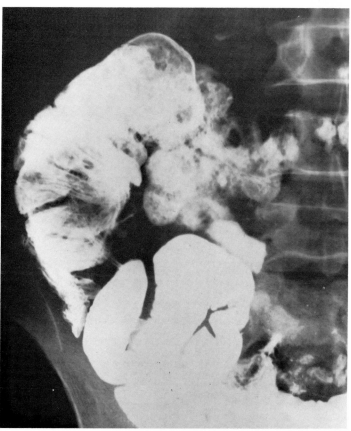

Figure 20–24 *Lymphosarcoma.* Less marked intussusception of a polypoid lymphosarcoma arising in the terminal ileum and extending into the right side of the colon.

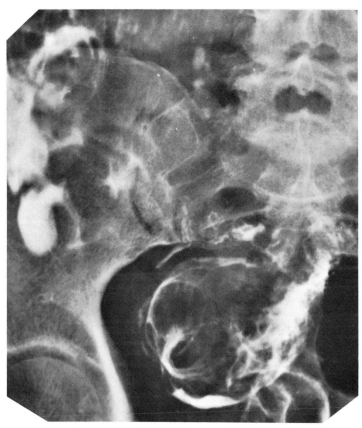

Figure 20–25 *Lymphosarcoma.* Large lobulated polypoid lymphosarcoma of the terminal ileum, seen after evacuation of a barium enema.

Endo-exoenteric Form with Excavation (Figs. 20-26 to 20-32)

In this instance a large irregular ulceration with multiple fistulas communicating with the adjacent bowel is seen. The roentgen findings are bizarre. Characteristically there is an extensive, irregular, amorphous patch of barium which does not conform to the intestinal lumen and communicates with the surrounding bowel. Adjacent loops are displaced by the large mass. This appearance is not pathognomonic of lymphosarcoma and has been observed in other sarcomatous tumors of the intestinal tract and in metastatic carcinoma. Fistulas are frequent. The earlier changes are seen less frequently. Before massive excavation occurs the tumor and the involved portion of the small intestine may be crisscrossed by many intercommunicating channels connecting the tumor with the lumen of the small intestine. These channels appear as amorphous barium streaks of varying caliber. In the early cases the presence of altered intestinal loops and fistulas may suggest regional enteritis. Subsequent events produce massive excavation of the involved area and indicate the presence of a necrotic neoplasm.

In lymphosarcoma many features may be combined and seen simultaneously. The lesion is usually multiple, and not infrequently the nodular type, the infiltrating and the endo-exoenteric forms may be seen at one time (Fig. 20-33).

(*Text continued on page 436.*)

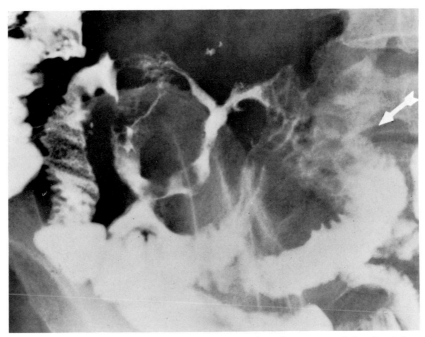

Figure 20–26 *Lymphosarcoma.* Endo-exoenteric lymphosarcoma of the distal ileum. The normal bowel lumen is replaced by many intercommunicating tortuous tracts throughout the tumor. The arrow points to the nodular mucosal pattern proximal to the mass. The lumen of this segment is not narrowed.

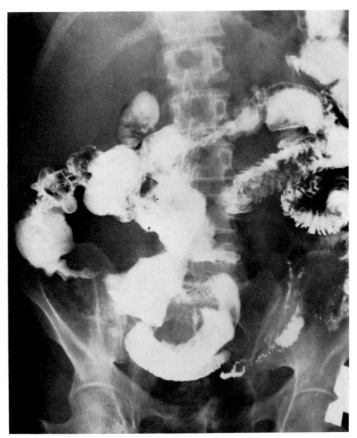

Figure 20–27 *Lymphosarcoma.* Same case three months later. There is a large irregular triangular excavated area within the lumen, containing an amorphous collection of barium. The mucosal pattern and the adjacent small intestinal loops are considerably thickened.

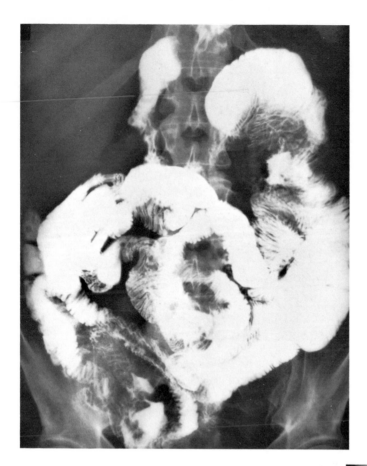

Figure 20–28 Lymphosarcoma. Multiple areas of irregular ulceration are seen in the small bowel.

Figure 20–29 Lymphosarcoma. In the distal jejunum there is a submucosal filling defect, associated with minimal dilatation. In the mid ileum a large irregular ulceration is identified.

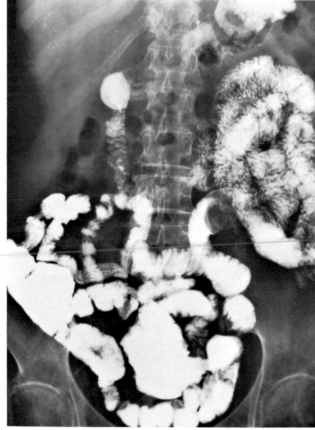

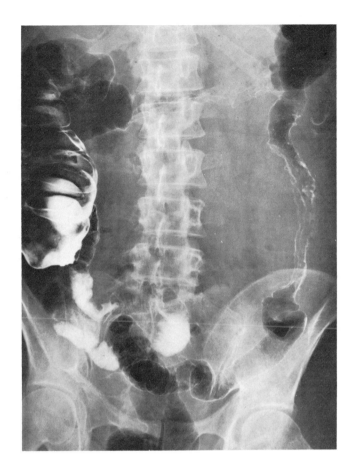

Figure 20–30   Lymphosarcoma. There is narrowing and evidence of extrinsic pressure on the mid descending colon.

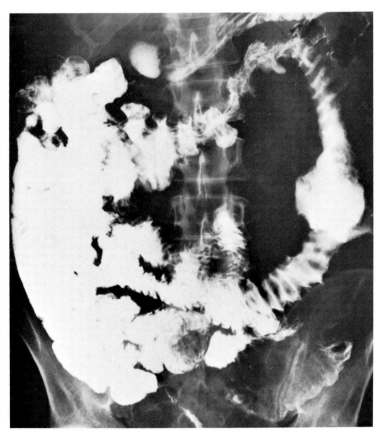

Figure 20–31   Same case as Figure 20–30, with a large irregular ulcer crater in the midjejunum. Proximal and distal to the crater there is a striking, symmetric thickening of the folds. Without the ulceration, a diagnosis of lymphosarcoma would be impossible.

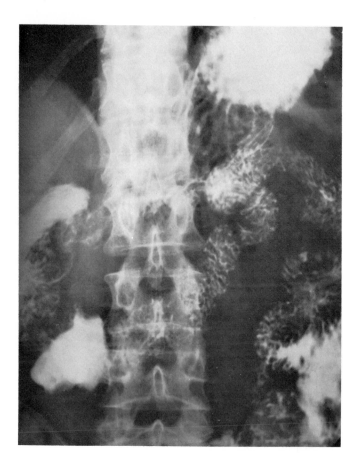

Figure 20–32   *Lymphosarcoma.* There is a large, irregular ulcer in the third portion of the duodenum. Other segments of small bowel are also involved.

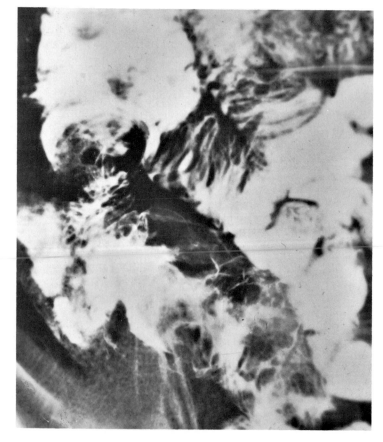

Figure 20–33   *Lymphosarcoma.* A markedly disorganized pattern produced by multiple polypoid masses with ulceration. Dilatation and numerous sinus tracts are also identified.

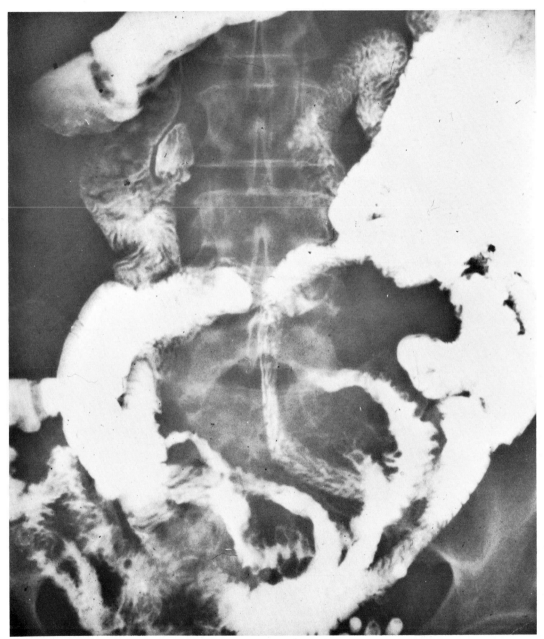

Figure 20–34 *Lymphosarcoma.* Multiple large masses compress and displace the intestinal loops.

Predominantly Invasive Form of Mesentery
(Fig. 20-35)

Large extraluminal masses are identified. The greater portion of the tumor grows centrifugally and produces tumors which can attain huge proportions and even extend into the retroperitoneum. These manifest themselves roentgenologically by displacement of the abdominal organs, pressure defects upon the adjacent viscera, and invasion of the intestinal wall. The presence of a mass alone is not diagnostic of lymphosarcoma unless mural alterations which characterize this type of growth are seen in the small intestine. Unlike metastatic carcinoma, the loops of intestine are not fixed, angulated, or obstructed. Also in contrast to metastatic carcinoma, the folds are not stretched, deformed, or separated.

In another form of the invasion of the mesentery, the sprue pattern is produced. This has already been discussed under Malabsorption (see page 22). Lymphosarcoma involving the duodenal bulb and duodenal loop reveals roentgen alterations similar to those seen in the small bowel (Figs. 20-36 to 20-38).

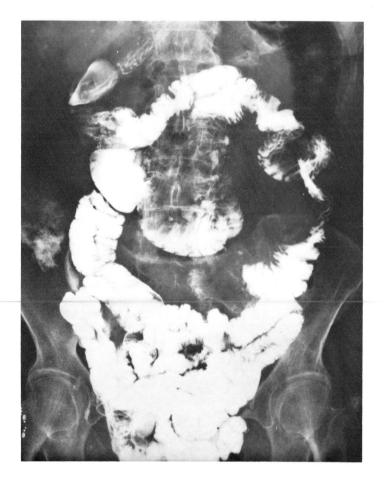

Figure 20–35 Lymphosarcoma. There is a large mass in the upper left quadrant causing compression and narrowing of the adjacent loops of bowel and slight obstruction. The presence of obstruction makes it difficult to exclude metastatic carcinoma.

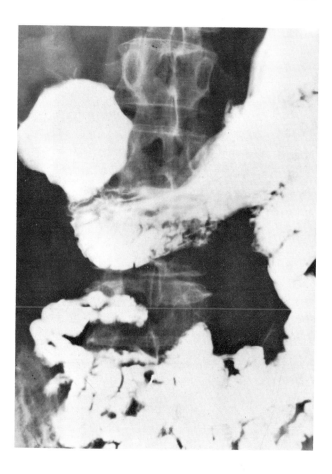

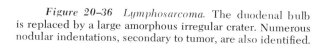*Figure 20–36 Lymphosarcoma.* The duodenal bulb is replaced by a large amorphous irregular crater. Numerous nodular indentations, secondary to tumor, are also identified.

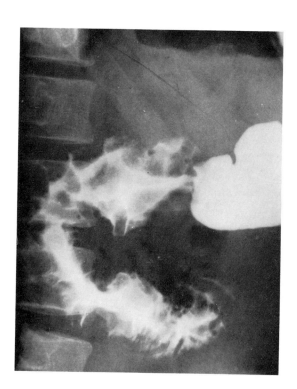

Figure 20–37 Lymphosarcoma. There is coarse, nodular irregularity of the folds in the duodenal bulb and duodenal loop.

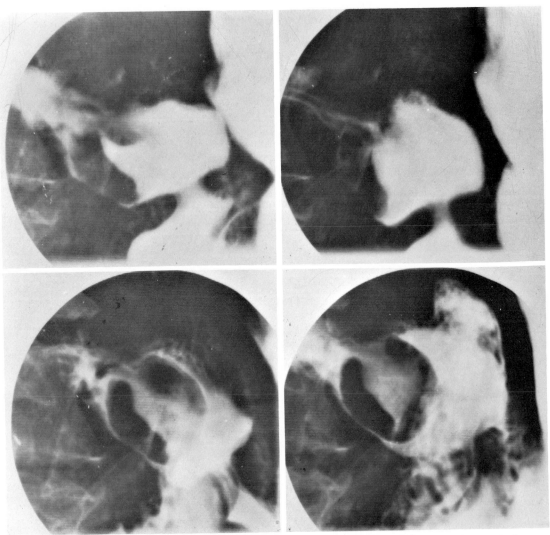

Figure 20–38   *Lymphosarcoma.* A smooth, circumscribed filling defect occupies most of the duodenal bulb. Within this defect there is a large, irregular ulceration. Any type of sarcoma may produce this finding.

HODGKIN'S DISEASE

Hodgkin's disease of the small bowel is less common than lymphosarcoma and more likely to be associated with systemic disease. Although Hodgkin's disease involving the small bowel shows many of the clinical and pathologic features of lymphosarcoma, the disease warrants a separate description from the roentgenologic point of view. Unlike lymphosarcoma, Hodgkin's disease can produce marked fibrosis of the bowel wall with constriction of the lumen.

Histologically Hodgkin's disease displays a more complex pattern than lymphosarcoma or reticulum cell sarcoma. A variety of cells is noted, including lymphocytes, granulocytes, monocytes, plasma cells, and the characteristic Reed-Sternberg giant cells. Fibroblasts are present and a variable degree of fibrosis may be seen. The architecture of normal lymphoid tissue is lost.

The prognosis for Hodgkin's disease involving the gastrointestinal tract appears to be more serious than for lymphosarcoma.[1, 5] As with gastrointestinal lymphosarcoma, surgical excision of the intestinal lesion is the treatment of choice.[6] Radiation therapy or chemotherapy is indicated when all evident disease cannot be removed.

Roentgen Features (Figs. 20-39 to 20-47)

Hodgkin's disease produces the same kinds of lesions of the small intestine as lymphosarcoma, but excavation, fistulas, and aneurysmal dilatation are not as frequent. Unlike lymphosarcoma, Hodgkin's disease can produce marked fibrosis of the bowel wall with constriction of the lumen. Roentgenographically, there is eccentric narrowing of the bowel lumen, which tapers in a fusiform manner. There are no overhanging edges at the margin of the lesion, which is frequently longer than that seen in carcinoma. The contour of the bowel lumen is irregular due to nodularity of the bowel wall. Because of the frequent narrowing associated with Hodgkin's disease, the differential diagnosis from other constricting lesions, such as inflammation, infarction, and carcinoma may be difficult. Another pattern noted in several cases of Hodgkin's disease is a ribbon-like appearance with some degree of rigidity, narrowing and evidence of extrinsic pressure. The folds adjacent to this segment are often thickened and blunted.

(Text continued on page 444.)

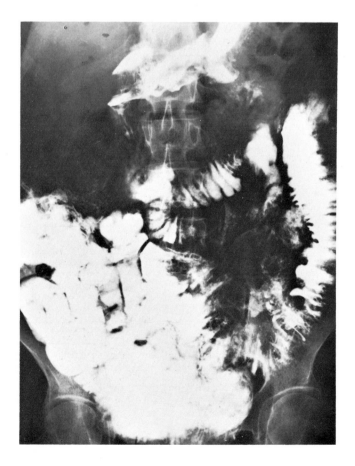

Figure 20-39 *Hodgkin's disease.* There is thickening and irregularity of the folds throughout the jejunum with minimal nodularity.

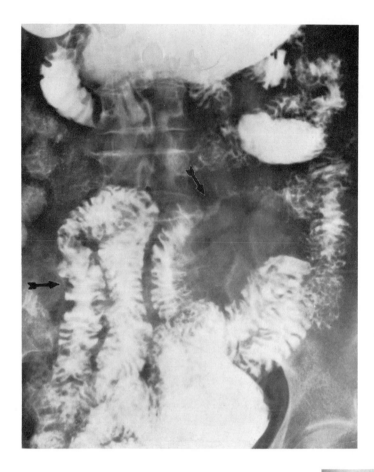

Figure 20–40   Hodgkin's disease. A segment of jejunum is narrowed and compressed by an extrinsic mass. An additional short segment reveals thickening and nodularity of the folds.

Figure 20–41   Hodgkin's disease. The terminal ileum is rigid, moderately narrowed and irregular.

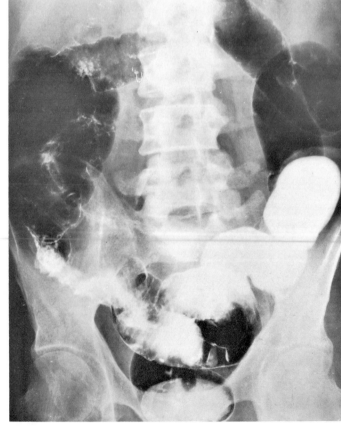

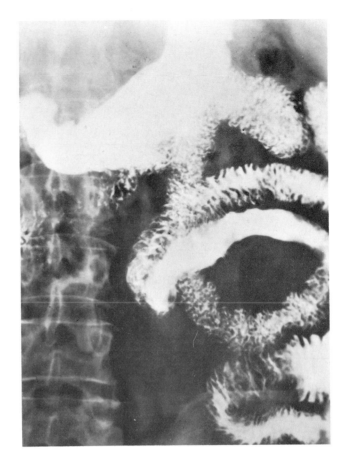

Figure 20-42 *Hodgkin's disease.* A segment of jejunum is compressed and displaced superiorly. The mucosa is effaced by the tumor.

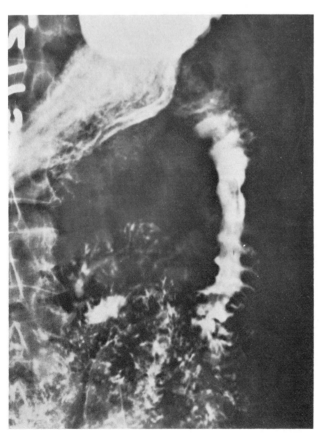

Figure 20-43 *Hodgkin's disease.* The proximal jejunum is narrowed and rigid. The folds are alternately thickened and effaced. The findings are produced by an intramural tumor involving the wall of the bowel.

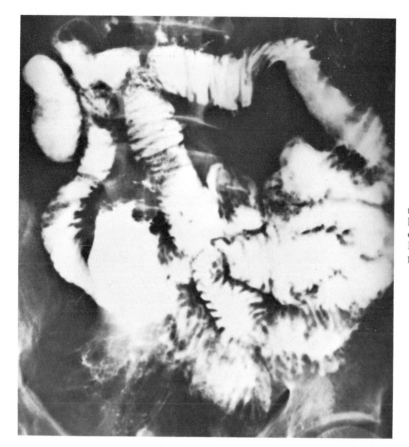

Figure 20-44   Hodgkin's disease. There are two segments of involvement. Proximally, the lesion simulates a long carcinoma except for lack of obstruction and proximal intestinal dilatation. Distally, the more usual characteristics of a lymphoma are seen with dilatation and perforation.

Figure 20-45   Hodgkin's disease. There are two short segments of eccentric narrowing with multiple dilated loops of bowel and thickened folds. Differential diagnosis from metastatic carcinoma is impossible.

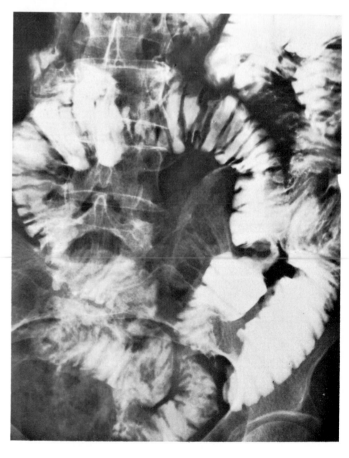

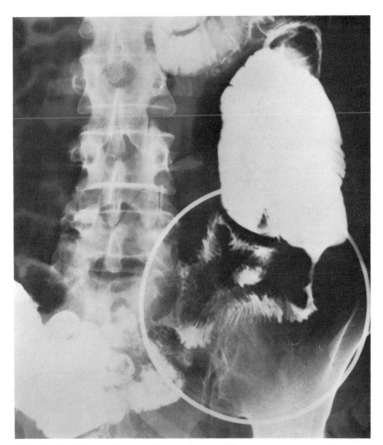

Figure 20–46 *Hodgkin's disease* of the jejunum. There is a narrow rigid segment producing obstruction to the barium column and dilatation. The contours are scalloped. No overhanging margins are seen. The lumen is eccentric. There is a fairly gradual transition between normal and abnormal bowel.

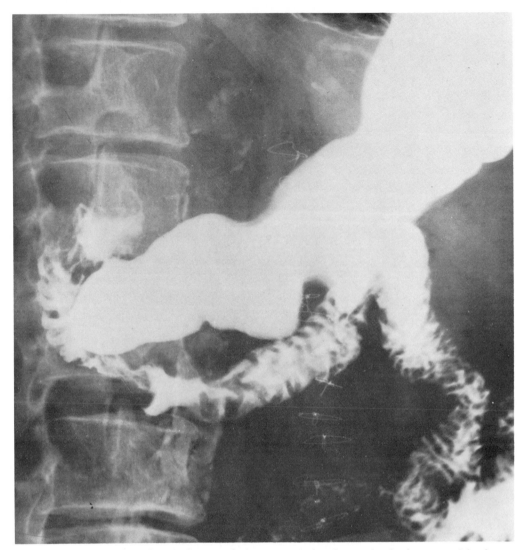

Figure 20–47 *Hodgkin's disease.* There is an irregular ulcer in the third portion of the duodenum. The diagnosis of Hodgkin's disease was made by peroral biopsy.

MELANOSARCOMA

Melanosarcoma (malignant melanoma) is a relatively uncommon cancer of the skin or eye. It enters into the discussion of small bowel lesions in terms of metastatic malignant melanoma. The tumor is considered here with lymphosarcoma because it is primarily a cellular tumor with little fibrotic reaction. The roentgen manifestations, therefore, resemble those of lymphosarcoma.

In patients dying from melanoma, metastases are found at autopsy widely spread throughout the body.[7] Almost three-fourths of patients have metastases in liver and lung, but involvement of the small bowel is also very common (58 per cent). In the same series, metastasis to stomach was found in 26 per cent and colon in 22 per cent.

Primary melanoma of the small bowel has been reported, but it must be exceedingly uncommon. It is difficult to establish a definite diagnosis of primary intestinal melanoma, because not infrequently metastases are the first clinical manifestations of an inconspicuous skin melanoma. The problem is further complicated by the observation that malignant melanoma may be pigmented or nonpigmented in either its primary or metastatic forms.

In the small bowel, melanosarcoma behaves clinically and radiologically like lymphosarcoma. The tumor commonly bleeds but may also intussuscept or obstruct. Treatment of the small bowel lesion is surgical, with resection of the involved area. Melanoma is ordinarily resistant to radiation therapy,[8] and effective chemotherapy awaits discovery of an appropriate agent.[9] The prognosis for the patient with melanoma metastatic to more than one lymphatic area or to the viscera is very poor. Ninety-nine per cent of such patients die of their disease within one year of the first clinical observation.[7]

Roentgen Features

Melanosarcoma (Figs. 20-48 to 20-53) has a propensity for metastasizing to the gastrointestinal tract, and produces multiple intraluminal or submucosal nodules. The tumors are cellular, grow rapidly in size, and encourage no desmoplastic reaction. There is a tendency to central necrosis and ulceration. Thus, a circular filling defect with a central ulceration is a well known hallmark of this disease and has been described in both the stomach and small bowel. As in lymphosarcoma, the tumor nodules produce dilatation, and differentiation

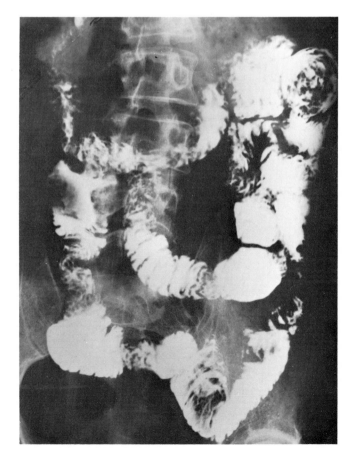

Figure 20–48   *Melanosarcoma.* There is a nodular filling defect in the jejunum with an eccentric lumen and no evidence of obstruction. An additional tumor, seen en face, is noted in the left upper quadrant.

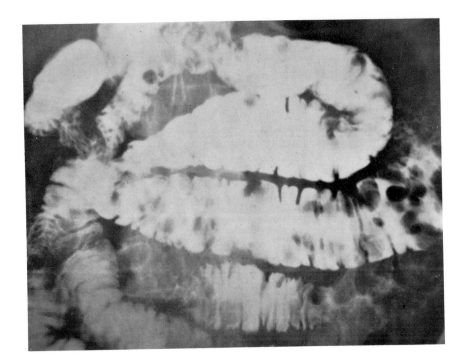

Figure 20–49 Melanosarcoma. Multiple polypoid and nodular defects, similar to lymphosarcoma, are identified. There is no definite evidence of ulceration within the tumor nodules. The lumen of the bowel is moderately dilated.

between the two lesions is often impossible. Early cases of melanosarcoma are similar to lymphosarcoma and demonstrate an eccentric lumen, slight dilatation, and no obstruction. Intussusception is not uncommon. Extensive necrosis of the tumor, sinus tracts, and fistulas may also be seen.

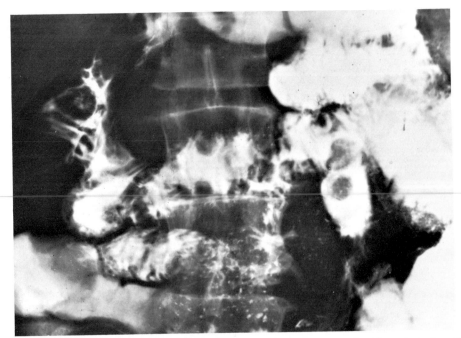

Figure 20–50 Melanosarcoma. Numerous filling defects associated with central ulceration are seen. This bull's-eye appearance is frequent in melanosarcoma; it may also be seen in lymphosarcoma and metastatic carcinoma.

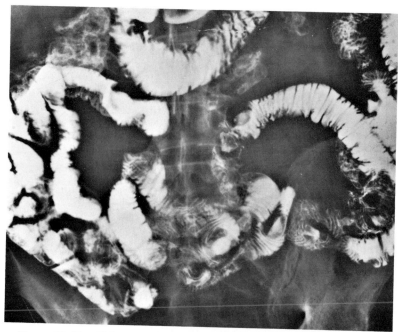

Figure 20–51 *Melanosarcoma.* Multiple large nodules are associated with central ulceration.

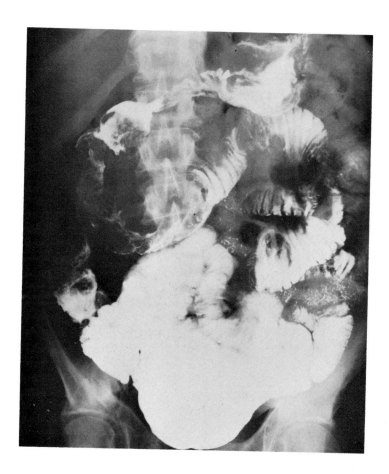

Figure 20–52 *Melanosarcoma.* Extensive irregular nodularity of the proximal small bowel due to melanosarcoma. A typical polypoid defect with a central ulceration is seen in the stomach.

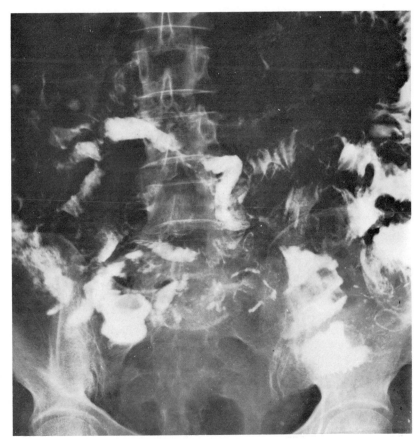

Figure 20–53 *Melanosarcoma.* Marked involvement of the small bowel with obvious metastatic nodules, many containing central ulcerations. The absence of obstruction is noteworthy.

LEUKEMIA AND MULTIPLE MYELOMA

Involvement of the intestine with leukemia has rarely been noted radiographically in our series. In a rare case, pea-sized nodules have been demonstrated in the terminal ileum associated with thickening of the folds. A diagnosis is impossible from the study of the small bowel itself.

Multiple myeloma rarely involves the small intestine. It may occur as multiple small filling defects involving the contour of the bowel, as seen in lymphosarcoma (Fig. 20-54), or in the form of an infiltrative lesion known as a plasmacytoma (Fig. 20-55). In the latter instance a long segment of bowel is involved with varying degrees of narrowing and rigidity and with tumor nodules simulating Hodgkin's disease. A specific diagnosis cannot be made. When multiple myeloma is associated with amyloid disease, the roentgen findings of intestinal amyloidosis may be present (see p. 62).

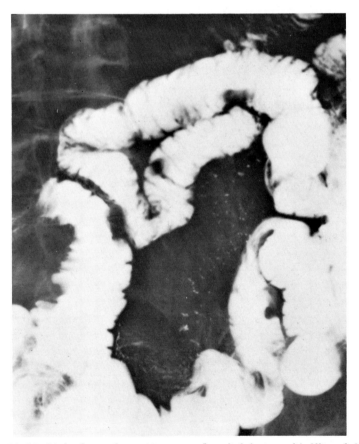

Figure 20–54   Multiple myeloma. Numerous flat, slightly irregular filling defects are seen along the contour of the bowel.

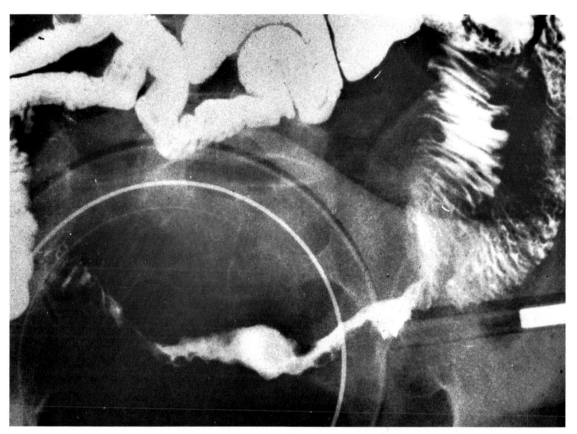

Figure 20–55   *Plasmacytoma.* There are irregular stenotic segments involving the mid-ileum. It is impossible to make the correct diagnosis in this case. The appearance suggests tumor rather than inflammatory or vascular disease.

NODULAR LYMPHOID HYPERPLASIA

Extensive nodular lymphoid hyperplasia may be related to lymphosarcoma, and differential diagnosis may be impossible (Fig. 20-3). (See Chapter 10, The Small Bowel in Immunoglobulin Deficiency Syndromes).

References

1. Dawson, I. M. P., Cornes, J. S., and Morson, B. C.: Primary malignant lymphoid tumors of the intestinal tract. *Brit. J. Surg.*, 49:80-89, 1961.
2. Rosenberg, S. A., Diamond, H. D., Jaslowitz, S., and Craven, L. F.: Lymphosarcoma: A review of 1269 cases. *Medicine*, 40:31-84, 1961.
3. Ullman, A., and Abeshouse, B. S.: Lymphosarcoma of the small and large intestines. *Ann. Surg.*, 95:878-915, 1932.
4. Sleisenger, M. H., Almy, T. P., and Barr, D. P.: The sprue syndrome secondary to lymphoma of the small bowel. *Amer. J. Med.*, 15:666-674, 1953.
5. Smith, D. C., and Klopp, C. T. The value of surgical removal of localized lymphomas. *Surgery*, 49:469-476, 1961.
6. Aisenberg, A. C.: Hodgkin's disease—prognosis, treatment, and etiologic and immunologic considerations. *New Eng. J. Med.*, 270:565-570, 1964.
7. McNeer, G., and Das Gupta, T.: Life history of melanoma. *Amer. J. Roentgen.*, 93:686-694, 1965.
8. McSwain, B., Riddell, D. H., Richie, R. E., and Crocker, E. F.: Malignant melanoma. *Ann. Surg.*, 159:967-975, 1964.
9. Nathanson, L., Hall, T. C., Vawter, G. F., and Farber, S.: Melanoma as a medical problem. *Arch. Intern. Med.*, 119:479-492, 1967.

21

The Small Bowel in Infants and Children

by JACK G. RABINOWITZ, M.D.
and JOHN E. MOSELEY, M.D.

Abnormalities of the small bowel in the neonatal period are predominantly congenital and present as intestinal obstruction. Congenital defects not causing significant neonatal obstruction may first become apparent in later infancy or childhood. Failure to recognize neonatal obstruction or undue delay in its surgical correction usually results in death of the infant.

The most important aids in the radiographic diagnosis of small bowel obstruction in the newborn are the supine, prone, and erect survey films of the abdomen. Air already present in the gastrointestinal tract or air injected after aspiration of fluid is all that is usually necessary for proper evaluation. Diagnostic criteria are based on the distribution and quantity of gas. Accurate interpretation of the findings requires an understanding of the normal intestinal gas pattern in newborn infants.

If there is no esophageal obstruction, air is usually present in the stomach immediately after birth.[1] This is due partly to swallowing and apparently also partly to crying which results in inspiratory movements against a closed glottis with relaxation of the superior esophageal sphincter.[2] Some gas can be seen in the small bowel within five to 30 minutes after birth, and the entire small intestine may contain gas after three hours. Gas usually reaches the ascending colon between three and four hours after birth, and the colon is outlined by gas in approximately five hours.[3] A film of the infant's abdomen made after 24 hours of life will normally show gas distributed throughout the entire gastrointestinal tract (Fig. 21–1). Generally the passage of gas through the intestinal tracts is more rapid in the premature than in the mature infant.

In infancy it is usual for gas to be distributed throughout the entire gastrointestinal tract, and the presence of gas and fluid levels in the small bowel under such circumstances is not abnormal. Usually the diffuse distribution of gas forms a polyhedral small bowel pattern which is characteristic (Fig.

451

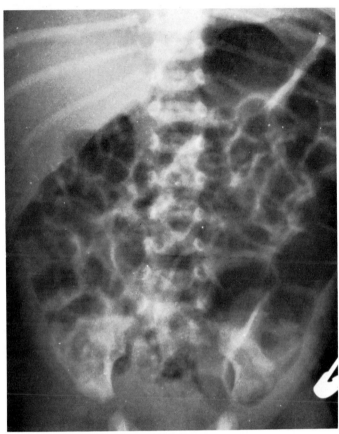

Figure 21-1 Normal abdomen in an infant approximately 24 hours old. Gas is distributed through entire small and large bowel, and no abnormal distention is visualized. Small bowel demonstrates a typical polyhedral configuration.

21-1). With increasing age and ambulation, decreasing quantities of gas are seen in the small intestine, and the intestinal gas distribution gradually approaches that seen in the older child and adult.

Occasionally the abdomen of the newborn is gasless or shows a significant paucity of gas several hours after birth. According to Singleton[3] this is sometimes the result of keeping the infant in a prone position during the interval between birth and the roentgen examination, but this appearance may be seen when there is respiratory depression, as in the premature or brain damaged infant. It may also be observed in infants born to mothers who have been heavily sedated or anesthetized during delivery. In recent years we have observed the same phenomenon in newborn infants of mothers addicted to narcotics and in infants requiring assisted respiration. Diarrhea and dehydration also may result in a gasless or relatively gasless abdomen.

Without the benefit of clinical information, and from a purely roentgenologic point of view, a gasless abdomen in the neonate should suggest the possibility of an esophageal atresia without a fistula between the trachea and the lower esophageal segment. It must not be forgotten, however, that in an occasional case of small bowel obstruction fluid may displace the gas, and especially in the supine position no gas may be demonstrable. In the erect position a small air-fluid level may be noted in the stomach or in both stomach and small bowel (Fig. 21-2). In such cases aspiration of gastric fluid and injec-

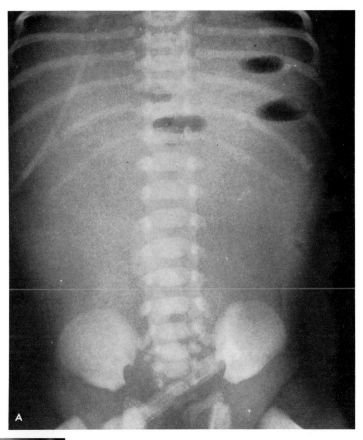

Figure 21-2 Jejunal atresia in a 36 hour old infant who presented with vomiting and abdominal distention. A, The abdomen is relatively gasless, although there are collections of gas in the right upper quadrant within the stomach and proximal small bowel. Abdomen is distended suggesting presence of fluid within the bowel or in the peritoneal cavity. These features are compatible with small bowel obstruction in which the gas is almost completely replaced by fluid.

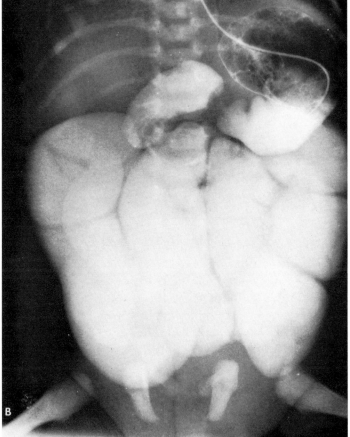

Figure 21-2 B, Injection of opaque material demonstrates marked small bowel distention. Air injection would be equally diagnostic. A low jejunal atresia was diagnosed and confirmed.

tion of an equal amount of air will usually outline the level of a high small bowel obstruction.

In high small bowel obstructions involving the duodenum or proximal jejunum it is the absence or marked decrease of intestinal gas distal to the gas-filled proximal bowel and stomach which characterize the condition. When obstruction involves the lower small intestine dilated loops of bowel may present a confusing gas pattern, and distinction between small and large bowel may be difficult. Although the configuration of the colon is not easily identified in this age group because of an underdeveloped haustral pattern, the ascending and descending colons are usually recognized by their vertical location along the abdominal flanks. In infants distention of the small intestine results in loss of its fold pattern. The polyhedral or honeycomb gas pattern seen under normal conditions is no longer observed, and in most cases multiple fluid levels are seen in the erect position. In those cases in which the obstruction is low and the abdomen is filled with smoothly outlined loops of bowel it is generally necessary to perform a barium enema to determine the location and character of the colon. Rarely is it necessary to resort to the use of oral contrast material to outline the point of obstruction. The use of water-soluble contrast media is not without risk because of their high osmolar activity, and there is some clinical evidence to indicate that infants undergoing investigation with such media may succumb to a severe state of hypovolemia.[4] The barium enema examination, on the other hand, is a strongly advised procedure in cases of suspected small bowel obstruction, because it not only reveals the location of the colon but also makes possible the distinction between small intestinal obstruction and colonic obstructions such as meconium plug syndrome and Hirschsprung's disease. In addition, a malrotated colon suggests the presence of malrotation of the small bowel and mid-gut volvulus. In cases of complete low congenital small bowel obstruction such as atresia of the terminal ileum, the barium enema will reveal a microcolon, which results from failure of succus entericus to pass through the colon in intrauterine life. Low small bowel lesions usually result in colons of smaller caliber than those observed with higher lesions, because in the latter instances the colon does act as a passageway for the succus entericus formed below the obstructing lesion.

DUODENAL ATRESIA AND STENOSIS

The most commonly encountered congenital obstructive lesions of the duodenum are those due to atresia, stenosis, annular pancreas, peritoneal band, and volvulus. The symptoms of atresia occur within the first 24 hours of life, usually after the first feeding. Vomiting is the most prominent feature, and since the atresia is most often distal to the ampulla of Vater the vomitus is usually bile-stained. Abdominal distention may not be marked, and it may be said that with high obstruction vomiting is more severe while with obstructions of the lower small bowel, distention is more prominent. There is a fairly high incidence of hyperbilirubinemia with duodenal and jejunal atresia. Boggs and Bishop[5] have found that 48 per cent of 48 infants with these conditions developed excessive total serum bilirubin concentrations. The primary cause for this is as yet not clearly defined. An association between hyperbilirubinemia and hypertrophic pyloric stenosis has also been discovered. The frequent association between Down's syndrome and duodenal atresia and annular pancreas is also noteworthy. The incidence of this syndrome is greater with duodenal atresia, where it occurs in about 30 per cent of cases. The radiologist would be well advised, therefore, when viewing the survey films of an infant with high intestinal obstruction to study the bones for evidence of the skeletal manifestations of this chromosomal abnormality (Fig. 21-3). There is no association between Down's syndrome and jejunal and ilial atresias.

Duodenal atresias are more commonly associated with other areas of atresia, e.g., esophagus and anus, as well as anomalies of the extremities and vertebrae, than are the jejunal and ilial atresias. This is reflected in the high mortality with these lesions and may be related to a difference in pathogenesis. Currently there are two outstanding concepts regarding the pathogenesis of intestinal atresias. It has been confirmed by several investigations that development of the human duodenum passes through a solid stage in some embryos owing to mucosal proliferation. This proliferation

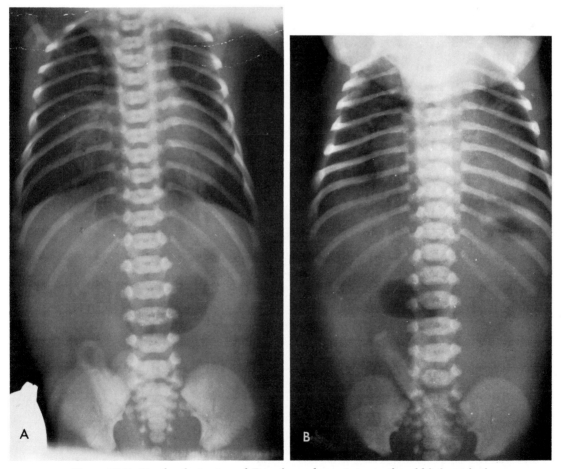

Figure 21-3 *Duodenal atresia and Down's syndrome* in a one day old baby girl who presented with vomiting. *A,* On a supine film of the abdomen air is seen within the stomach. In addition there is cardiac enlargement associated with increased pulmonary vascular markings. Flaring of the iliac wings is also noted.

B, Upright film of abdomen reveals a double bubble. The distended duodenal bulb is seen as a large air collection with an associated air-fluid level in the right upper quadrant. Air in fundus of stomach represents the second part of the double bubble. This case demonstrates the importance of studying the chest and skeleton in cases of duodenal atresia.

leads to obliteration of the lumen in the fifth and sixth weeks. The lumen is reformed by vacuoles which coalesce and reestablish the lumen by the eighth week of intrauterine life.[6] Complete or partial failure of vacuolation and recanalization could result in atresia or stenosis. It is also considered that interruption of the blood supply to a bowel segment with resulting infarction may cause disintegration and eventual disappearance of the affected segment.[7] The development of the jejunum, ileum and colon only rarely passes through a solid stage, and it is tentatively considered that while some cases of duodenal atresia may be due to failure of recanalization (Tandler's theory), atresias of the jejunum, ileum, and colon more likely result from vascular accidents occurring later in fetal life.

Radiographically, duodenal atresia is characterized by gaseous distention of the stomach and that portion of the duodenum proximal to the site of atresia, and absence of gas distally. When atresia involves the second portion of the duodenum a characteristic "double bubble" sign is formed by gas in the fundus of the stomach and in the duodenal bulb, with a total absence of gas in any other portion of the abdomen (Figs. 21-3B and 21-4). Two large bubbles of this type are seen with duodenal atresia and with some cases of annular pancreas associated with duodenal atresia (Fig. 21-5). Obstructions of the duodenum by stenosis, peritoneal bands, volvulus, or annular pancreas without atresia usually do not produce such considerable dilatation of the duodenal bulb.

Rarely, because of an associated anomaly of the common bile duct, gas may be detected in the distal small bowel. In this anomaly, the terminal portion of the bile duct divides into two and inserts both above and below the area of atresia, allowing for passage of air around the obstruction.[8] Gas within the biliary

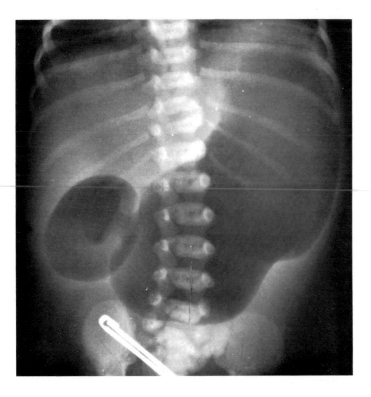

Figure 21-4 Duodenal atresia. A hugely distended stomach and duodenal bulb are noted. The large circular collection of air in right upper quadrant is the duodenal bulb, through which the distal part of the antrum can be seen.

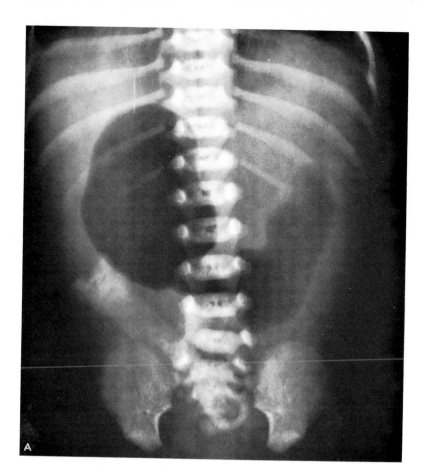

Figure 21-5 *Annular pancreas and associated duodenal atresia* in a newborn. *A,* Supine film demonstrates marked distention of the duodenal bulb within right upper quadrant as well as air within stomach.

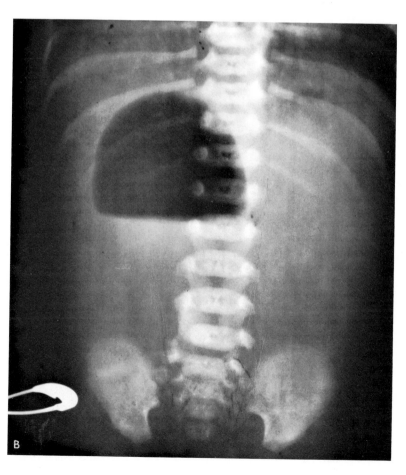

Figure 21-5 *B,* The huge duodenum with an associated air-fluid level is again seen in the upright film. The stomach contains a considerable amount of fluid and only a small air-fluid level is noted in left upper quadrant.

457

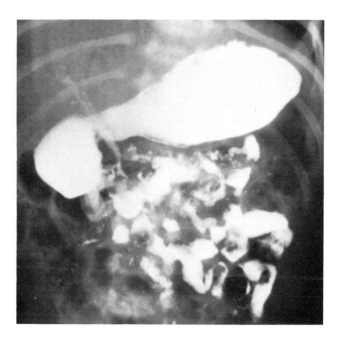

Figure 21-6 *Duodenal stenosis with reflux into the biliary system.* Upper gastrointestinal examination demonstrates a markedly dilated stomach and proximal duodenum. The distal duodenum and small bowel are collapsed, indicating duodenal stenosis. Barium can be seen refluxing into the common duct (arrow). Air can also be detected within the more distal hepatic branches.

tree has also been encountered in cases of severe duodenal obstruction, e.g., atresia or stenosis. Excessive dilatation of the duodenum results in a patulous papilla of Vater that allows for easy reflux of air into the common duct (Fig. 21-6).

Stenosis implies partial obliteration of the intestinal lumen. While multiple areas of atresia are not uncommon (15 to 25 per cent) multiple areas of involvement by stenosis are relatively rare. Clinical distinction between stenosis and atresia is based on the degree of obstruction. Severe stenosis may present as early as atresia and the obtruction may be marked (Fig. 21-7). When

Figure 21-7 *Severe duodenal stenosis* in a newborn. The stomach and duodenum are dilated and contain residual opaque material from a previous study. No gas is seen distal to the distended duodenum, and differentiation between duodenal atresia and stenosis in this situation would be impossible.

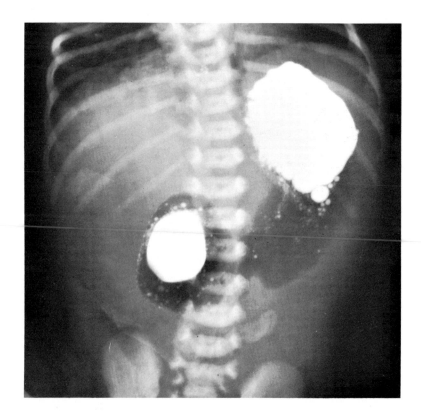

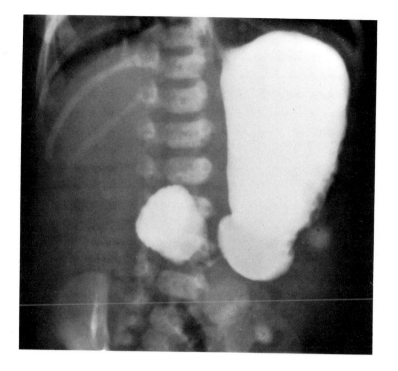

Figure 21-8 Duodenal stenosis. Dilated stomach and duodenum are outlined by opaque material. Distal to the obstructed duodenum, small air collections are present within both small and large bowel. This feature indicates the presence of an incomplete duodenal obstruction compatible with stenosis, annular pancreas, or an extrinsic process.

stenosis is less severe, clinical symptoms are milder and may, in fact, be delayed for days or weeks or may be intermittent. In some instances the clinical picture may resemble that seen with milk allergy or other feeding problems. When the stenosis is minimal there may be no symptomatology until much later in life.

Radiographically duodenal stenosis, unlike atresia, results in the appearance of an incomplete obstruction. The stomach and duodenal bulb may show variable degrees of distention, but characteristically some gas will be seen distal to the dilated proximal duodenum (Fig. 21-8). More often than not, much of the small bowel will contain collections of gas without distention.

ANNULAR PANCREAS

Annular pancreas is a band of pancreatic tissue which arises from the head of the pancreas and forms a partial or complete ring around the second portion of the duodenum. When the ring is incomplete it takes the form of two arms extending from the head of the pancreas, partially engulfing the duodenum but leaving a space on its ventral surface, which is filled with loose fibrous tissue.[9] When complete, it may be associated with an underlying duodenal atresia.

The clinical manifestations of annular pancreas depend upon the degree to which the lesion obstructs the duodenum. Complete obstructions present with the same clinical and roentgenographic appearance as duodenal atresia. With incomplete obstructions symptoms tend to be delayed until later in childhood or even until adulthood, and usually consist of intermittent nausea, vomiting, and epigastric pain. When there is no obstruction, symptoms referable to annular pancreas may be absent throughout life, the lesion being discovered only incidentally at autopsy.

The roentgen findings in annular pancreas are related to the degree of obstruction. When the obstruction is complete or associated with atresia there is considerable distention of the duodenal bulb and stomach, which present as the "double bubble" identical to that described in duodenal atresia (Fig. 21-5). In some cases, however, the obstruction is almost but not quite complete. In these instances small bubbles of gas may be seen distal to the site of obstruction. While this appearance excludes duodenal atresia it cannot be differentiated from partial obstruction due to stenosis or an extrinsic process. In these circumstances barium studies should be performed to exclude malrotation as a cause of the obstruction. While there are no pathognomonic roentgen signs of annular pancreas this condition should be included in the differential diagnosis of all complete obstructions of the second portion of the duodenum. In those cases in which the duodenal obstruction is mild, permitting passage of significant amounts of gas to outline the small bowel, further examination with the aid of contrast material is justified. In such examinations annular pancreas is usually seen as a concentric narrowing or a smooth compression of the right side of the second portion of the duodenum.

MALROTATION

In order to appreciate the effects of malrotation it is important to understand the normal rotation of the intestines which occurs during fetal life. The superior mesenteric artery is the main fulcrum around which the intestines rotate. Initially the intestinal tract is a straight tube lying in front of the superior mesenteric artery. As the small bowel, right colon, and part of the transverse colon extend outside the abdomen into the cord, the duodenum begins to curve downward and to the right of the artery. At about the 25 mm. stage the duodenum lies beneath the artery, completing a rotation of 180 degrees. At approximately the tenth week or the 40 mm. stage the intestines begin their return to the abdomen. The small intestine migrates inward initially and pushes the duodenum and jejunum to the left, completing a 270 degree turn around the vessel. The rotation corresponds to a 270 degree turn in a counterclockwise direction. The right colon returns last to the abdomen and is therefore located on the left side of the artery. The cecum then continues to migrate above and anterior to the vessel in a counterclockwise direction to attain its normal position on the right side of the superior mesenteric artery. Completing this process, it similarly has undergone a 270 degree turn. To summarize, intestinal rotation consists mainly of two segments: the duodenojejunal and the cecocolic. The return and rotation of each segment is sequential, not simultaneous, and can occur independently of each other. Arrest of rotation at any one time may therefore affect either or both of these segments.

Variations in the rotation and fixation of the intestines result in numerous anomalies, the radiographically most important of which are non-rotation, incomplete rotation, reversed rotation, and normal rotation with inadequate mesenteric peritoneal fusion.[10] Volvulus of the mid gut or obstruction due to bands may complicate any of these varieties. It will aid in the radiologic evaluation of these conditions if one keeps in mind the final anatomic pattern associated with these anomalies. In non-rotation the entire mid gut returns to the peritoneal cavity without completing its rotation around the superior mesenteric artery. The small bowel then comes to lie in the right abdomen and the colon in the left abdomen (Fig. 21-9). In incomplete rotation or malrotation, the pre-

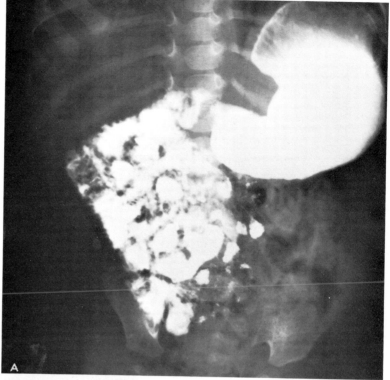

Figure 21-9 *Nonrotation of the mid gut.* A, Gastrointestinal series demonstrates the small bowel to be lying completely within the right side of the abdomen.

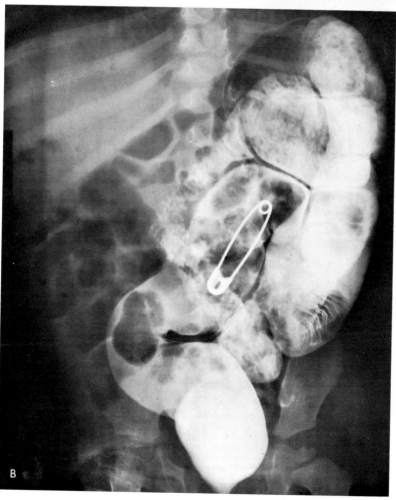

Figure 21-9 *B,* Barium enema performed on the same patient reveals the entire colon located on the left side of the abdomen. Cecum and terminal ileum are situated within the left upper quadrant. This child had recurrent bouts of abdominal pain and, shortly after these studies were performed, entered the hospital in acute distress. A mid-gut volvulus was reduced at surgery.

arterial segment is usually in a normal position, but the colon usually terminates prematurely with the cecum lying in the left abdomen, the epigastrium, or high on the right side. In some cases only an abnormal mobile cecum may be present. As a result of this incomplete process, the usual peritoneal attachment of the right colon forms bands, the so-called "Ladd's Bands," which extend from the right colon across the duodenum to the right upper quadrant, a situation predisposing to duodenal obstruction.

Failure of the jejunum to rotate normally under the superior mesenteric artery results in an abnormal attachment of the mesentery of the small bowel to the posterior wall. Consequently the only line of attachment is a small narrow area around the superior mesenteric artery. The small bowel is then exceedingly mobile, and volvulus occurs easily. Isolated incomplete rotation of the duodenum is also known to occur. In this rare abnormality, the distal duodenum passes either beneath but to the right of, or anterior to the superior mesenteric vessels. In no instance is it located in its normal position to the left of these vessels.[11] Bands and adhesions form across portions of the duodenum with resulting obstruction. An unusual and rare form of rotation is the passage of the cecum underneath the artery. This is termed reversed rotation. As a result, the position of the duodenum and the colon is reversed, i.e., the duodenum overlies the colon and is separated from it by the superior mesenteric artery.

Congenital diaphragmatic hernias and omphaloceles by nature of their embryologic development are forms of nonrotation. Following repair of the primary process, the possibility of volvulus occurring is always present. Other rare manifestations related to rotation are the presence of right and left paraduodenal hernias. These hernias are rarely encountered in childhood and represent imprisonment of the small bowel within the mesentery of the large bowel.

Clinical manifestations resulting from nonrotation or malrotation of the intestinal tract are due to complete, partial or intermittent obstructions associated with peritoneal bands, mid-gut volvulus, or both. Although the second portion of the duodenum or the more distal parts of the small bowel may be affected, the third portion of the duodenum is usually the site of the obstruction. In the neonatal period the obstruction is usually complete or at least severe. The predominant symptom is vomiting. If the vascular supply of the bowel is compromised, venous or lymphatic obstruction or eventual necrosis of bowel occurs. As a result melena or chylous ascites are part of the clinical presentation. Should the obstruction involve a site lower in the small bowel, significant degrees of abdominal distention will be noted. The more usual involvement of the third portion of the duodenum is not associated with distention, or is associated with distention of the upper abdomen only. Vomiting may occur on the first day of life, but in incomplete obstructions it may be delayed for a week or so or even later in childhood when it may be intermittent in character, simulating cyclic vomiting or an allergic disorder. As a matter of fact, it should be noted that in later childhood malrotation may give rise to symptoms and signs similar to those of celiac disease. In such cases torsion of the small bowel is considered to result in partial obstruction of the superior mesenteric vein with resulting intramural edema, congestion, and malabsorption. It is also possible that twists in the bowel may result in chronic or intermittent obstructions at the terminal ileum. At any rate these children do present with chronic or intermittent abdominal distention, signs of malabsorption, and constipation or diarrhea.

In the neonatal period complete obstruction of the duodenum because of bands, mid-gut volvulus, or both presents roentgenologic findings similar to those of other complete duodenal occlusions (Fig. 21-10). It is more likely, however, that obstructions resulting from these lesions will be located in the third portion of the duodenum, and although there is dilatation of the proximal duodenum the degree of dilatation of the duodenal bulb seen in duodenal atresia is usually not present in obstructions due to malrotation anomalies (Fig. 21-10 and 21-11). Currently, it appears that the diagnostic procedure of choice

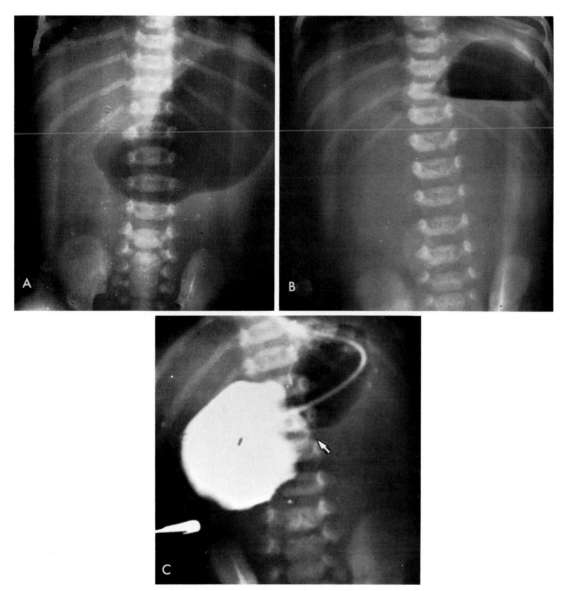

Figure 21-10   *Malrotation and mid-gut volvulus* in a three day old infant who was vomiting bile-stained material.

A, Supine film of abdomen reveals a dilated stomach and duodenal bulb with no visible air distal to this area.

B, On the upright film of the abdomen a large air-fluid level is present within the stomach with minimal air noted within the duodenal bulb. These findings are compatible with a duodenal obstruction, and the differentiation between duodenal atresia and mid-gut volvulus may be difficult. However, the duodenum is only minimally dilated, a feature not associated with atresia.

C, With the injection of opaque material the obstruction is demonstrated at the level of the ligament of Treitz (arrow). At surgery malrotation with minimal volvulus was present, and the third portion of the duodenum was obstructed by peritoneal bands.

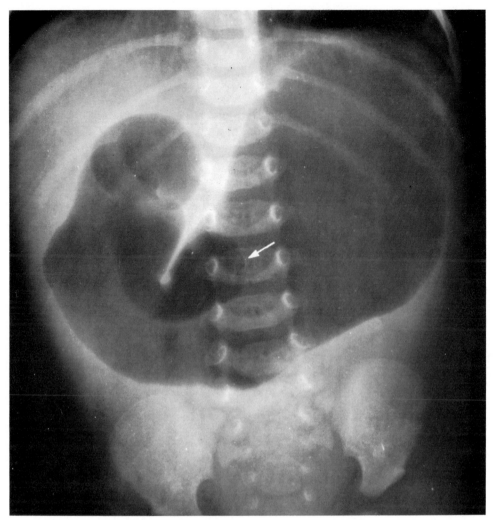

Figure 21-11 *Malrotation and mid-gut volvulus* in a six week old infant with recent onset of bile-stained vomiting.

Stomach and duodenum are distended. The obstructed distal third of duodenum (arrow) is visualized through the gastric antrum. No air is seen distally.

Findings at surgery were malrotation with mid-gut volvulus. In addition a peritoneal band extended across and obstructed the duodenum.

following abdominal studies is an examination of the upper gastrointestinal tract. This study is easily performed, carries little morbidity, and not only localizes the site of obstruction but often indicates its nature, e.g., band or volvulus. The bowel in the latter assumes a twisted or corkscrew appearance at the point of obstruction. In addition, the presence or absence of internal occlusion of the bowel caused by a coexisting duodenal diaphragm can be determined. This anomaly occurs in approximately 10 per cent of cases with malrotation and volvulus, and if left uncorrected at the time of the original surgery results in recurrent obstruction. The barium enema examination is still a worthwhile procedure. In many institutions it is the preferred study, performed either by itself or in conjunction with the upper gastrointestinal examination. Evidence on the enema films of malposition of the cecum is suggestive of malrotation with peritoneal bands, mid-gut volvulus, or both. This procedure, nevertheless, has some inherent diagnostic limitations since it demonstrates neither the precise

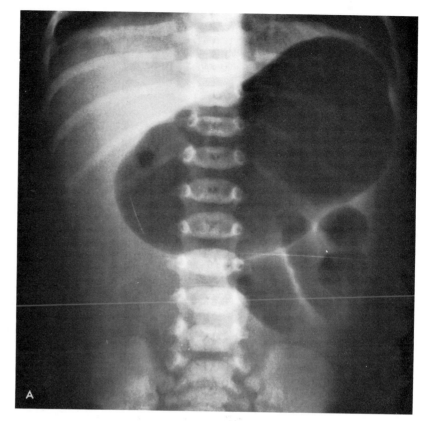

Figure 21-12 *Malrotation and midgut volulus* in a four day old infant who on the first day of life passed a large bloody meconium stool and began to vomit shortly afterward.

A, Supine film of abdomen reveals a distended stomach as well as some dilated loops of small bowel within left upper quadrant. These findings suggest a small bowel obstruction, most likely jejunal.

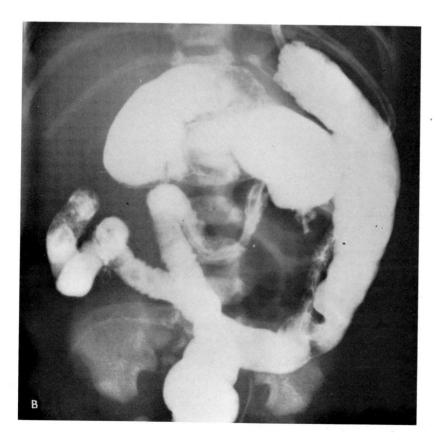

Figure 21-12 B, On barium enema examination the colon is completely located within the left abdomen indicating the presence of a malrotation and probable mid-gut volvulus. These findings were confirmed at surgery. (Courtesy of Dr. H. Grossman, New York, New York.)

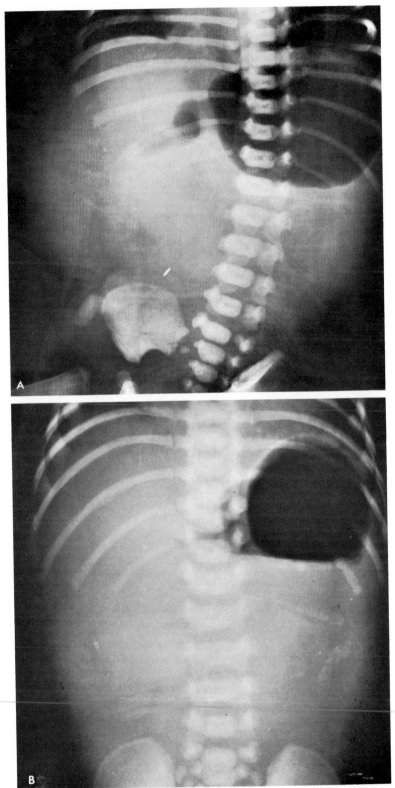

Figure 21-13 *Malrotation, mid-gut volvulus, and meconium peritonitis* in a newborn who presented with abdominal distention and vomiting.

A, Stomach and duodenum are moderately dilated, and only a portion of the duodenal sweep is visualized. No air is seen distally. However, there is a soft tissue mass in the right upper quadrant displacing the duodenal sweep. The mass represents fluid-filled infarcted small bowel.

B, On the upright film an air fluid level is seen within the stomach. In addition mottled calcifications indicating meconium peritonitis are present in left part of the abdomen. Findings at surgery were malrotation, mid-gut volvulus, and meconium peritonitis.

diagnosis, the presence of intrinsic disease, nor isolated incomplete rotation of the duodenum. The latter anomaly is frequently accompanied by a normally positioned colon.[11]

Where malrotation has resulted in an incomplete obstruction, moderate dilatation of the proximal duodenum will be associated with variable amounts of gas in the lower small bowel. The appearance will be similar to that of duodenal stenosis. The site of obstruction in malrotation with mid-gut volvulus is not always at the third portion of the duodenum, however, and may occur in the jejunum or the ileum (Fig. 21-12). Barium enema studies will facilitate diagnosis by indicating an abnormal position of the cecum consistent with some form of malrotation. Rarely, malrotation and mid-gut volvulus will present as duodenal obstruction associated with fluid filled loops of small bowel (pseudo-tumor) (Fig. 21-13).

JEJUNOILEAL ATRESIA AND STENOSIS

Atresia and stenosis of the jejunum and ileum are less often associated with other important congenital anomalies than are the duodenal occlusions, and they have no particular relation to the occurrence of Down's syndrome. Louw[12] found the most serious abnormalities associated with jejunoileal occlusions to be meconium peritonitis and omphalocele. As with duodenal occlusions, hyperbilirubinemia is often found associated with obstructing jejunal lesions. Louw[12] found five of his 17 cases to be deeply jaundiced, three of them requiring exchange transfusions. A rare phenomenon associated with high jejunal atresia is agenesis of the dorsal mesentery. In this anomaly, the primary mesenteric branches to the ileum and jejunum are absent and the blood supply to the distal jejunum is via the ileocecal and marginal arteries. The remaining distal small bowel is spiraled around a vascular stalk and has been termed "apple peel small bowel" or "Christmas tree deformity."

High jejunal lesions may present a clinical picture similar to that of duodenal obstruction, but the lower the obstruction in the small bowel the more prominent is the abdominal distention and the less frequent the vomiting. Delay in the diagnosis of jejunal or ileal atresias and severe stenosis is particularly dangerous because increasing distention of the bowel wall leads to vascular changes and eventual perforation.

Atresia, which is more commonly encountered than stenosis, presents radiographically as a complete obstruction of the small bowel with distention of the small intestine proximal to the site of obstruction (Figs. 21-14 and 21-15). There is no gas demonstrable in the large bowel or rectum. When the obstruction is in the jejunum the gas-filled loops of intestine tend to be localized to the upper abdomen in the erect position. Occlusions involving the more distal portions of the small bowel frequently present more difficult diagnostic problems because a greater length of bowel becomes distended and the infant abdomen becomes crowded with gas-filled loops with no characteristic markings or position, making differentiation between small bowel and colon practically impossible on the survey films. In this circumstance a barium enema examination will indicate the position and condition of the colon, making it possible to differentiate between small bowel and colonic obstruc-

(*Text continued on page 471.*)

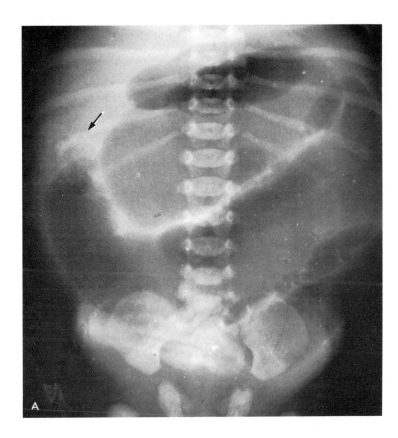

Figure 21-14 *Jejunal atresia and meconium peritonitis* in a two day old infant with vomiting. A, The small bowel is markedly dilated. The valvulae conniventes are still detected within a large loop of jejunum located in the mid-portion of the abdomen. In the right upper quadrant are the calcifications (arrow) indicating the presence of meconium peritonitis.

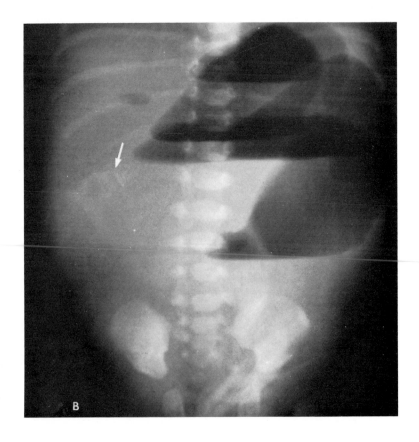

Figure 21-14 *B*, Upright film of abdomen demonstrates huge air fluid levels and peritoneal calcifications (arrow). At surgery, jejunal atresia was present with a small perforation just proximal to the atresia.

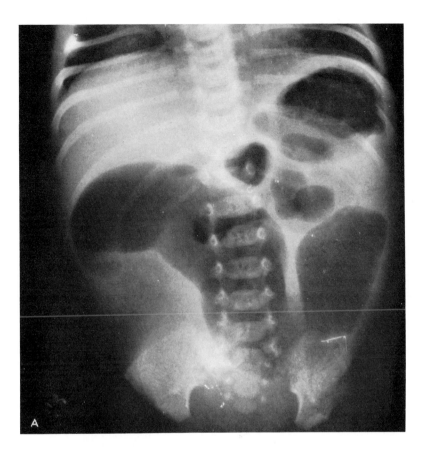

Figure 21-15 Jejunal atresia. A, Distended loops of small bowel are noted.

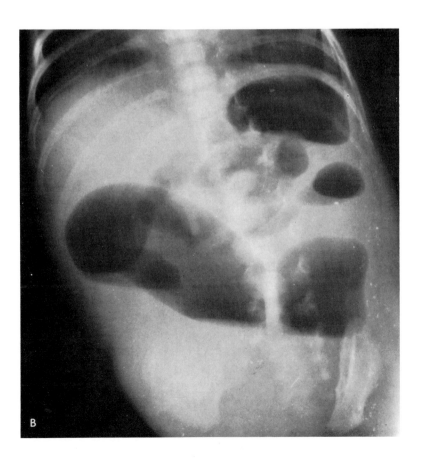

Figure 21-15 B, Upright film, same patient, demonstrates air fluid levels within the small bowel. Although no characteristic bowel markings are maintained, the predominant location within the upper abdomen and the limited number of distended loops suggest jejunal atresia.

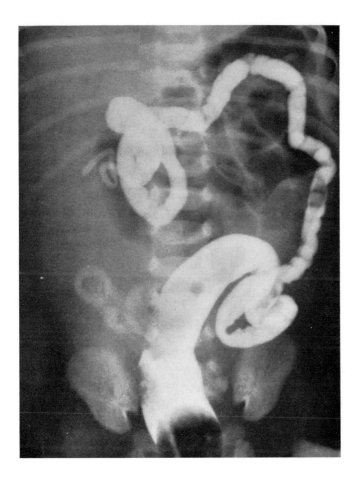

Figure 21-16 Ilial atresia, malrotation, and volvulus in a one day old infant presenting with abdominal distention. The original study of the abdomen demonstrated distended small bowel loops. Barium enema reveals a microcolon extending from the sigmoid to the cecum, which is located in the right upper quadrant. There are also dilated small bowel loops, and a mass is present in the right lower quadrant.

Ilial atresia and malrotation were diagnosed by the presence of a microcolon and an abnormally located cecum. A mass in the right lower quadrant suggested an associated volvulus. All findings were confirmed at surgical exploration.

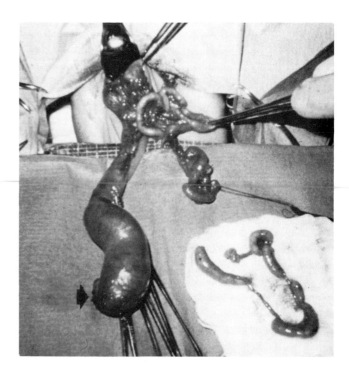

Figure 21-17 Multiple small bowel atresias. Operative specimen demonstrates the markedly dilated proximal loop (arrow). The distal bowel is collapsed, with multiple areas of atresia (note resected specimen).

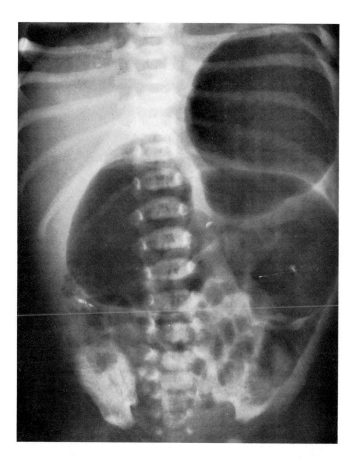

Figure 21-18 Jejunal stenosis. The jejunum is markedly distended, although gas is present distal to the dilated bowel. The features indicate an incomplete small bowel obstruction. At surgery the obstruction was found to be caused by a membrane with a small pinpoint opening.

tion. As noted, distal small bowel atresia is associated with microcolon, since little or no meconium has passed through the colon (Fig. 21-16). Higher levels of atresia are associated with larger colons because of the passage of quantities of meconium formed below the site of obstruction. Consequently, multiple atresias of the small bowel (Fig. 21-17) may be suspected when a high jejunal atresia is encountered on the abdominal study associated with a microcolon on the barium enema examination. Small bowel stenosis presents as an incomplete obstruction, and variable quantities of gas will be seen distal to the point of obstruction (Fig. 21-18).

DUPLICATIONS

Duplications of the intestinal tract may cause complete or partial obstruction of the small bowel. While this usually does not occur until late infancy or early childhood, it may develop in early infancy. Duplications may arise from any portion of the alimentary tract, from the tongue to the anus; but these congenital anomalies are most common in the ileum and esophagus. Gross et al.[13] found that of 39 duplications involving the small intestine the distribution was as follows: four in the duodenum, four in the jejunum, 20 in the ileum, and eight at the ileocecal junction. Three others arising from the duodenum or jejunum extended as a tubular structure through the diaphragm into the thorax. Duplications are usually spherical or tubular in shape, have a

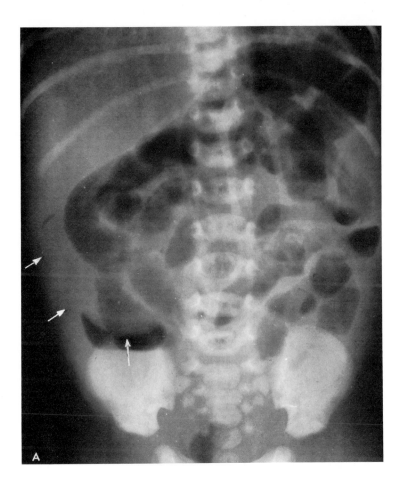

Figure 21-19 Ileocecal duplication in a newborn. *A,* A large mass is present within the right lower quadrant (arrows) and is outlined along its lateral and inferior margins by air within the bowel. The small bowel is moderately dilated although gas is seen within the rectum.

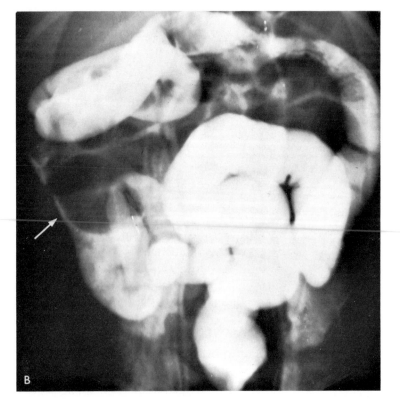

Figure 21-19 B, Barium enema study again outlines the mass in the right lower quadrant (arrow).

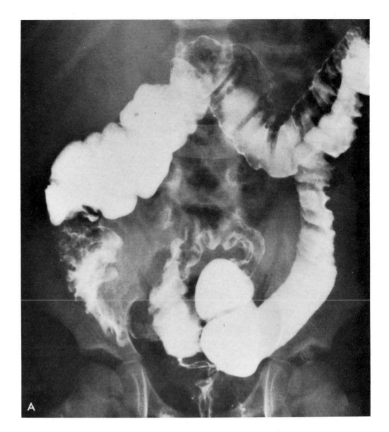

Figure 21-20 *Ileal duplication* in a young boy who presented with right lower quadrant pain of one month's duration. *A*, Mass is seen displacing medial part of cecum as well as the adjacent small bowel.

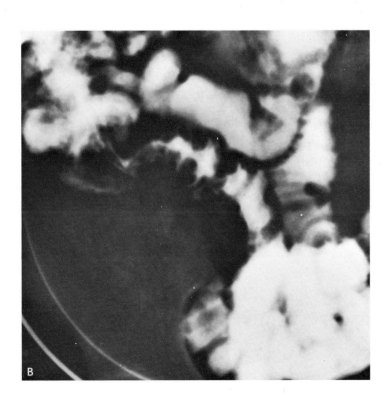

Figure 21-20 *B*, Spot film of terminal ileum obtained during a small bowel study reveals the extrinsic nature of the mass as well as its mobility. The mucosa of the terminal ileum is altered but not destroyed or infiltrated. (Courtesy of Dr. H. Grossman, New York, New York.)

well developed smooth muscle layer, and are lined with a mucous membrane. The type of mucosa is not always similar to that of the adjacent intestine, and on occasion there may be two or three different types of mucosa in a single structure.

It is considered that duplications arise during the stage of recanalization of the intestinal tract. The solid core of epithelial cells which have obliterated the lumen is recanalized by vacuoles which coalesce to reestablish a lumen. If one vacuole fails to coalesce with the re-formed lumen it may persist as a duplication. In a recent study of 39 enteric duplications, Favara et al. noted that 19 cysts were located within the small bowel. All were intimately associated with areas of small bowel atresia, and mesenteric defects. The authors postulate that the development of enteric duplication may also be an end result of intra-uterine bowel infarction.[14]

Duplications of the small bowel usually present clinically as partial or complete intestinal obstruction. This results from compression of a segment of intestine by a noncommunicating adjacent duplication which has become distended by the accumulation of secretions within it. In some instances, the duplication may obstruct by intussusception or by torsion with small bowel volvulus. Pain may result from overdistention of the duplication. When there is a lining of gastric mucosa and a communication between the duplication and the adjacent intestine, pain may result from peptic ulceration within the duplication or the adjacent communicating bowel segment. Bleeding is associated with ulceration or with interference of the vascular supply of the bowel by the distended duplication.

Duplications are only rarely filled by barium and can be appreciated on survey films if they are quite large (Fig. 21-19). Should a communicating duplication in the distal bowel be visualized with barium, its radiographic differentiation from Meckel's diverticulum would most likely not be possible. The usual radiographic features of duplications are those of partial or complete bowel obstruction. These may occur at any level of the bowel although they are most commonly seen in the ileum and at the ileocecal region. Barium studies may reveal displacement of the adjacent bowel by a sharply defined extrinsic mass (Figs. 21-19 and 21-20). The intestinal mucosa will appear stretched with no demonstrable ulcerations. If a duplication is the cause of intussusception, it will be difficult to differentiate from other mass lesions.

Duplications which arise in the small bowel and extend through the diaphragm into the thorax appear as spherical or tubular soft tissue densities in the posterior mediastinum. They are usually associated with anomalies of the lower cervical or upper dorsal spine. Gross[13] found that in all such lesions there was communication with the intestine at the site of origin of the duplication. In some cases the anomalous structure may be coiled upon itself in the thorax, presenting a radiographic appearance difficult to distinguish from diaphragmatic hernia. The coexistence of a duplication extending into the thorax with a diaphragmatic hernia has been reported.[13, 15]

MECONIUM ILEUS

Meconium ileus is a common cause of intestinal obstruction in the newborn period. It is one of the protean manifestations of cystic fibrosis (mucovisci-

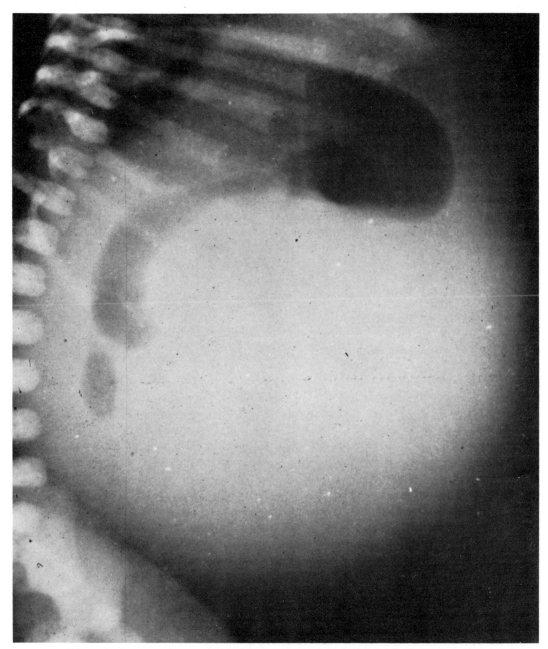

Figure 21-21 *Pseudocyst, meconium ileus.* Lateral film of the abdomen in a newborn with meconium ileus demonstrates a huge cystic mass. Surgical exploration revealed this to be necrotic intestine filled with meconium. (Courtesy of Dr. H. Grossman, New York, New York.)

dosis) and occurs in approximately 20 per cent of all patients with that disorder. In meconium ileus the intestine is obstructed by abnormal meconium which becomes inspissated in the distal ileum. For some time it was considered that this abnormal meconium was the result of deficient enzyme production due to fibrosis of the pancreas. Recent pathologic studies,[16] however, indicate that altered small intestinal glands are primarily responsible for the development of meconium ileus and that pancreatic lesions are of secondary, if any, importance in the pathogenesis of this condition.

Introduction of new surgical techniques has increased the surgical survival rate (50 per cent) in uncomplicated cases, but meconium ileus is frequently accompanied by the intra-abdominal complications of volvulus, gangrene, atresia, and perforation. Atresia or volvulus without gangrene or peritonitis does not appear to alter the survival rate significantly, but perforation, peritonitis, and gangrene are ominous developments which gravely affect the chance for survival.[17] These secondary complications unfortunately are quite common and occur when the grossly distended meconium-filled loops twist upon themselves. In some cases vascular compromise leads to gangrene, which in turn may progress to necrosis and perforation. At times there may be formation of a cystic mass of necrotic intestine containing fluid meconium. Santulli[18] has referred to this as a "pseudocyst" (Figs. 21-21 and 21-22). In meconium ileus, atresias are considered to be the result of volvulus and of "inflammation and fibrosis."[17]

Although the clinical picture is essentially that of any neonatal low small bowel obstruction there are some suggestive features which may be noted. The abdomen is distended. Rubbery loops of bowel which pit on pressure may be palpated through the abdominal wall, and rectal examination usually reveals an unusually small anus and rectum. About one-third of the patients will have a family history of cystic fibrosis or meconium ileus.

In some cases the radiographic appearance is indistinguishable from low small bowel obstructions due to other causes. In many cases, however, there are roentgen features which provide reliable clues to the correct diagnosis. Characteristically, in many cases the gas-filled loops of small bowel show a significant variability in size. Some may be considerably distended while others are only moderately dilated or practically normal in caliber (Fig. 21-23).

Neuhauser[19] first called attention to a ground-glass or soap bubble pattern of the meconium in the bowel as seen on the survey film (Fig. 21-23). This

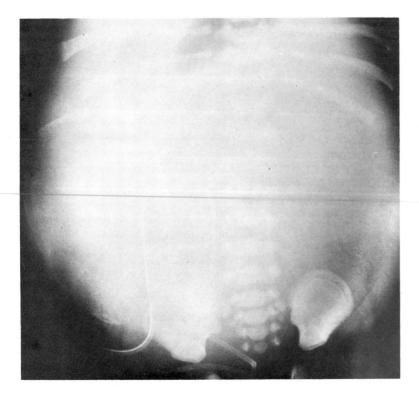

Figure 21-22 Pseudo-cyst, meconium, meconium peritonitis and bony stress lines. Total body opacification (obtained during intravenous pyelography) reveals a huge cystic mass occupying the center of the abdomen. Stress lines can be seen in the left iliac crest, suggesting meconium peritonitis, although peritoneal calcifications are not distinctly visualized. At surgery, a huge necrotic mass containing meconium, ileal atresia, and meconium peritonitis was found.

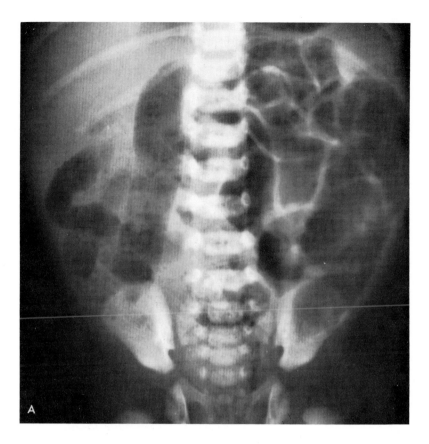

Figure 21-23 Meconium ileus. A, Small bowel is markedly dilated. The small bowel on the left is considerably more dilated than that located on the right. A ground-glass appearance due to the presence of meconium within the bowel is also observed on this side. Associated with this are multiple bubbles of air of variable sizes.

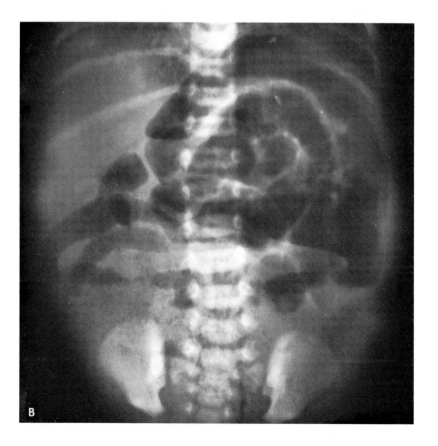

Figure 21-23 B, Upright film of same patient demonstrates poorly defined and irregular air-fluid levels. Air bubbles are still apparent, since most of the air still remains mixed with meconium.

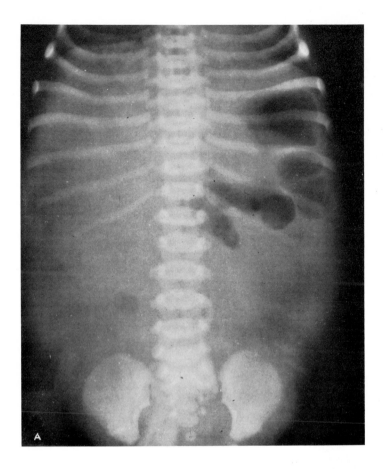

Figure 21-24 Meconium ileus. A, Supine film of abdomen taken during the first day of life shows marked abdominal distention and discrepancy in small bowel distention. Within the left upper quadrant some dilated loops of small bowel are noted, and little gas is present on the right side.

Figure 21-24 B, Barium enema was performed the following day, and the film demonstrates a typical microcolon. Also at this time there has been marked increase in small bowel distention. A ground-glass appearance is observed within the right lower quadrant.

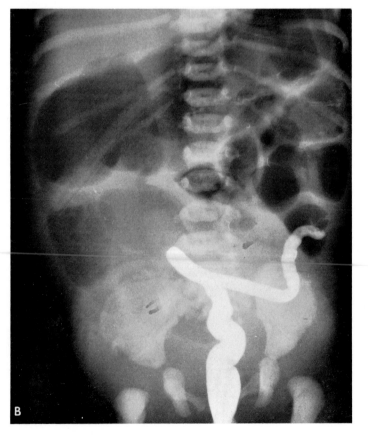

·characteristic pattern is considered to be due to a mixture of air with thick inspissated meconium. While this soap bubble pattern of meconium in the obstructed small bowel of a neonate should strongly suggest meconium ileus, the same pattern occasionally may be seen in patients with ileal atresia or aganglionic involvement of the terminal ileum.

Another roentgen feature of some cases is the absence of fluid levels in the erect position,[20] presumably due to the viscosity of the intestinal contents and the inhibition of intestinal secretion by the adherence of viscid meconium to the bowel wall. Absence of fluid levels in the erect position is not a feature of all cases, however, and the presence of fluid levels does not necessarily mitigate against the diagnosis. The lack of fluid levels on the other hand is a strong clue in favor of meconium ileus. When present, fluid levels tend to form slowly with changes in the infant's position. In some cases a huge mass filling much of the abdomen and representing a large pseudocyst may be seen (Figs. 21-21 and 21-22).

As with other low small bowel obstructions, differentiation between small and large bowel may be impossible, and a barium enema will reveal the position and character of the colon. In meconium ileus, the colon is usually very small in caliber (microcolon) (Fig. 21-24). Although small or hypoplastic colons may be demonstrable in other forms of small bowel obstruction, Singleton[10] has found that the smallest colons are seen with meconium ileus. The calibre of the colon, however, is not determined by the amount of swallowed amniotic fluid, gastric juice, or bile pigments but by the amount of succus entericus and the ability of the small bowel to propel the succus into the colon.[21] Despite the presence of a microcolon, residue may still be apparent in some colons. Meconium ileus is presumed to be a third trimester event, following which fluid is resorbed from the colon.

There is presently a great trend to treat uncomplicated meconium ileus with cleansing water soluble contrast enemas.[22, 23] The previous use of hydrogen peroxide enemas for this purpose has been discontinued because of the frequent deaths resulting from gas embolism. However, the introduction of water soluble contrast enemas for this purpose appears to be more successful and safe if done with careful monitoring of the infant's state of hydration. Sodium or sodium methylglucamine diatrizoate solutions can be refluxed through the microcolon into the dilated obstructed loop. The hyperosmolar solution exerts a strong hydroscopic action within the bowel lumen. The added fluid then not only softens the meconium but provides a fluid medium between the meconium and the bowel wall. The use of supportive intravenous fluids is essential, as stated, to counteract the development of hemoconcentration.

Complicating volvulus or atresia is usually first appreciated at surgery. Peritoneal calcifications indicative of prenatal meconium peritonitis may be noted, especially localized around the peripheral regions of the peritoneal cavity. Calcifications may also be seen in the bowel wall. Associated congenital anomalies are relatively rare in meconium ileus.[17]

MECONIUM ILEUS EQUIVALENT

Meconium ileus equivalent may occur in older infants and children and has been reported in patients ranging in age from 7 months to 15 years. The clinical features of this condition are those of mechanical intestinal obstruction occurring in a child known to have cystic fibrosis of the pancreas. Frequently the meconium ileus equivalent has been associated with inadequate dosage, cessation, or omission of pancreatic enzymes in treatment. Cardonnier and Izant[24] have called attention to certain aids in the diagnosis of this condition, which must be differentiated from other forms of intestinal obstruction, particularly intussusception and postoperative adhesions. Often a soft, indentable mass of impacted material in the intestine can be palpated through the abdomen or rectum. Radiographically, the flat film of the abdomen may show the cecum and ascending colon and the distal ileum to be filled with a soap bubble pattern of intestinal content similar to the soap bubble pattern of meconium in meconium ileus of the neonate. A contrast enema, preferably with a water-soluble contrast medium, will sometimes demonstrate the intraluminal nature of the obstruction and the dilated proximal intestine and will make possible the exclusion of an intussusception.

MECONIUM PERITONITIS

Meconium peritonitis is a nonbacterial, chemical peritonitis resulting from a perforation of the gastrointestinal tract during intrauterine or early neonatal life. Should the perforation remain patent after birth, a secondary bacterial peritonitis results. In some cases, no sign of perforation can be found at operation, indicating that perforation during intrauterine life was sealed off before birth. Meconium peritonitis is usually due to an intestinal obstruction resulting from thick inspissated meconium in patients with fibrocystic disease of the pancreas, or to intestinal atresia (Fig. 21-14), and in some cases to a combination of both. In general, however, 40 per cent of all cases of meconium peritonitis are associated with fibrocystic disease. Less commonly the condition may result from intestinal stenosis, volvulus (Fig. 21-13), bands, or rupture of a Meckel's diverticulum. In those infants who do not present with associated meconium ileus, the prognosis is more favorable, provided that the condition is diagnosed and treated prior to the onset of superimposed bacterial infection.

When the perforation has occurred in utero without an associated obstruction and with sealing of the defect before birth, the patients are asymptomatic and the disease is discovered fortuitously on films of the abdomen made for some unrelated reason. In general, however, meconium peritonitis is associated with an intestinal obstruction. Abdominal distention, vomiting, and obstipation are the usual clinical features. In some cases there may be variable degrees of pneumoperitoneum.

The roentgen diagnosis of meconium peritonitis is based on the identification of calcium within the peritoneal cavity on abdominal roentgenograms. Meconium in contact with the peritoneal fluid shows a marked propensity to calcify, and calcification may occur in some cases as early as 24 hours after extrusion of the meconium into the peritoneal cavity. The intra-abdominal calcium deposits may appear as a single cluster (Fig. 21-14), a few small scattered clusters, or as long linear calcium shadows which tend to be localized to the periphery of the abdomen (Fig. 21-25). These lie on the peritoneal surface and are seen to be situated anteriorly or posteriorly in the lateral projection or at the flank in the anteroposterior projection. On occasion calcium deposits may be

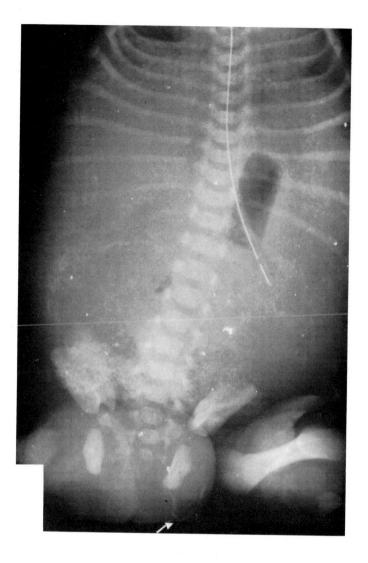

Figure 21-25 Meconium peritonitis in a newborn presenting with marked distention and scrotal swelling. There is very little gas distributed throughout the small bowel. Plaques and linear strands of calcification outline the abdominal flanks. In addition the scrotal sac is distended, and there is a linear calcification within it (arrow).

seen within the scrotal sac, extruded meconium having spilled into the scrotum through the communication between the peritoneal cavity and the processus vaginalis (Fig. 21-25).

Although the calcific meconium salts in meconium peritonitis are easily identified when they lie peripherally or in the scrotal sac, it may be difficult to differentiate calcifications on the serosa of the bowel from intraluminal or intramural calcification (Fig. 21-26). Intraluminal calcifications within inspissated meconium may occur in association with obstructions. The calcification in these instances is likely to appear as multiple rounded densities or occasionally as concentric rings, in contrast to the cluster-like plaques or peripheral calcium lines of meconium peritonitis. Intraluminal calcifications, however, may also appear in a linear arrangement, in which case their location is suggested by their more central position in the abdomen as seen in the anteroposterior and lateral projections.

Intramural calcification apparently represents an incomplete form of perforation and occurs when meconium is extruded into the wall of the intestine through an ulceration. This has been described in rare instances in association with small bowel atresia, volvulus, and fibrocystic disease of the pancreas.

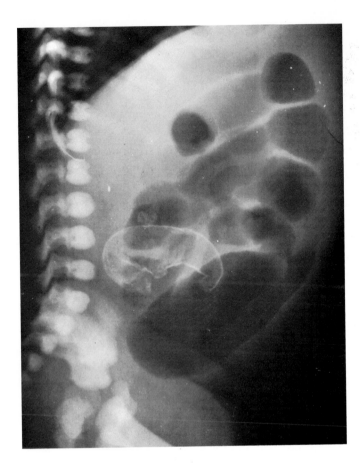

Figure 21-26 Meconium peritonitis and ileal atresia. Lateral film of abdomen shows intramural calcification within a loop of ileum. Somewhat superior to this is a mottled collection of calcifications. The small bowel is distended proximally, indicating ileal atresia.

Meconium peritonitis apparently can cause interrupted bone growth, manifested at the ends of the long and flat bones as metaphyseal bands.[25] These bands or stress lines present as opaque stripes separated from the epiphysis by a zone of lucency (Fig. 21-22). Recognition of these stress lines provides a valuable adjunct in diagnosing meconium peritonitis in infants with intestinal obstruction, even in the absence of calcifications.

DISEASE SIMULATING SMALL BOWEL OBSTRUCTION

Because it is difficult in many cases to differentiate between distended small bowel and colon on survey films of the neonatal abdomen, lesions of the large bowel may simulate low small bowel obstruction. The clinical manifestations are also similar and usually provide no reliable means for differential diagnosis. In this instance it is always worthwhile to examine the abdomen in the lateral projection, since in this view the long sweep of the descending colon may occasionally be identified in the prevertebral area.[26] When the colon cannot be so identified, a barium enema examination is imperative to exclude a large bowel obstruction. The study should be performed with a straight catheter. The use of a Foley catheter is to be avoided since it obscures the calibre of the rectum. Care must also be given to the type of enema utilized. If Hirschsprung's disease is suspected, physiologic saline should be used to prevent unnecessary absorption of fluid from the colon. Water soluble contrast enemas must be used with care since they behave as a cathartic, stimulating evacuation, and thus distort the diagnosis.

Hirschsprung's disease (aganglionosis) in the neonate presents as intestinal obstruction.[27] The disease is rarely seen in the premature and affects the male more commonly than the female by a ratio of approximately 4:1. An increased incidence has also been noted in Down's syndrome. The rectum and distal sigmoid colon are the most common sites of involvement and pathologic studies of these tissues reveal absence of ganglion cells within the sub-mucosal and muscle layers. Although initially well, infants with this disorder usually become distended and vomit bile-stained material within the first 36 or 48 hours of life. The passage of meconium is frequently delayed. Survey films of the distended abdomen may show numerous gas-filled loops of intestine with air-fluid levels (Fig. 21-27). Differentiation between small bowel and colon is usually difficult or impossible and barium contrast examination of the colon is necessary. In some instances the barium enema films may show a transitional zone in the colon, representing a change from the narrower distal aganglionic segment to a dilated ganglionic portion. The aganglionic segment usually extends somewhat proximal to the actual site of transition, as demonstrated radiographically. In many instances, however, the colon in the newborn will show a normal caliber throughout, with no evidence of a transitional zone. In either case the microcolon seen in distal small bowel atresia (or meconium ileus) is excluded, and a normal position of the cecum rules against a malrotation with small bowel volvulus. When the barium enema shows a colon of uniform caliber, delayed films are of the utmost importance since patients with aganglionosis show very poor evacuation on films made 24 and 48 hours after the enema study (Fig. 21-28). In the neonate, radiographic diagnosis of Hirschsprung's disease may be made on the basis of this colonic stasis alone. Hope et al.[28] have stressed the diagnostic importance of irregular, bizarre contractions of the aganglionic segment and believe that these indentations, which are irregular in both spacing and extent are the result of dysrhythmia produced by the aganglionosis. It is their experience that in early infancy these irregular contractions are a more frequent finding than a well demarcated transitional zone. This has also been our experience, but in those instances in which there are neither bizarre contractions nor a transitional zone, persistent colonic stasis may be relied upon as a major diagnostic feature.

Long-segment Hirschsprung's disease, i.e., aganglionosis involving the entire colon and the terminal ileum, presents during the first three months of life as an intermittent small bowel obstruction. This form of Hirschsprung's disease is found in 10% of the cases, has a definite family incidence and an equal sex ratio. The diagnosis, at times, may be difficult to establish since barium enema examination may reveal varying features within the colon. The colon in some patients may appear completely normal both in length and in calibre; in others, it may be of normal calibre but shorter in length, e.g., the usual redundant sigmoid colon seen in a comparable newborn is foreshortened;[29] and in some patients it may present as a microcolon.[30] Rectal biopsy to demonstrate absent ganglion cells is required in cases where any of these roentgenographic features are associated with undiagnosed small bowel obstruction.

The meconium plug syndrome may also simulate neonatal small bowel obstruction. In this syndrome, a functional disturbance of the colon results in

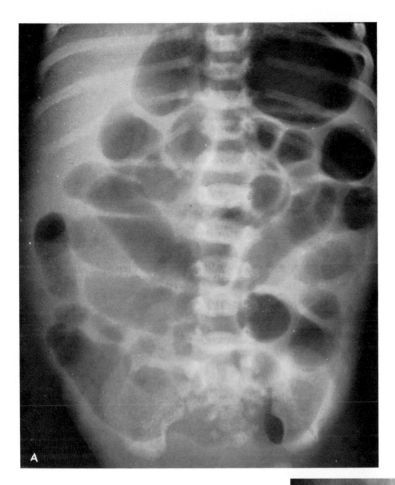

Figure 21-27 Hirschsprung's disease. A, The abdomen is distended, with dilated loops of bowel. Differentiation between small and large bowel in this instance is difficult.

Figure 21-27 B, A minimal amount of contrast material was inserted into the rectum and a transitional zone was observed (arrow).

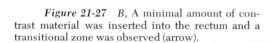

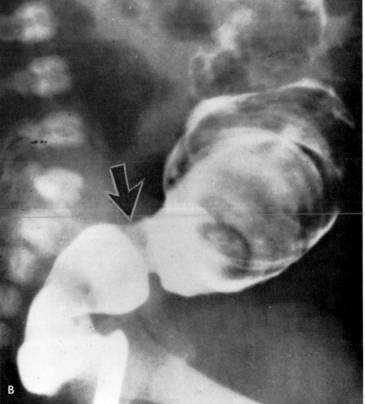

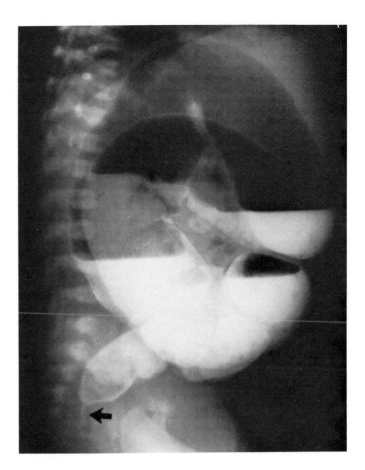

Figure 21-28 *Hirschsprung's disease* diagnosed on delayed films. This film is a delayed study demonstrating a narrowed rectum and a grossly dilated proximal colon.

excessive water absorption with the meconium becoming dry and hard. As a result, the presence of air fluid levels in the colon on x-ray are uncommon. In contrast to Hirschsprung's disease, there is relief of the obstructive symptoms after digital examination of the rectum or a cleansing enema which dislodges a meconium plug. Barium enema examination in these patients often discloses a long plug of obstructing meconium high in the colon and a small caliber collapsed left colon. When the meconium plug extends to the rectum the colon may be of normal caliber (Fig. 21-29). Subsequent barium studies performed after the plug has been extruded show a normal colon with normal evacuation and no bizarre contractions. This is imperative in order to exclude the presence of Hirschsprung's disease. Hirschsprung's disease as well as fibrocystic disease has been associated with the meconium plug syndrome and proper studies to exclude either are justified.[31]

Davis et al.[32] have recently described 19 patients with what they termed the "Neonatal Small Left Colon Syndrome." Pathologic studies in these patients revealed many small cells of immature neuronal elements. The clinical presentation, radiographic appearance, and outcome of the disease strikingly resemble those of the meconium plug syndrome. Although it is possible that both diseases may be one and the same, Clatworthy et al.,[33] in their original description of the meconium plug syndrome, demonstrated normal ganglion cells in the colon.

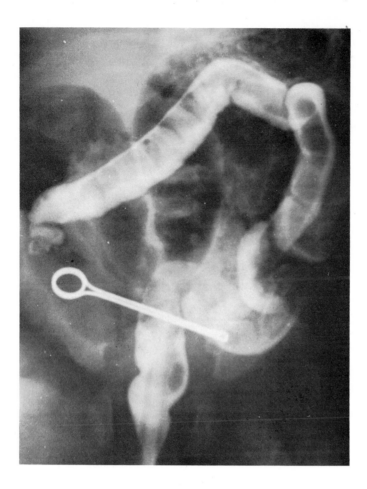

Figure 21-29 Meconium plug syndrome. A long filling defect, representing a meconium plug, extends from the hepatic flexure to the rectum. The barium-filled colon is of normal caliber. There is, however, a marked degree of small bowel obstruction. The plug was promptly extruded, and the patient became and has remained asymptomatic.

ENTEROCOLITIS

Entercolitis is a highly fatal disease that presents in infancy and childhood as a complication of prematurity, intestinal obstruction, and other causes. Its association with Hirschsprung's disease is well known, and there is little doubt that some infants who die from "diarrhea" have in fact died from this frequent complication of Hirschsprung's disease.[27]

Since the clinical manifestations of enterocolitis are the same regardless of the underlying cause, it is imperative to differentiate enterocolitis occurring in the premature infant from that associated with Hirschsprung's disease. In the latter situation, nonoperative therapy is often inadequate. Since Hirschsprung's disease is rarely found in the premature infant, all full-term infants with enterocolitis should be considered to have this disease until proven otherwise. Recently improved diagnostic and surgical techniques for Hirschsprung's disease have resulted in a decrease in this fatal complication.

The pathogenesis of enterocolitis in Hirschsprung's disease is unknown, but it is related in some way to obstruction. Although this enterocolitis may be of viral or bacterial origin, in most instances no enteric organisms can be cultured during the acute episode.

Enterocolitis in Hirschsprung's disease may start at any age. It may appear as early as the first or second day of life with explosive diarrhea (often bloody), fever, distention, and prostration. In some instances, constipation and bilious vomiting may be the presenting symptoms. If and when the disease occurs in the newborn it may be difficult to distinguish from sepsis or other forms of necrotizing enterocolitis, and a barium enema must be performed to exclude Hirschsprung's disease as the underlying cause of the enterocolitis (Figs. 21-30 and 21-31).

The clinical presentation of necrotizing enterocolitis in the premature is quite similar although its occurrence in premature infants usually weighing less than 1500 gm. is typical. It may also present, however, in full-term infants, who seem to have a better chance of survival than do premature infants.

The etiology of necrotizing enterocolitis in the premature also remains obscure, although multiple theories have been proposed, e.g., maternal and

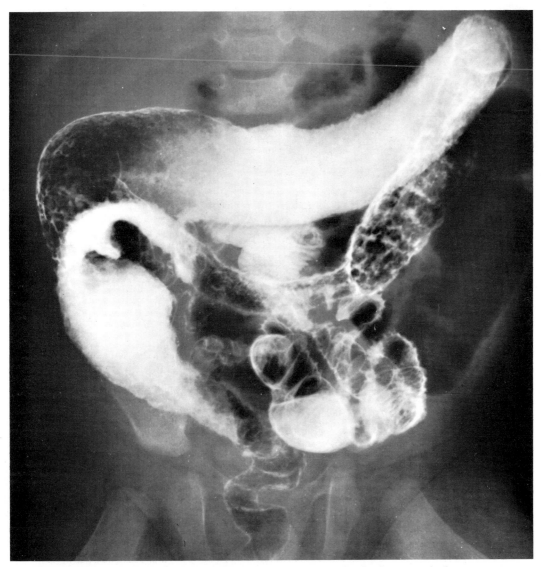

Figure 21-30 *Enterocolitis in Hirschsprung's disease.* Multiple mucosal ulcerations are seen, involving the entire colon. Although the colon is normally devoid of haustra at this age, the entire appearance and contour of the colon is abnormal. The rectum is narrowed, and a transition zone is present in the rectosigmoid region. The latter finding is typical for Hirschsprung's disease. The remainder of the colon demonstrates necrotizing colitis. (The features of the latter strongly resemble ulcerative colitis.)

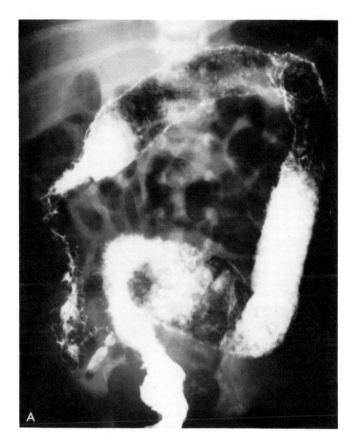

Figure 21-31 *Enterocolitis in Hirschsprung's disease.* A, The contour of the colon is irregular and severely involved with deep ulcerations.

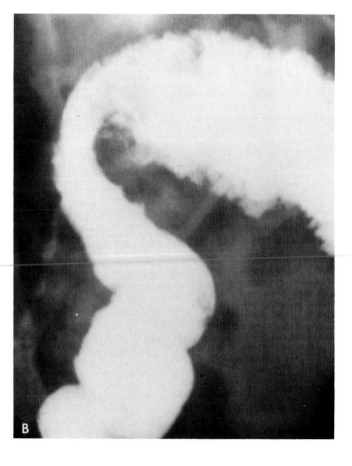

Figure 21-31 B, Spot film of the rectum demonstrates a transition zone at the junction of the rectosigmoid colon and deep ulceration of the sigmoid. Prior to this study the diagnosis of Hirschsprung's disease was unsuspected.

fetal infection with endotoxins exciting a local immune bowel reaction, sepsis, deficient lysozymes, and so forth. Santulli[34] indicates three conditions that must be present for the susceptible infant to develop the disease: feeding, injury to intestinal mucosa, and bacteria. The question of feeding is interesting since it appears that infants rarely develop the disease before being fed. In addition, recent investigations[35] suggest that the use of hyperosmolar formula may be responsible for damaging the mucosal wall and allowing for bacterial overgrowth and gut wall invasion. This situation may be prevented by feeding the susceptible infant breast milk, which contains large amounts of macrophages, lymphocytes, and antibodies. This is nature's way of providing immunity to the premature until he is able to establish his own defense mechanism.

Mucosal damage also occurs following periods of stress, particularly hypoxia. A physiologic reflex, the so-called "Diving Seal Reflex," is instigated and results in the selective shunting of blood away from the gastrointestinal tract to areas of greater need, e.g., heart and brain. The viscera are thus poorly perfused and as a result the intestinal mucosa, along with its protective mucus coating, is injured. Autodigestion by proteolytic enzymes is the end result.

To summarize, the main underlying pathogenetic feature in necrotizing enterocolitis is mucosal damage caused by multiple factors, resulting in an immune deficient bowel that allows for bacterial overgrowth and mural invasion.

The pathologic picture is principally that of mucosal necrosis and ulceration followed by pseudomembranous covering of the denuded friable surface. This is complicated frequently by perforations with resulting local or generalized peritonitis. In addition, intramural gas within the submucosa and subserosa occurs in approximately 50 per cent of the cases. The subsequent transport of gas into the portal circulation is an ominous sign. Thrombosis of small vessels and coagulation necrosis have been found at the periphery of the diseased bowel and it is conceivable that the entire pathologic process may be related to vascular ischemia.

Roentgenographically, the findings are typical and represent the composite picture of all the pathologic findings. The presence in an infant of diffuse small bowel distention associated with either a distended abdomen, acidosis, or non-bloody diarrhea has been observed by us to be the earliest manifestation of enterocolitis. This combination of clinical and radiographic features was present in 9 out of 12 patients in whom abdominal studies were available well before the clinical onset of the disease.[36] As the disease progresses, however, diffuse distention of both small and large bowel is found. When peritonitis is present, the presence of fluid within the peritoneal cavity imparts an overall grayness to the abdomen. Free air related to perforation will be detected over the liver, or within the abdomen as an oval collection of air resembling a football (Fig. 21-32). On the upright films air collects under both diaphragms (Fig. 21-33). However, in 50 per cent of our cases of perforation diagnosed at surgery or on post-mortem studies, no obvious free air could be detected on x-ray. The perforation was obviously sealed over by adjacent bowel. Early findings of enterocolitis may be localized to the right lower quadrant where bubbles of air may be seen outlining the wall of the ileum or cecum (Figs. 21-32 and 21-33).[38] The presence of air cysts throughout the intestine facilitates the diagnosis. These may present as localized bubbles of air or large lucent linear streaks dissecting along the bowel wall (Fig. 21-34). When viewed on end, they appear as rings. Al-

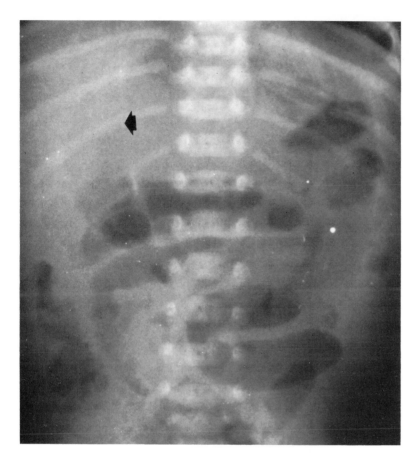

Figure 21-32 Pneumoperitoneum (football sign) in necrotizing enterocolitis. Abdominal film exposed in the supine position demonstrates an oval configuration of free intraperitoneal air that resembles a football. Linear density in right upper quadrant (arrow) is the falciform ligament. Small collections of air in a bubbly pattern are present within the cecum.

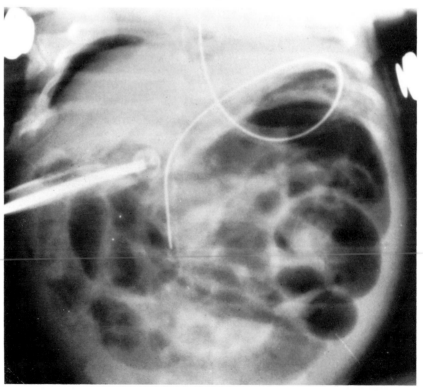

Figure 21-33 Pneumoperitoneum in necrotizing enterocolitis. Free air is collected over the liver and beneath the right diaphragm. Intramural air in both a bubbly and linear pattern outlines the ascending and proximal transverse colon.

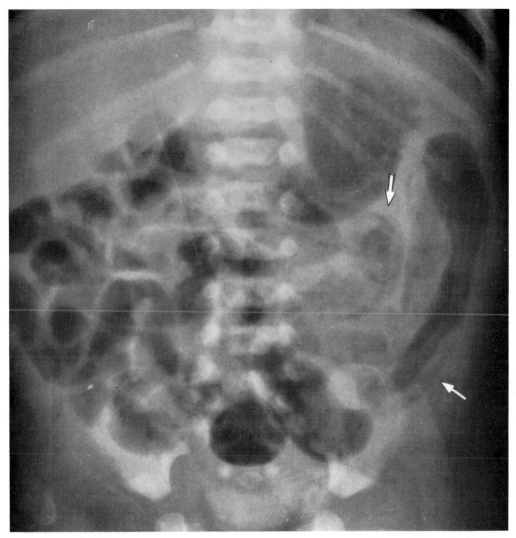

Figure 21-34 *Necrotizing enterocolitis* in the newborn. The abdominal film reveals distention of both small and large bowel with no specific obstruction. Linear lucencies are seen in the wall of the major portion of both the transverse and descending colon (arrows). The distal transverse colon has a bubbly appearance, which may represent intramural air, intraluminal bloody contents, or both.

though the presence of intramural air is an excellent diagnostic sign of enterocolitis, it is by no means specific for this disease. In fact, pneumatosis intestinalis in the neonatal period has been seen associated with several disease processes. Occasionally, obstruction or distention alone, e.g., Hirschsprung's disease, can produce air within the bowel wall because of mucosal breakage. In contrast to necrotizing enterocolitis, this is often self-limiting and uneventful. Pneumatosis following umbilical artery or vein catheterizations signifies necrotic bowel resulting from vascular occlusion.[38] Other causes associated with pneumatosis intestinalis have been pneumomediastinum and peroxide enemas.

The presence of air within the bowel wall by itself no longer imparts a fatal prognosis. Many patients with enterocolitis or with other underlying diseases accompanied by pneumatosis intestinalis have survived. The presence of air within the portal venous system (Fig. 21-35), however, is far more grave and must be distinguished from air within the biliary system. Portal venous gas is

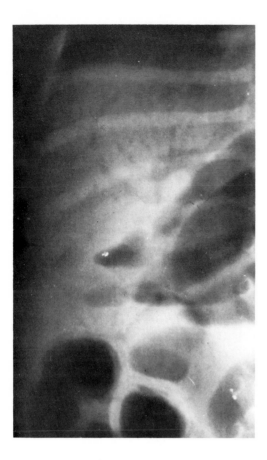

Figure 21-35 *Portal venous gas in necrotizing enterocolitis.* Massive collections of air outline almost the entire intrahepatic portal system. The air in this condition is transported peripherally to the edge of the liver. Linear collections of air (pneumatosis) also outline the bowel wall below the liver.

transported peripherally by the portal flow and is therefore recognized along the margins of the liver. Portal venous gas has also been associated with malpositioned umbilical catheters and has been noted in septic infants who at autopsy demonstrated normal to only mildly diseased bowel.[39] Gas in the biliary system is rare in this age group but may accompany severe duodenal obstructions (Fig. 21-6). The accumulation of peritoneal fluid following the appearance of intramural air is, however, strong radiologic evidence of clinical deterioration.[40]

The diagnosis of enterocolitis with aganglionosis is simplified once the presence of a transitional zone in the colon is demonstrated on the barium enema (Figs. 21-30 and 21-31). Above this zone, the colon is dilated, with loss of haustral markings. The underlying mucosa is ulcerated and the appearance resembles that of ulcerative colitis.

Necrotizing enterocolitis in the newborn is presently associated with an improving survival rate owing to the aggressive care given these infants. As a result, late complications and alterations of bowel are being discovered. Subsequent barium studies in infants who have survived have revealed two major findings; a transitory diffuse nodular mucosal pattern (Fig. 21-36) and colonic strictures (Fig. 21-37).[41] In the former, morphologic sections have revealed markedly redundant mucosal folds as well as distinct polypoid nodules.[42] The nodules on microscopic section are composed of large localized aggregations of lymphoid tissue which probably represent a late reaction to the inflammatory process. Radiographically and pathologically the changes resemble the benign lymphoid hyperplasia associated with dysgammaglobulinemia. The colonic strictures, in all probability, occur as an end result of the underlying ischemic process.

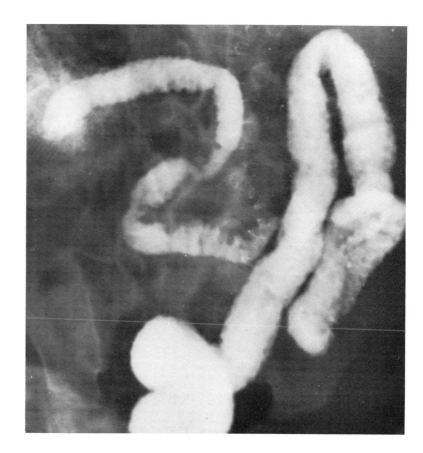

Figure 21-36 Barium enema taken at the age of six months in one patient following necrotizing enterocolitis in the neonatal period reveals multiple nodular defects throughout the entire colon. On biopsy these proved to be large submucosal aggregates of lymphoid tissue.

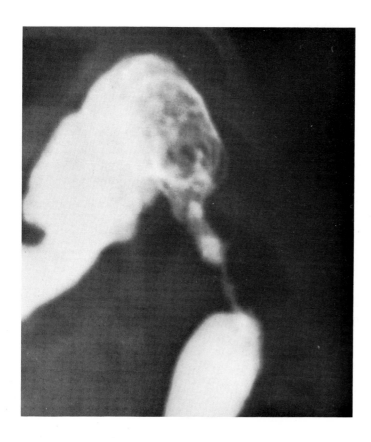

Figure 21-37 Spot film of splenic flexure taken in another patient at the age of one month following a bout of necrotizing enterocolitis reveals a stricture within the proximal portion of the descending colon.

INTUSSUSCEPTION

Intussusception results from invagination of one portion of the intestine into another. The condition occurs in three principal forms: enteroenteric, ileocolic and colocolic. Ileocolic intussusception is by far the most common, occurring in approximately 75 per cent of cases.[43] The disorder occurs most often during the first three years of life, with its peak incidence between the third and twelfth months of the first year. The onset is usually sudden, with crampy abdominal pains that cause the child to flex his thighs and thrash about. Although the initial episode may abate promptly, repeated bouts of abdominal colic occur with increasing severity, and sooner or later vomiting begins. The bowel movements may be normal at the onset but soon become bloody and may contain mucus. Clinical examination of the abdomen usually reveals a palpable sausage-shaped mass situated in the lateral or upper regions of the abdomen.

In approximately 95 per cent of infants below the age of two years the cause of the intussusception remains undetermined. The most likely mechanism is considered to be related to functional changes associated with the increased amount of fat and lymphoid tissue characteristic of the infant bowel. In addition, the change from a liquid to a solid diet with subsequent increased peristaltic activity may be an important precipitating factor. In about half of the children over two years of age a demonstrable lesion responsible for the intussusception is found. Although the direct causes of intussusception vary and include such factors as hypertrophied Peyer's patches, lymphoma, enlarged mesenteric nodes, and duplications, the most commonly encountered causative lesions are Meckel's diverticulum and polyp.[44] In patients with cystic fibrosis, intussusception is caused by the presence of thick putty-like material within the terminal ileum and cecum.[45]

Roentgen diagnosis of intussusception on the basis of survey films of the abdomen alone may be very difficult.[46] As a matter of fact in many cases the distribution of intestinal gas may be quite normal. In some cases there may be a poorly defined density, corresponding to the area of a palpable mass, or there may be an absence of the gas shadow of the right colon, this being replaced by loops of small bowel (Fig. 21-28). Probably the most commonly found diagnostic sign is a soft tissue mass, the convex edge of which protrudes into a gas shadow in the colon distal to the intussusception. The soft tissue mass represents the leading point of the intussusception. This is usually seen in the right abdomen or in the epigastrium, although occasionally it may be noted more distally. When there is frank intestinal obstruction or peritonitis the roentgen features of these conditions may be observed.

In the absence of clinical and roentgenologic evidence of intestinal obstruction or peritonitis, the use of a barium enema examination is advisable to demonstrate the lesion. The retrograde flow of barium will stop abruptly at the leading head of the intussusception, which will often produce a concave configuration in the barium column (Fig. 21-39). Some of the barium may flow in between the intussusceptum and the intussuscipiens, producing the characteristic "coiled-spring" appearance of intussusception (Fig. 21-40). The use of a barium enema for therapy depends not on the duration of symptoms but rather on whether or not there is any clinical or roentgen evidence of intestinal obstruction or peritonitis, both of which are contraindications to the use of a barium enema. There should be surgical exploration in all cases, regardless of the time

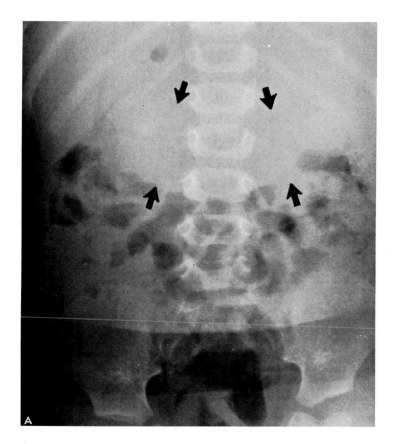

Figure 21-38 A, Flat film of the abdomen in an infant reveals an elongated soft tissue mass extending across the epigastrium (arrows). There is also an apparent absence of colon within the right lower quadrant. Minimal distention of small bowel is present throughout the remaining portion of the abdomen.

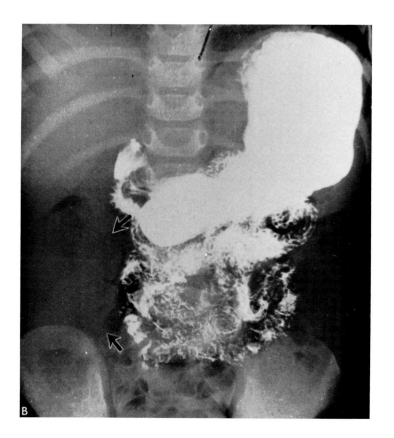

Figure 21-38 B, Flat film of the abdomen taken during a G.I. series on a patient with recurring abdominal pain reveals a huge soft tissue mass (arrows) within the right abdomen. This proved to be an area of intussusception caused by multiple cecal polyps.

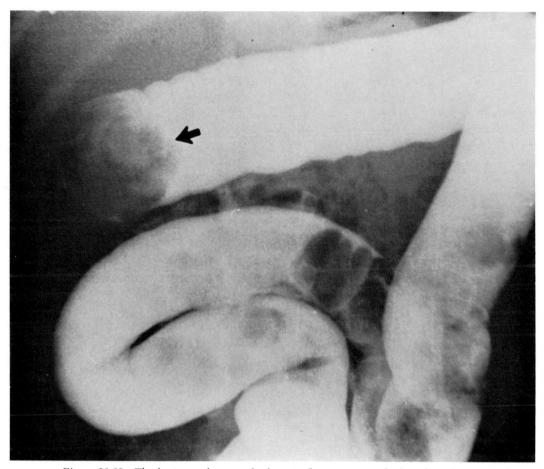

Figure 21-39   The barium column at the hepatic flexure surrounds the edge of a mass and assumes a concave contour outlining the intussusceptum. Filling defects in the distal portion of the colon are feces.

of onset, when intestinal obstruction or peritonitis is present. The technique of hydrostatic reduction is more or less similar in most institutions. At the beginning of the procedure the patient should be mildly sedated. A Foley catheter, approximately size 16, is then introduced into the rectum and inflated. The buttocks are held together tightly, either manually or with adhesive tape. The barium container is placed no more than 3 feet above the table top, to allow contrast material to run freely and without external abdominal pressure. The barium column frequently flows easily to the level of the intussusceptum and continued hydrostatic pressure will displace the intussusceptum proximally along the colon until it reaches the ileocecal valve. Reduction is often delayed at this level, and persistent hydrostatic pressure is required for a successful reduction. Singleton[10] recommends repeated emptying and refilling of the colon by lowering and raising the container beyond the level of the table. Once complete reduction is achieved, an adequate amount of ileum must be filled to exclude the possibility of an ileoileal intussusception or an organic causal lesion. A postevacuation film is also taken to obtain further proof of complete reduction. Occasionally following reduction a persistent defect representing edema or inflammatory swelling is seen at the ileocecal valve.

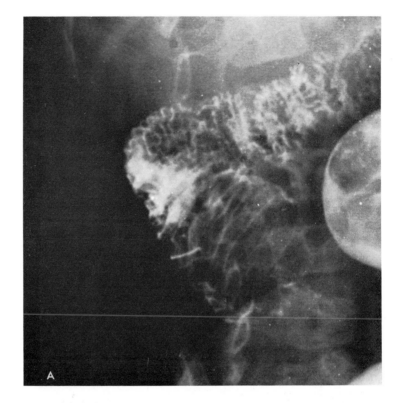

Figure 21-40 Coiled-spring appearance. A, An evacuation film shows the barium surrounding the intussusceptum and producing a ringlike appearance. The diameter of the colon in this area is increased by the intraluminal mass.

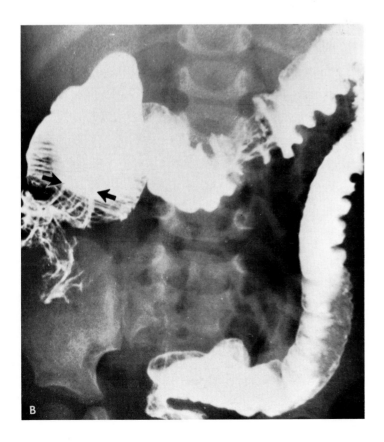

Figure 21-40 B, Further demonstration of a coiled-spring appearance. Barium surrounds the invaginated bowel. This in turn is also filled with barium (arrows).

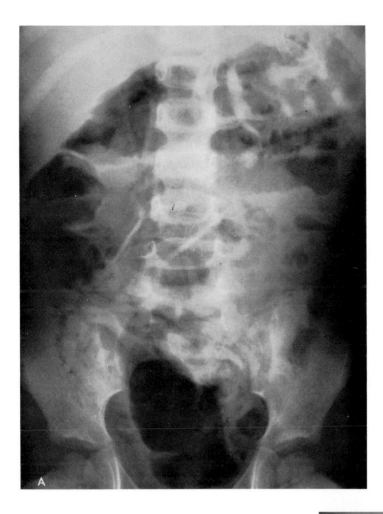

Figure 21-41 Ascariasis. A, A flat film of the abdomen reveals masses of worms present within the right lower quadrant. The worms are recognized as lengthy soft tissue masses outlined by the air within the bowel.

Figure 21-41 B, Long tubular defects are present within the small bowel. In addition, thin elongated channels of barium outline the intestinal tracts of the worms. These channels are more easily seen on delayed films, since ingestion of barium by the worm is slower, and barium remains within the worm over a longer period of time.

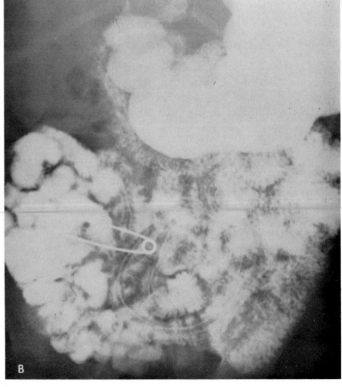

PARASITIC INFECTION

Ascaris lumbricoides is the most common parasite to involve small bowel. Infection begins after the ingestion of contaminated vegetables, water, or soil. The larvae hatch in the small bowel and begin a complicated migration that carries them through the bowel wall to the lung via veins or lymphatics. From here they emerge into the alveoli and ascend the tracheobronchial tree to reach the glottis. They then descend the esophagus to ultimately reach the small bowel, their original point of origin, where they eventually mature into adult worms.

Transient episodes of pneumonia with hemoptysis may occur when the larvae migrate through the lungs. More frequently, the infestation is asymptomatic. However, an overwhelming infestation of bowel may give rise to obstructive symptoms.

Although roentgenograms of the abdomen occasionally demonstrate masses of coiled worms contrasted by the intestinal gas (Fig. 21-41A), a barium examination is more definitive. The worms are easily seen as elongated radiolucent filling defects measuring approximately 3 to 5 mm. in width and 15 to 35 cm. in length. In a patient fasting for more than 12 hours, the worm may ingest the barium and the gastrointestinal tract of the worm will be seen as a thin longitudinal line bisecting the length of the filling defect[47] (Fig. 21-41B). Delayed films demonstrate retention of barium within the worm as a thin curved line.

Other common parasitic infestations of the small bowel are caused by *Ancylostoma duodenale* (hookworm) and *Strongyloides stercoralis.* The larvae in both these infestations have a similar migration through the lungs before reaching their final destination, the duodenum and small bowel, where they undergo maturation. Rarely the stercoralis larvae remain in the lung, causing hemorrhage, granulomas, and fibrosis. Ancylostoma involves predominantly the mucosa of the duodenum and incites a superficial inflammatory reaction evidenced by thickened edematous mucosal folds. Strongyloides, however, invades the wall more profoundly, but in the early stages of infestation results in an inflammation resembling that caused by *Ancylostoma duodenale.* As the parasite burrows into the wall it is accompanied by a more chronic granulomatous reaction. The mucosa is thick, coarse, and nodular, demonstrating an appearance resembling Crohn's disease of the duodenum.[48] An interesting feature in this disease is the presence of free reflux into the common duct because of an incompetent sphincter of Oddi caused by the rigidly fixed duodenal wall. As would be expected, this feature has also been sporadically observed in cases of Crohn's disease of the duodenum.

Tapeworm infestations have also been described radiologically,[49] and the worms may appear as thin radiolucent lines within the barium-filled small bowel.

References

1. Boreadis, A. G., and Gershon-Cohen, J.: Aeration of respiratory and gastrointestinal tracts during first minute of neonatal life. *Radiology,* 67:407, 1956.
2. Maddock, W. G., Bell, J. L., and Tremaine, M. J.: Gastrointestinal gas: observations on belching during anesthesia, operations and pyelography and rapid passage of gas. *Ann. Surgery,* 130:512, 1949.
3. Singleton, E. B.: Radiologic evaluation of intestinal obstruction in the newborn. *Radiol. Clin. N. Amer.,* 1:571, 1963.

4. Harris, P. D., Neuhauser, E. B. D., and Gerth, R.: The osmotic effect of water soluble contrast media on circulating plasma volume. *Amer. J. Roentgen.*, 91:694, 1964.

5. Boggs, T. R., and Bishop, H.: Neonatal hyperbilirubinemia associated with high intestinal obstruction in the small bowel. *J. Pediat.*, 66:349, 1965.

6. Louw, J. H.: Congenital intestinal atresia and stenosis in the newborn: observations on its pathogenesis and treatment. *Ann. Roy. Coll. Surg. Eng.*, 25:209, 1959.

7. Louw, J. H.: Investigations into the etiology of congenital atresia of the colon. *Dis. Colon Rectum* 7:471, 1964.

8. Astley, R.: Duodenal atresia with gas below the obstruction. *Brit. J. Radiol.*, 42:359, 1969.

9. Hope, J. W., and Gibbons, J. F.: Duodenal obstruction due to annular pancreas. *Radiology*, 63:473, 1954.

10. Singleton, E. B.: X-ray diagnosis of the alimentary tract in infants and children. Chicago, Year Book Publishers, Inc., 1959.

11. Firor, H. V., and Harris, V. J.: Rotational abnormalities of the gut. Re-emphasis of a neglected facet, isolated incomplete rotation of the duodenum. *Amer. J. Roentgen.*, 120:315, 1974.

12. Louw, J. H.: Jejunoileal atresia and stenosis. *J. Pediat. Surg.*, 1:8, 1966.

13. Gross, R. E., Holcomb, G. W., and Farber, S.: Duplications of the alimentary tract. *Pediatrics*, 9:449, 1952.

14. Favara, D. E., Franciosi, R. A., and Akers, D. R.: Enteric duplications: 37 cases: vascular theory of pathogenesis. *Amer. J. Dis. Child.*, 122:501, 1971.

15. Neuhauser, E. B. D., Harris, G. B., and Benett, A.: Roentgenographic features of neurenteric cysts. *Amer. J. Roentgen.*, 79:235, 1958.

16. Thomaidis, T. S., and Avery, J. B.: Intestinal lesions in cystic fibrosis of pancreas. *J. Pediat.*, 63:444, 1963.

17. Holsclaw, D. S., Eckstein, H. B., and Nixon, H. H.: Meconium ileus. *Amer. J. Dis. Child.*, 109: 101, 1965.

18. Santulli, T. V.: In *Pediatric Surgery*, Mustard et al. (eds.) Chicago, Year Book Medical Publishers, 1969, Vol. 2.

19. Neuhauser, E. B. D.: Roentgen changes associated with pancreatic insufficiency in early life. *Radiology*, 46:319, 1946.

20. White, H.: Meconium ileus: new roentgen sign. *Radiology*, 66:567, 1956.

21. Berdon, W. E., Baker, D. H., Santulli, T. V., Amoury, R. A., and Blanc, W. A.: Microcolon in newborn infants with intestinal obstruction. *Radiology*, 90:878, 1968.

22. Noblet, H. R.: Treatment of uncomplicated meconium ileus by gastrografin enema. A preliminary report. *J. Pediat. Surg.*, 4:190, 1969.

23. Frech, R. S., McAlister, W. H., Ternberg, H., and Strominger, D.: Meconium ileus relieved by 40% water soluble contrast enemas. *Radiology*, 94:341, 1970.

24. Cardonnier, J. K., and Izant, R. J.: Meconium ileus equivalent. *Surgery*, 54:667, 1963.

25. Wolfson, J. J., and Engel, R. R.: Anticipating meconium peritonitis from metaphyseal bands. *Radiology*, 92:1055, 1969.

26. Berdon, W. E., and Baker, D. H.: The roentgenographic diagnosis of Hirschsprung's disease in infancy. *Amer. J. Roentgen.*, 93:432, 1965.

27. Moseley, J. E.: Radiological notes: pediatric radiology. *J. Mount Sinai Hosp. N.Y.*, 31:64, 1964.

28. Hope, J. W., Boins, P. F., and Berg, P. K.: Roentgenologic manifestations of Hirschsprung's disease in infancy. *Amer. J. Roentgen.*, 95:217, 1965.

29. Berdon, W. E., Koontz, P., and Baker, D. H.: The diagnosis of colonic and terminal ileal aganglionosis. *Amer. J. Roentgen.*, 91:680, 1964.

30. Sane, S., and Girdany, B. R.: Total aganglionosis coli: clinical and roentgenographic manifestations. *Radiology*, 107:397, 1973.

31. Pochachevsky, R., and Leonidas, J. C.: Meconium plug syndrome. *Amer. J. Roentgen.*, 120:342, 1974.

32. Davis, W. S., Parker-Allen, R., Favara, B. E., and Slovis, T. L.: Neonatal small left colon syndrome. *Amer. J. Roentgen.*, 120:322, 1974.

33. Clatworthy, H. W., Jr., Howard, W. H. R., and Lloyd, J.: The meconium plug syndrome. *Surgery*, 39:131, 1956.

34. Santulli, T. V.: Acute necrotizing enterocolitis: recognition and management. *Hosp. Prac.*, p. 129, 1974.

35. Risemberg, H., Mazzi, E., Nishida, H., and White, J. J.: Hyperosmolar neonatal enterocolitis. Presented at the Annual Meeting Amer. Acad. Pediat., Oct. 19, 1974, San Francisco, Cal.

36. Siegle, R. L., Rabinowitz, J. G., Karones, S., and Eyal, F.: Early diagnosis of necrotizing enterocolitis. Presented at the Annual Meeting Radiol. Soc. N. Amer., Dec. 4, 1974, Chicago, Ill.

37. Berdon, W. E., Grossman, H., Baker, D. H., Misrahi, A., Barlow, O., and Blanc, W. A.: Necrotizing enterocolitis in the premature infant. *Radiology*, 83:879, 1964.

38. Robinson, A. E., Grossman, H., and Brumely, G. W.: Pneumatosis intestinalis in the neonate. *Amer. J. Roentgen.*, 120:333, 1974.

39. Arnon, R. G., and Fishbein, J. F.: Portal venous gas in the pediatric age group. *J. Pediat.*, 79:255, 1971.

40. Leonidas, J. C., Krasna, I. H., Fox, H. A., and Broder, M. S.: Peritoneal fluid in necrotizing enterocolitis: radiologic sign of clinical deterioration. *J. Pediat.*, 82:672, 1973.

41. Rabinowitz, J. G., Wolf, B. S., Feller, M. R., and Krasna, I.: Colonic changes following necrotizing enterocolitis in the newborn. *Amer. J. Roentgen.*, 103:359, 1968.

42. Leonidas, J. C., Krasna, I., Strauss, L., Becker, J. M., and Schneider, K. M.: Roentgen appearance of the excluded colon after colostomy for infantile Hirschsprung's disease. *Amer. J. Roentgen.*, 112:116, 1971.

43. Perrin, W. S., and Linsay, E. C.: Intussusception. A monograph based on 400 cases. *Brit. J. Surg.*, 9:46, 1921.
44. Ponka, J. L.: Intussusception in infants and adults. *Surg. Gynec. Obstet.*, 124:99, 1967.
45. Holsclaw, D. S., Rocmans, C., and Swachman, H.: Intussusception in patients with cystic fibrosis. *J. Pediat.*, 48:51, 1971.
46. Levine, M., Schwartz, S., Katz, I., Burko, H., and Rabinowitz, J. G.: Plain film findings in intussusception. *Brit. J. Radiol.*, 37:678, 1964.
47. Moseley, J. E.: Radiological notes. Case No. 109. *J. Mount Sinai Hosp. N.Y.*, 27:466, 1960.
48. Berkman, Y. M., and Rabinowitz, J. G.: Gastrointestinal manifestations of the strongyloidiasis. *Amer. J. Roentgen.*, 115:306, 1972.
49. Margulis, A. R., and Burhenne, H. J.: Alimentary tract roentgenology. St. Louis, C. V. Mosby Co., 1973.

22

Uncommon Lesions of The Small Intestine

by ARTHUR R. CLEMETT, M.D.

The conditions considered here are rare, except for cystic fibrosis. Many are systemic illnesses with important intestinal manifestations. One feature is common to these conditions: all cause significant roentgen abnormalities of the small intestine.

ABETALIPOPROTEINEMIA (BASSEN-KORNZWEIG SYNDROME)

The principal features of this syndrome, first described in 1950, are neuromuscular disturbances, retinal abnormalities, acanthocytosis, steatorrhea, and virtual absence of serum betalipoprotein.[1, 2] The neuromuscular disorder is progressive and may simulate Friedreich's ataxia. The retinal lesions have been described as atypical retinitis pigmentosa, retinitis punctata albescens, and myopic choroiditis. Examination of fresh undiluted blood reveals the red cells to have a thorny appearance. In addition to the absence of betalipoprotein, serum cholesterol is markedly reduced, as are other serum lipids. The combination of steatorrhea and a very low serum cholesterol is believed to be unique to this condition.[3] The disease is hereditary and is probably transmitted by an autosomal recessive gene with variable penetrance. Many degrees of betalipoprotein deficiency exist, even in symptom-free patients, and only when the betalipoprotein is virtually absent do the characteristic features appear. The steatorrhea is due to the lack of betalipoprotein essential to transport of fat from the gut.[4] Increased amounts of lipid have been demonstrated in mucosal cells, and diets high in fat intensify the diarrhea and steatorrhea.

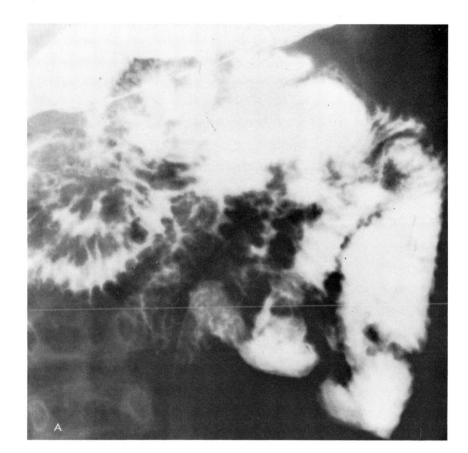

Figure 22-1 Beta-lipoprotein-emia. A, There is moderate thickening of the mucosal folds in the jejunum.

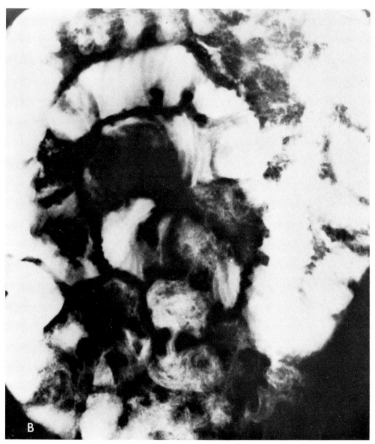

Figure 22-1 B, Segmentation of the barium column is present in the ileum, and the bowel is slightly dilated with thickening of the mucosal folds. (Courtesy of Dr. John W. Loop, Seattle, Washington.)

The prolonged malabsorption and malnutrition may cause retarded growth and development.[5]

Roentgen examination of the small intestine has shown dilatation of the bowel with mild to moderate thickening of mucosal folds of the duodenum and jejunum.[3, 6, 7, 8] Since segmentation and flocculation of the barium meal frequently occur (Fig. 22-1), these cases are commonly confused with sprue, but intestinal biopsy and failure to respond to a gluten-free diet should prevent this. Correct diagnosis depends on recognition of the distinctive clinical and laboratory features of abetalipoproteinemia.

CYSTIC FIBROSIS

Abdominal symptoms are prominent in many patients with cystic fibrosis, especially in older children and adults in whom pulmonary disease is not severe or has been controlled by appropriate therapy.[9] These symptoms may be due to a variety of gastrointestinal complications of the disease. Most but not all patients have pancreatic achylia with resultant maldigestion. This causes steatorrhea and contributes to the malnutrition which may occur despite a ravenous appetite. About 10 per cent of patients with cystic fibrosis have meconium ileus in the neonatal period. Thick, putty-like intestinal contents may cause mechanical obstruction in older patients.[10, 11, 12] This "meconium ileus equivalent" frequently follows a change in diet or cessation of pancreatic enzyme therapy. In

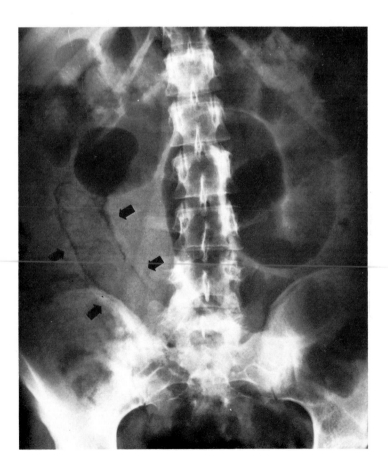

Figure 22-2 A 19 year old girl with meconium ileus equivalent as the initial manifestation of cystic fibrosis. There is marked small bowel distention due to obstruction of the fecal mass in the ileum (arrows). (Courtesy of Dr. Robert Berk, Dallas, Texas).

rare cases it may be the initial clinical manifestation of the disease in an older patient (Fig. 22-2).[13] Some patients develop fecal masses which adhere to the mucosa of the ileum or cecum and may cause intermittent intussusception.[14, 15] At times, these have been confused with tumors and appendiceal abscesses. The insidious development of multilobular biliary cirrhosis with portal hypertension complicates a few cases. This often becomes apparent when there is hemorrhage from unsuspected esophageal varices. The rare occurrence of pancreatic calculi or pancreatitis may account for abdominal pain in some patients with cystic fibrosis.[16]

Some of these patients have morphologic changes in the intestinal mucosa which may be visualized on roentgen examination. The features of these mucosal lesions are increased numbers of goblet cells and dilatation of mucosal glands, which are distended with inspissated mucus.[17] There are all gradations of severity of this "mucosis." Extreme cases exhibit a goblet cell metaplasia of the intestinal epithelium, and adherent mucus may coat the mucosal surface and fuse with luminal contents (Figs. 22-3 and 22-4).

The mucosal pathology explains the redundant, hyperplastic-appearing colon mucosa observed in some patients with cystic fibrosis. This feature is best appreciated on evacuation films (Fig. 22-5). Some examinations show fixed marginal defects resembling polyps, which are caused by adherent mucus partially extruded into the bowel lumen (Fig. 22-6). The margins of the colon may

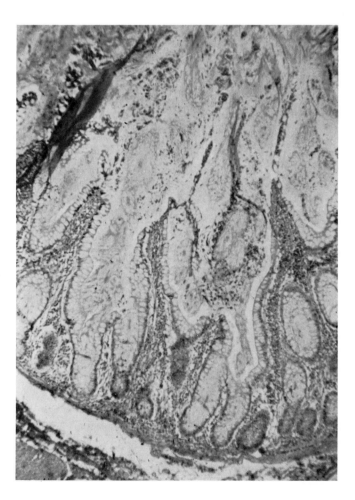

Figure 22-3 Marked mucosal disease of the small intestine in cystic fibrosis. The epithelium of the villi and crypts is almost completely replaced by goblet cells. Acidophilic secretions distend the mucosal glands, coat the surface, and fuse with the luminal contents.

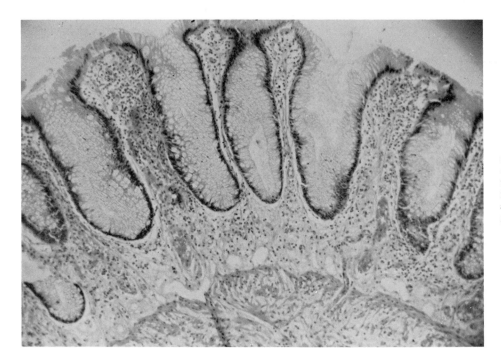

Figure 22-4 Mucosal lesion of the colon in cystic fibrosis. The epithelium is taller than normal and appears stratified in some areas. The glands are greatly dilated and have gaping orifices.

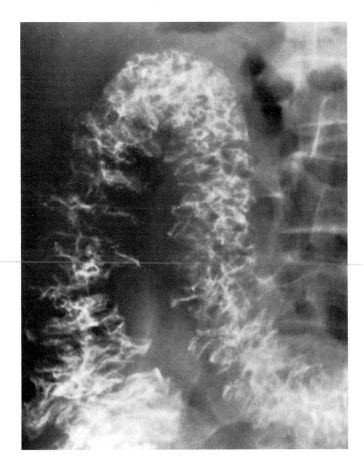

Figure 22-5 Cystic fibrosis. Evacuation film. The colon mucosa is redundant and hyperplastic in appearance. This finding occurs in over half of all patients, and its incidence increases with advancing age.

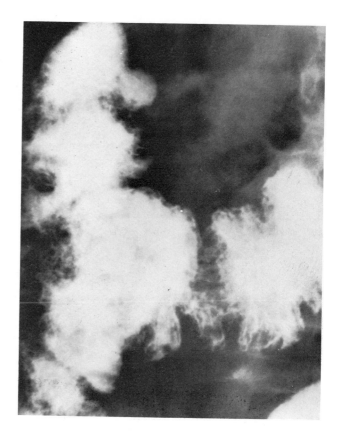

Figure 22-6 *Cystic fibrosis.* There are numerous filling defects simulating small polyps. These are caused by adherent mucus which has been extruded into the bowel lumen.

have a striking spiculated appearance due to barium filling the dilated mucosal glands.[18] Rectal biopsies, advocated and used as diagnostic aids in cystic fibrosis, have now provided enough pathologic material to confirm these interpretations.[19]

By contrast, small bowel histologic material is scarce. This makes radiologic correlation speculative. Small bowel biopsies in some cases have been normal while others have shown increases in plasma cells, goblet cells, and mucus as well as mild chronic inflammation. These mucosal changes may contribute to the roentgen abnormalities, but it has been suggested that duodenal muscle dysfunction secondary to irritation from unbuffered gastric acid is the major cause.[20] It is of interest that the duodenal pattern in cystic fibrosis may mimic that found in the Zollinger-Ellison syndrome.

In the typical case the proximal duodenum has a smooth, smudged character with absence of mucosal folds (Fig. 22-7). Peculiar indentations or invaginations of the duodenal wall are present in some cases (Figs. 22-8 and 22-10). The distal duodenum and jejunum show a transition from this appearance to one of marked thickening and distortion of the folds (Fig. 22-8). The distal small bowel often lacks a regular pattern of delicate valvulae conniventes.

One study revealed changes in the duodenum of some degree in 84 per cent of cystic fibrosis patients and abnormalities of the mesenteric small bowel in 27 per cent.[20] Another study revealed these abnormalities in 38 per cent of older cystic fibrosis patients.[21] With one exception, the duodenum was affected in all positive cases, and at times it was the only abnormal segment. The exception was a young adult who had thickening of the ileal mucosa associated with similar changes throughout the colon (Fig. 22-9). Only one-fifth of the

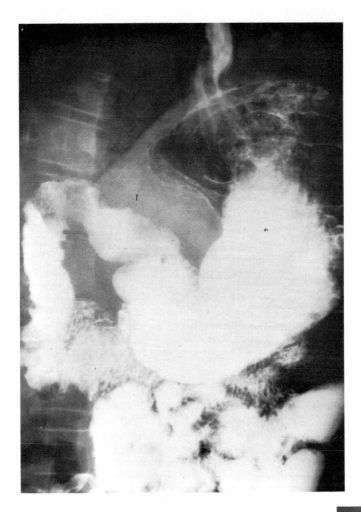

Figure 22-7 Cystic fibrosis. The mucosal surface of the first and second parts of the duodenum has a smudged appearance. This patient was bleeding from small esophageal varices secondary to multilobular biliary cirrhosis.

Figure 22-8 Cystic fibrosis. The defects in the contours of the second duodenum are caused by small invaginations of the thickened mucosa. These are transient and change from film to film. Jejunal mucosal folds are thickened and distorted. The bowel is not dilated.

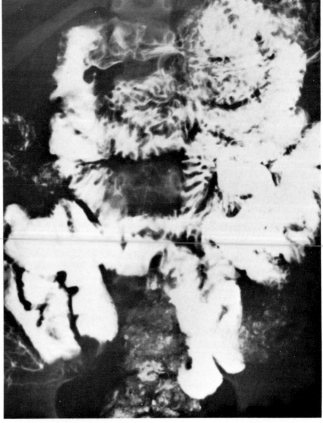

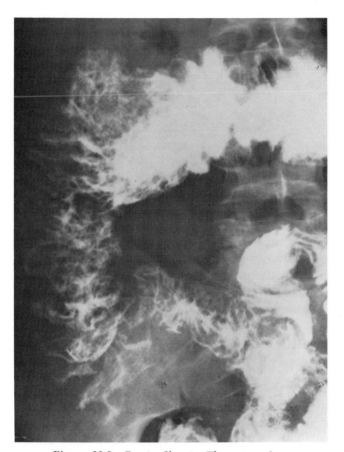

Figure 22-9 Cystic fibrosis. There is a hyperplastic mucosa in the terminal ileum with similar changes
in the colon. The proximal small intestine of this patient
was normal.

positive cases had dilatation of the small bowel (Fig. 22-10). This suggests that differential diagnosis from sprue is possible on roentgen evidence alone.

Figure 22-11 illustrates a remarkable case where the duodenal and colonic changes were the major abnormalities in a man who was 50 years old at the time the diagnosis of cystic fibrosis was first established.

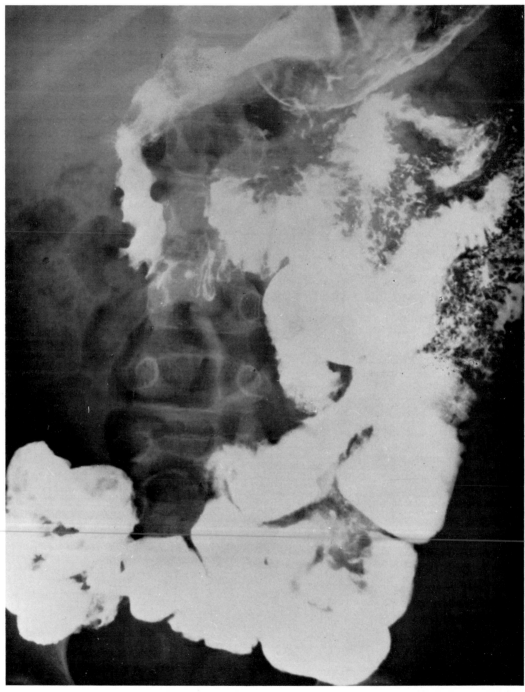

Figure 22-10 *Cystic fibrosis*. Dilatation of the small bowel in this case makes roentgen differential diagnosis from celiac disease difficult.

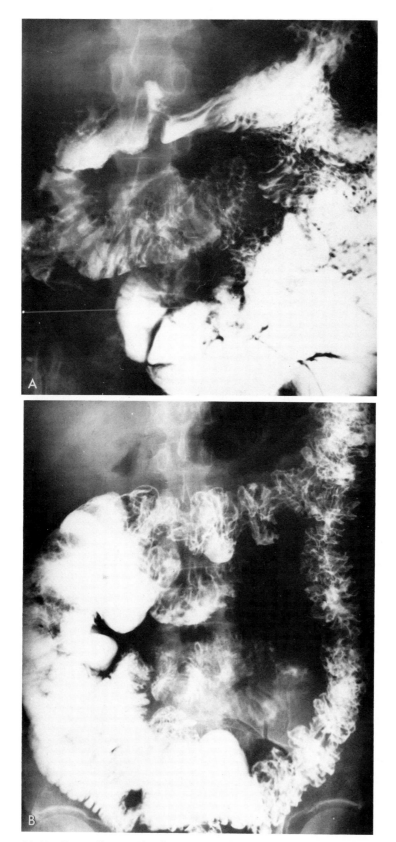

Figure 22-11 *Cystic fibrosis.* The diagnosis was first established in this man at the age of 50 when he was evaluated for steatorrhea. His major radiological abnormalities were the thick folds in the duodenum and proximal jejunum (*A*) and the hyperplastic colon mucosa (*B*). (Courtesy of Dr. Ross Hill, Montreal, Canada.)

DEGOS' DISEASE

Degos' disease is a rare entity with a characteristic skin lesion which presages an eventual abdominal catastrophe.[22, 23] Victims of this fatal condition have ranged in age from 14 to 59 years, but this is predominantly a disease of young adult males. One instance of familial occurrence has been reported.[24] The onset is innocent and heralded by the development of the typical skin lesion, malignant atrophic papulosis. This descriptive term indicates the ominous prognosis, for within a few weeks to a few years most patients exhibit evidence of systemic involvement. The gastrointestinal tract is affected in almost all cases and most patients have died of peritonitis secondary to intestinal perforation. Other reported causes of death have been intestinal hemorrhage and multiple cerebral infarcts. No effective therapy is known.

The fundamental lesion is a progressive occlusive fibrosis of small and medium sized arteries. In acute lesions a cellular infiltrate of lymphocytes, histiocytes, and a few neutrophils may be found, but the predominant lesion is an acellular subendothelial fibrosis. In some instances veins are also affected by this process. The arterial lesions are accompanied by small focal areas of tissue necrosis with little inflammatory reaction. At times the arterial lesions are accompanied by acute thromboses, and regional infarcts then occur.

The etiology of Degos' disease is unknown. One case has been reported with coexistent malignant atrophic papulosis and progressive systemic sclerosis and attention called to the similarity of the histological blood vessel changes in the two diseases.[25] In another series of cases elevations of serum IgA and fibrinogen were noted in the patients, but the significance of these abnormalities remains uncertain.[26]

The skin lesions are distinctive. They occur in crops on the trunk and extremities and sometimes affect the mucous membrane and sclerae. They begin as small red papules which within a few days become umbilicated and develop a white center covered by a thin, easily removable dry white scale. The fully developed lesion seldom exceeds 10 mm. in diameter. The periphery is red and elevated and may show slight telangiectasia (Fig. 22-12). Histologically, the epidermis is markedly thinned and atrophic, and the underlying dermis contains acellular collections of fibrous tissue. Similar collections of fibrous tissue may surround the small arteries containing the vascular lesion.

The gastrointestinal lesions are similar to the skin lesions in many respects. In some cases acute necrosis and ulceration have been noted in the serosa and mucosa.[27] Collections of acellular fibrous tissue in the form of small plaques may occur in the serosa and the submucosa of the bowel. Submucosal edema has been described, as well as acute bowel infarctions.

Most case reports of Degos' disease mention normal roentgen examinations of the gastrointestinal tract. The patient illustrated in Figure 22-13 had

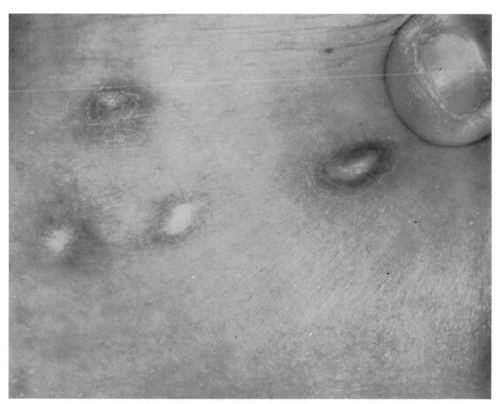

Figure 22-12 *Degos' disease*. Typical skin lesions have a porcelain-white center covered by a thin scale which is easily removable. The elevated red margins show slight telangiectasia.

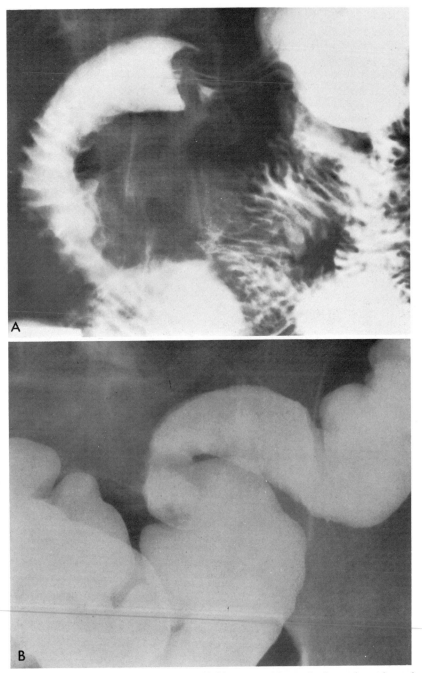

Figure 22-13 *Degos' disease* in a 25 year old woman. Mucosal edema throughout the duodenum (A) and small punctate colonic ulcers (B) were found during an episode of ill-defined abdominal pain. Repeat examination after the abdominal pain subsided was normal.

edema of the duodenal mucosa and punctate colon ulcerations when examined during an exacerbation of abdominal pain. Previous and subsequent examinations when the patient was free of abdominal symptoms were normal. Figure 22-14 illustrates positive findings in another case which has been previously reported.[28] This patient also had malabsorption and chylous ascites. At laparotomy the entire serosal surface of the intestinal tract was studded with gray-white patches similar to his skin lesions. The submucosa of the small intestine was thickened by acellular fibrous tissue, and there was some fibrosis in the muscularis. The patient succumbed to peritonitis secondary to a spontaneous perforation of the jejunum. Autopsy revealed vascular lesions in the intestinal submucosa as well as the stomach, colon, pancreas, kidneys, adrenals, heart, meninges, retroperitoneal soft tissues, and skin.

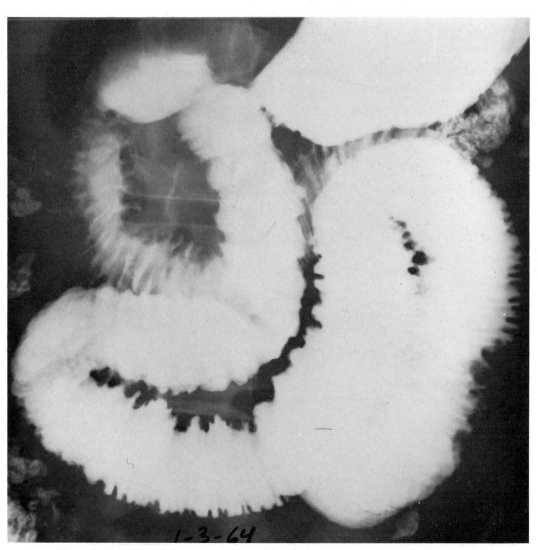

Figure 22-14 Degos' disease complicated by chylous ascites and malabsorption. There is diffuse edema of the duodenum. The jejunum is dilated and exhibits focal areas of mucosal and submucosal edema, interspersed with areas in which the mucosal folds remain normal in thickness. (Courtesy of Dr. Kurt J. Isselbacher, Boston, Massachusetts.)

EOSINOPHILIC GASTROENTERITIS

The roentgen features of eosinophilic gastroenteritis have been recorded several times in recent years.[29] In this disease there is a diffuse infiltration of mature eosinophils in one or more segments of the alimentary tract. The etiology is unknown, but a history of allergy is common. Eosinophilic gastroenteritis should be distinguished from "granuloma with eosinophils," which is also known as "inflammatory fibroid polyp." The latter is a focal lesion found in the stomach but known to occur in the colon and small bowel.

Eosinophilic gastroenteritis is characterized clinically by recurrent episodes of abdominal pain accompanied by vomiting, diarrhea, or both. The course may run for months or years. Peripheral blood eosinophilia is a common

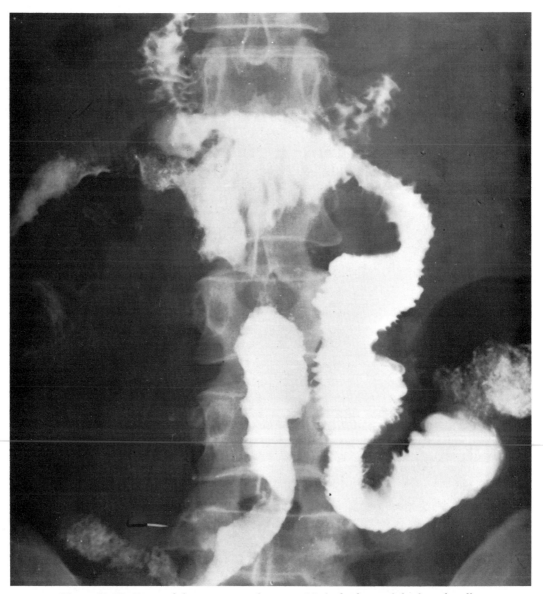

Figure 22-15 *Eosinophilic enteritis and ascites.* Marked edema of the bowel wall causes thickening and blunting of the valvulae conniventes and irregular narrowing of the bowel lumen in some areas. The patient had eosinophilia and an allergic history. (Courtesy of Dr. H. Joachim Burhenne, San Francisco, California.)

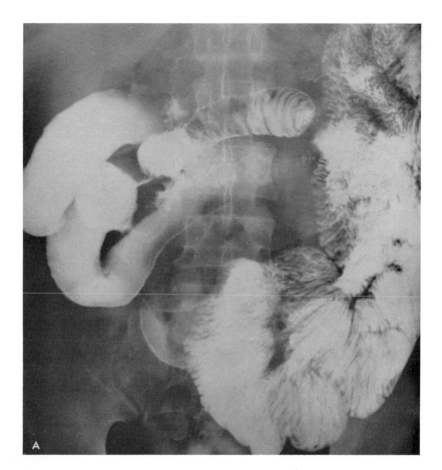

Figure 22-16 *A, Eosinophilic enteritis.* There is thickening of the wall and effacement of the folds in a segment of proximal ileum.

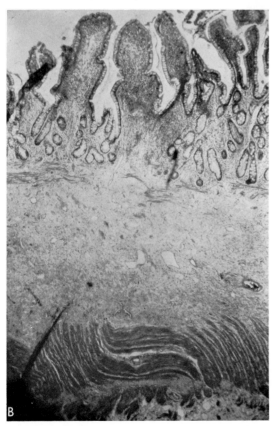

Figure 22-16 *B,* Histologic section shows all layers of the bowel to be infiltrated with mature eosinophils. There is thickening of the submucosa due to accumulation of edema fluid. The eosinophilic infiltrate in the muscularis propria may account for the moderate dilatation of the involved segment of small bowel. (Courtesy of Dr. Barry T. Held, New York, New York.)

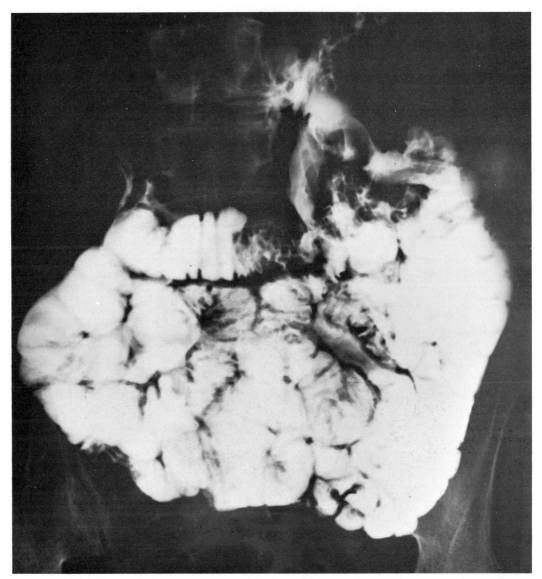

Figure 22-17 *Eosinophilic enteritis.* The proximal jejunum is narrowed and moderately rigid, and the folds are thickened or effaced. The patient had 60 per cent eosinophils. After steroid therapy there was resolution of this process.

but not invariable feature, and the eosinophil count may fluctuate with the clinical symptoms. Some cases have excessive gastrointestinal protein losses.[33, 34, 35] Diagnosis has usually been made on surgical biopsy. The course of the disease is benign; spontaneous remissions occur, and a response to steroid therapy is the rule.[30, 36]

As the name implies, the stomach and small bowel are affected in most cases, although colonic lesions can occur. The gastric lesion is usually confined to the antrum. At times the pathologic process is limited to the small intestine, which may be affected diffusely or in a segmental fashion.[37] Pathologically, the gastric antrum and affected bowel are diffusely thickened and usually edematous.[38] There is an infiltration of chronic inflammatory cells, predominantly mature eosinophils.

In some cases the infiltration is perivascular in location. Hypertrophy of the muscularis with an eosinophilic infiltrate extending between muscle bundles is a frequent feature. Occasionally, serosal infiltration is accompanied by ascites, and the fluid may contain large numbers of eosinophils.

The roentgen features of eosinophilic gastroenteritis are variable and depend upon the sites of disease and the severity and extent of the infiltrate.[39] Thickening and rigidity of the wall of the gastric antrum narrow the lumen and simulate carcinoma. The mucosa has a "cobblestone" appearance in some instances. Residual pliability and the presence of some peristalsis may suggest its benign nature.

The wall of affected small bowel segments is thickened. The mucosal folds are widened, blunted, and sometimes completely effaced in the presence of submucosal edema (Fig. 22-15). Edema and infiltration produce narrowing of the bowel lumen in some instances whereas in others extensive infiltration of the muscularis causes slight dilatation of the affected segment (Fig. 22-16). These lesions might be confused with regional enteritis, but ulceration, fistulas, and stricture have not been noted roentgenologically, even though small ulcerations are present in some surgical specimens. Although the roentgen changes are nonspecific, the possibility of eosinophilic gastroenteritis should be considered when an infiltrative lesion of the distal stomach, small bowel, or both are encountered in a patient with eosinophilia and an allergic history (Fig. 22-17).

HEREDITARY ANGIONEUROTIC EDEMA

Hereditary angioneurotic edema is a rare familial disease transmitted by an autosomal dominant gene. It is characterized by recurrent attacks of circumscribed subepithelial edema of the skin and the mucous membranes of the respiratory and gastrointestinal tracts. The other varieties of angioneurotic edema differ in that they respond well to treatment with epinephrine and antihistamines and have an excellent prognosis for life. In hereditary angioneurotic edema there is no response to these agents and death from acute laryngeal edema is common.[40]

Normal serum contains an alpha$_2$ globulin which is an inhibitor of the activated first component (C'1) of complement, an esterase. The basic biochemical fault in hereditary angioneurotic edema is a deficiency of or a defect in this alpha$_2$ globulin. In most of these patients there are abnormally low levels of the inhibitor, and the levels fall even farther during attacks. In some kindreds of hereditary angioneurotic edema the inhibitor protein is present in normal quantities but is nonfunctional. In reality, therefore, hereditary angioneurotic edema represents two genetic diseases having the same phenotype.[41]

The reasons for the periodic activation of the complement system in hereditary angioneurotic edema are unknown. Local trauma and pressure seem to be the only consistent precipitating factors.[40] The onset of clinical disease has ranged from infancy to the fourth decade but usually occurs in mid-childhood. Thereafter most patients have recurrent episodes of abdominal pain and edema of the skin and the pharyngo-laryngeal area for the rest of their lives. Acute

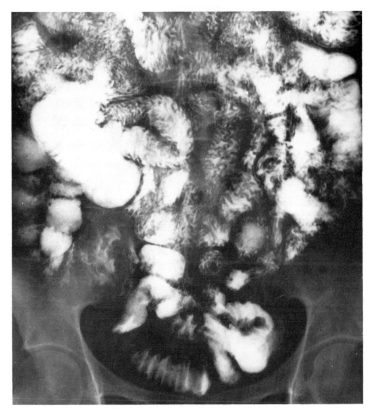

Figure 22-18 Hereditary angioneurotic edema. There is edema of a segment of ileum in the pelvis. At this time the patient had cutaneous edema, abdominal pain, vomiting, and diarrhea. (Courtesy of Dr. Robert Berk, Dallas, Texas.)

laryngeal edema is a frequent and dreaded complication. In one review this was the cause of death in 77 per cent of these patients, with such deaths occurring at an average age of 35 years.[40]

The diagnosis of hereditary angioneurotic edema is usually based on a positive family history and recognition of the typical clinical features. In addition to the skin swellings, which may last for 1 to 3 days, almost all patients have episodes of abdominal pain. These usually accompany the skin lesions, but either manifestation may occur alone or even precede the other by years.[42] There are a few reports of radiologic examinations demonstrating focal areas of edema of the stomach,[43] duodenum,[44] small bowel, [40, 45] or colon.[46, 47] The latter site seems to be the least frequently involved.

Radiologic recognition of this focal submucosal edema in the small bowel is not difficult (Fig. 22-18). The findings, however, will be indistinguishable from focal edema or hemorrhage resulting from numerous other causes, such as the early stages of segmental infarction, intramural hemorrhage, and eosinophilic enteritis. It should be stressed that the changes are transitory and are likely to be found only while the patient is symptomatic. With resolution of symptoms, the radiologic abnormalities quickly disappear (Fig. 22-19).

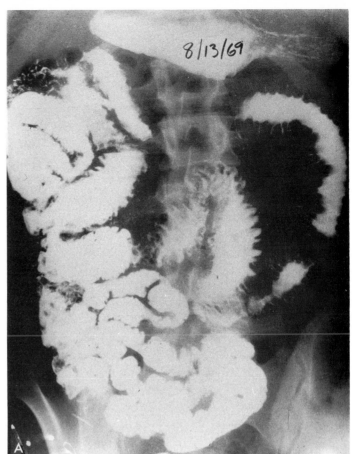

Figure 22-19 *Hereditary angioneurotic edema.* A, There is severe segmental edema in the proximal jejunum when the patient is symptomatic.

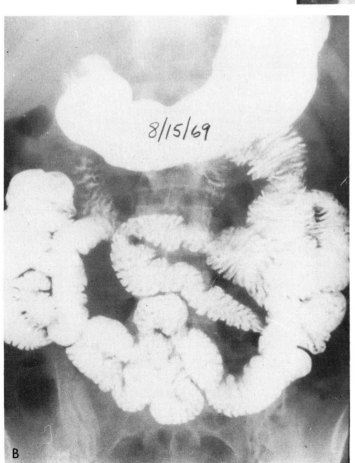

Figure 22-19 B, This has resolved less than 48 hours later when abdominal symptoms have subsided.

521

HISTOPLASMOSIS

The disseminated form of histoplasmosis is rare, and pulmonary and reticuloendothelial lesions predominate. Gastrointestinal symptoms occur and in some cases dominate the clinical picture.[48, 49] Focal ulcerative granulomatous disease of the gastrointestinal tract occurs, but the usual case has multiple lesions of small bowel and colon.[50] Spontaneous perforation of small bowel ulcers has been noted as well as obstruction due to ileal stenosis.[51, 52] Some of the ulcerated histoplasma granulomas present as small polypoid lesions, and roentgenologically this form has been confused with neoplasms of the small intestine and colon.[53] The granulomatous lesions of the small bowel and right colon are indistinguishable from Crohn's disease, although the tendency to inflammatory pseudopolyps suggests the possibility of histoplasmosis (Fig. 22-20).

One unique case of histoplasmosis has been reported in which the disease presented as a diffuse lesion confined to the small intestine.[54] The patient had mild diarrhea and was edematous due to a secondary protein-losing enteropathy. Roentgen examination revealed diffuse thickening of the valvulae conniventes throughout the small bowel (Fig. 22-21), and the mucosal surface was studded with punctate filling defects. Inspection of the small bowel biopsy revealed that these were enlarged individual villi which measured up to 1.0 mm. in height and 0.5 mm. in width. Histologic examination demonstrated an edematous lamina propria infiltrated with macrophages containing histoplasma organisms. The surface epithelium was flat with loss of the brush border, but there was no evidence of ulceration. The morphology of the intestinal lesion, both roentgenologically and pathologically, is similar to Whipple's disease. Identification of the organism on tissue section and a response to treatment with amphotericin B confirmed this case as an example of histoplasmosis.

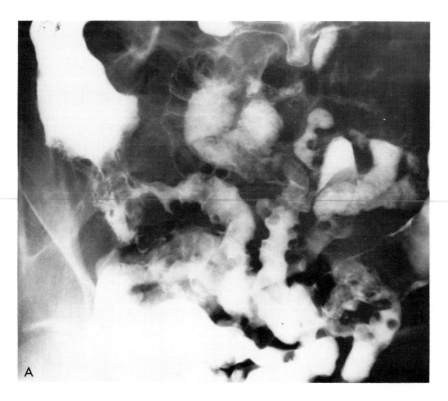

Figure 22-20 Histoplasmosis. There is extensive granulomatous disease of the ileum (*A*) and right colon (*B, C*) that is indistinguishable from Crohn's disease, although the marked pseudopolyposis in the ileum would be unusual in regional enteritis. (Courtesy of Dr. Ross Hill, Montreal, Canada.)

Figure 22-20 B.

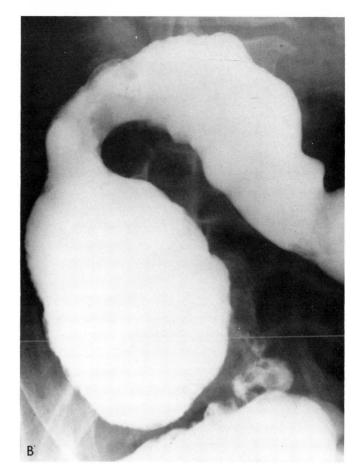

B

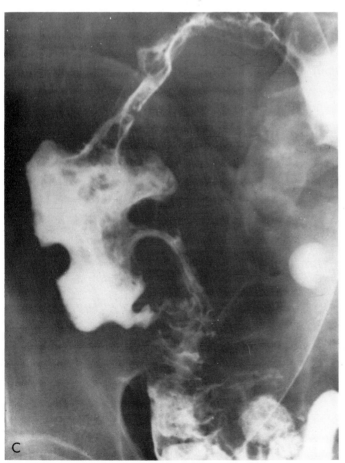

C

Figure 22-20 C.

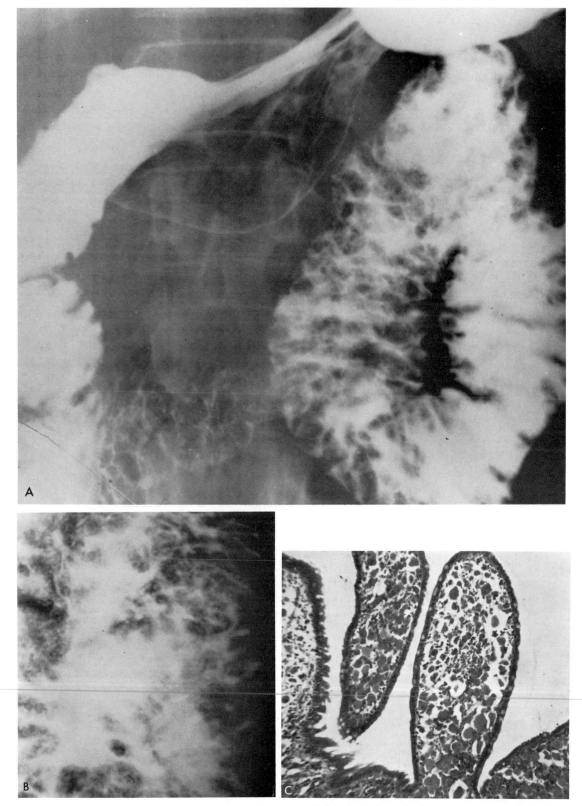

Figure 22-21   *A,* Diffuse histoplasmosis of small intestine. The valvulae conniventes of the jejunum are thickened. *B,* Photographic enlargement shows the mucosal surface to be studded with punctate filling defects. *C,* Histologic examination reveals these defects to be swollen villi measuring 1.0 mm. in height and 0.5 mm. in width. The lamina propria is edematous and infiltrated by large macrophages containing Histoplasma organisms. (Courtesy of Dr. S. Bank, Cape Town, South Africa.)

MASTOCYTOSIS

Urticaria pigmentosa is an uncommon but distinctive skin disease in which there is infiltration of the dermis by tissue mast cells. In some of these cases, more properly designated mastocytosis, there is mast cell proliferation in the reticuloendothelial system as well. One or more organs may be involved, and the disease runs an indolent course.

The pathology of mastocytosis is unique. The biochemically potent mast cells contain histamine, heparin, hyaluronic acid, and other biologically active substances. Mast cell proliferation seems to stimulate fibrosis and nonspecific cellular infiltrations. Sometimes the mast cells diminish in number or eventually disappear during these reactions. Myelofibrosis, periportal fibrosis, and splenic fibrosis may be found in the late stages of mastocytosis with or without striking mast cell infiltration.

The clinical manifestations of the disease are variable. Urticaria pigmentosa presents as a red-brown macular rash. The skin is sensitive, and exposure to heat, cold, or slight trauma produces localized urticaria and pruritus. Skin lesions are present in almost all cases, but systemic mastocytosis occurs without involvement of the skin. About half of the patients have hepatomegaly, splenomegaly, or sclerotic bone lesions. These are usually diffuse, giving the picture of myelofibrosis, but focal lesions indistinguishable from osteoblastic metastases are noted in some cases.

Nausea, vomiting, abdominal pain, and diarrhea are common symptoms. The incidence of peptic ulcer is high but only partially explains the gastrointestinal symptoms which plague most of these patients. In recent years, small bowel disease has been recognized with increasing frequency, and a few

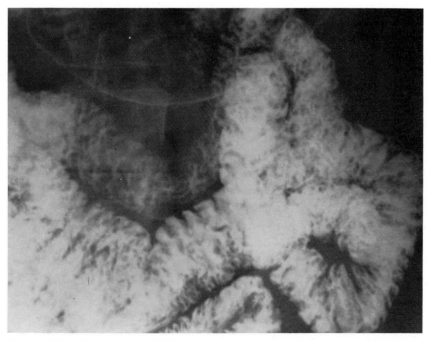

Figure 22-22 *Mastocytosis.* Ill-defined mucosal nodules are present throughout the jejunum. Partial villous atrophy, edema of the lamina propria, and mast cell infiltration were found on intestinal biopsy.

of these patients with small bowel lesions have presented with severe malabsorption.[55, 56] The patients frequently have an intolerance to alcohol and in one instance alcohol was shown to cause an exacerbation of symptoms accompanied by pylorospasm and increased gastric and intestinal secretions.[57]

Knowledge of the small bowel pathology is limited. Cellular infiltration of the lamina propria of the intestinal mucosa has been present in all cases. The mast cell component of the infiltrate has been variable and some specimens do not show increased numbers of mast cells. Edema of the mucosa and submucosa has been noted. Partial villous atrophy has been found in some cases, normal villi being seen in others. Marked variability of villous architecture was a feature in one specimen (Fig. 22-24).

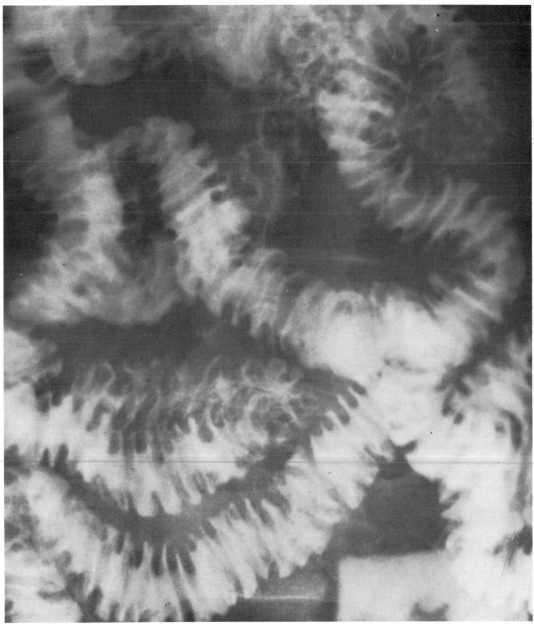

Figure 22-23   Mastocytosis. Diffuse thickening of the valvulae conniventes of the jejunum is the predominant feature in this case.

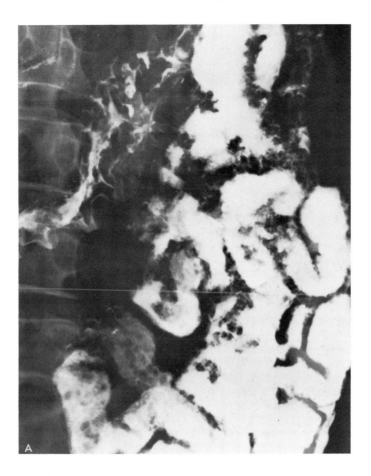

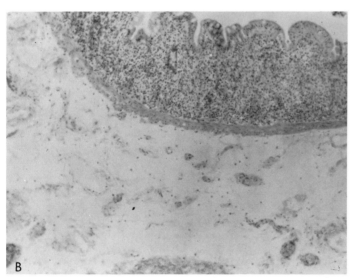

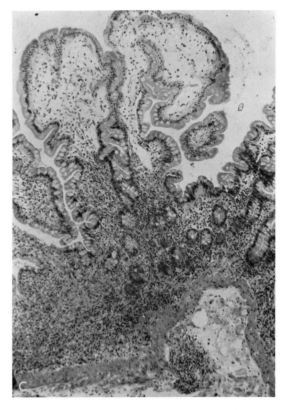

Figure 22-24 *Mastocytosis with malabsorption. A,* Mucosal nodules are present in some areas, and the valvulae conniventes are thickened or effaced. This gives the bowel its rigid, tubular character. *B,* One section of the intestinal biopsy shows villous atrophy, a marked cellular infiltrate in the mucosa, and edema of the submucosa. *C,* Tall villi with focal areas of edema were present in other portions of the same biopsy specimen.

Roentgen examination of the small intestine shows thickening of the bowel wall, mucosal nodularity, or both[58, 59] (Figs. 22-22 and 22-23). The cellular infiltrate and edema cause diffuse thickening of the valvulae conniventes, especially in the jejunum. In the more severe cases, marked mucosal edema may efface the folds and give the bowel a rigid, tubular appearance (Fig. 22-24). The mucosal nodules measure 2 to 5 mm. in diameter. When small, they may be ill-defined. They occur in short segments of jejunum but have been noted in the ileum as well. It has been suggested that the nodules represent urticarial lesions of the mucosa, but their precise nature has not been determined.

RETRACTILE MESENTERITIS

This unusual disorder of the mesentery causes significant roentgen abnormalities of the small bowel. It is a fibro-fatty thickening of the mesentery with chronic inflammation of the mesenteric fat. First described by Jura in 1924, this lesion has since been reported in the literature under a variety of names, the most important of which are retractile mesenteritis,[60, 61] mesenteric panniculitis,[62-64] and isolated lipodystrophy of the mesentery.[65-67] These diagnoses reflect the outstanding features of a given case—fibrosis, inflammation, or fatty infiltration. To a greater or lesser extent, all three are present in most reported cases. The etiology of the condition is unknown.

Retractile mesenteritis affects both sexes, and patients have ranged in age from eight to 80. There is no distinctive clinical picture. The most frequent

(*Text continued on page 532*)

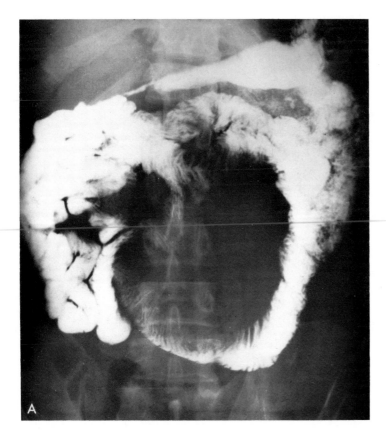

Figure 22-25 Retractile mesenteritis or mesenteric fibromatosis in a patient with Gardner's syndrome with previous subtotal colectomy. *A*, The large mesenteric mass displaces and distorts small bowel loops.

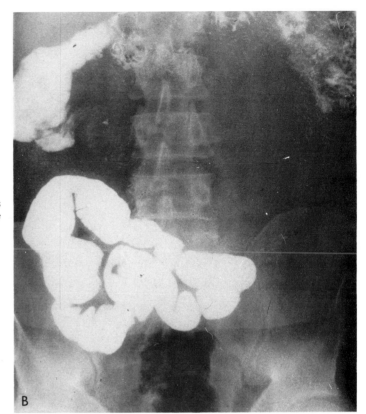

Figure 22-25 Continued B, On the late film gas is present in the rectal stump, which contains multiple polyps.

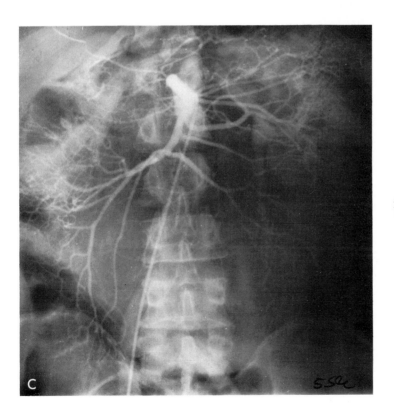

Figure 22-25 C, Selective superior mesenteric arteriogram shows stretching and distortion of jejunal branches but no tumor vessels or encasement.

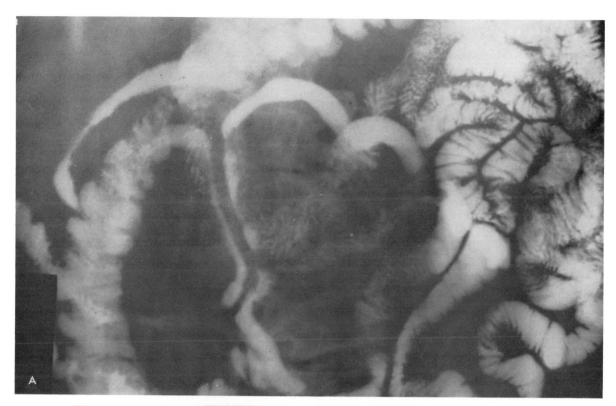

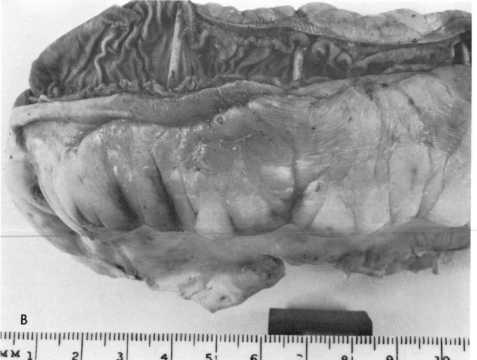

Figure 22-26 A and B   *See legend on opposite page.*

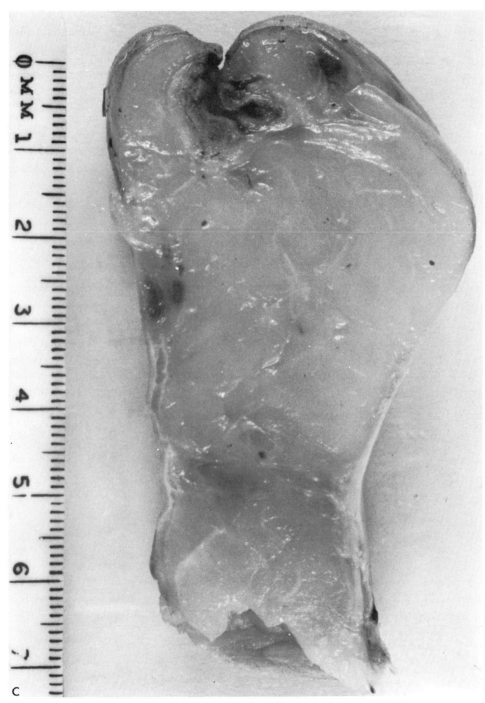

Figure 22-26 *Retractile mesenteritis. A,* The diffuse mesenteric mass causes separation of ileal loops with kinking and angulation of the bowel. The affected loops are narrowed and stretched. Fluoroscopy revealed normal peristalsis, and no intrinsic bowel abnormality could be detected. *B,* Lipomatous projections of mesenteric fat almost encircle the bowel. *C,* Cross section reveals the thickened mesentery which is composed of fat with interlacing strands of fibrous tissue. There is subperitoneal fibrosis at the root of the mesentery.

symptom is abdominal pain, and this may be accompanied by nausea, vomiting, diarrhea or constipation, malaise, and low-grade fever. An ill-defined abdominal mass is often palpable and occasionally is found in asymptomatic patients. The disease has a benign course, and once diagnosis is established, no treatment is indicated or required as a rule. Steroids have occasionally been employed to control abdominal pain. It is generally agreed that surgical resection of the mesenteric lesion should not be attempted.

The disease process originates in the root of the mesentery, which is invariably thickened and usually lobulated or nodular. Lipomatous projections from the main mass are frequent. The fat has a firm or rubbery consistency, and red-brown discoloration is frequently described. The nonspecific inflammatory reaction varies from sparse collections of lymphocytes in some cases to dense infiltrations of lymphocytes, plasma cells, lipid-laden macrophages and foreign body giant cells in others. Fat necrosis is common and may result in microscopic calcification. The fibrotic reaction extends diffusely through the mesenteric fat but tends to be most severe in the subperitoneal tissue at the root of the mesentery. Retraction of the mesentery is seldom marked, and the mechanical bowel obstruction which complicates a few cases is usually due to adhesions between bowel loops. The disease process is confined to the mesentery, and there is no intrinsic abnormality of the intestine or mesenteric blood vessels,[68, 69] although mesenteric venous thrombosis may be a rare complication.

A benign, non-neoplastic fibrous proliferation of the mesentery occurs in some cases of familial polyposis, most of which seem to be examples of Gardner's syndrome.[70-73] This lesion, designated "mesenteric fibromatosis," appears identical to retractile mesenteritis and has been reported as such.[74] In Gardner's syndrome the fibromatous mesenteric masses almost always occur after abdominal surgery, which in most cases is a total or subtotal colectomy (Fig. 22-25).

The roentgen abnormalities (Fig. 22-26) in retractile mesenteritis are determined by the extent and severity of the mesenteric lesion.[75] Small tumefactions of the mesenteric root may go undetected. Somewhat larger lesions displace bowel loops from a central location and may compress and distort the distal duodenum. Mesenteric cysts or neoplasms present identical changes. The more extensive lesions cause separation of the bowel loops, one from another, which indicates diffuse thickening of the mesentery. When the mesenteric disease extends to the bowel margins, kinking and angulation of intestinal loops occurs. The affected bowel segments are often stretched and distorted, but no intrinsic abnormality can be demonstrated on careful fluoroscopic examination. This combination of roentgen features should confirm, or at least suggest, the diagnosis of retractile mesenteritis.

WALDENSTRÖM'S MACROGLOBULINEMIA

First described by Waldenström in 1944, this is a primary proliferative disease of the lymphoreticular system, the cardinal feature of which is marked increase in the IgM or macroglobulin fraction of serum proteins.[76] Diagnosis is established by serum ultracentrifugation and serum immunoelectrophoresis. The abnormal macroglobulins are produced by cells of the lymphocyte-plasma cell series, variously designated as lymphocytoid plasma cells or plasmacytoid lymphocytes. These cells diffusely infiltrate lymph nodes, spleen, liver, bone marrow, and in some instances other tissues as well. The various manifestations of the disease are attributable to both the cellular infiltrates and the serum protein abnormality.

The disease occurs in later adult life and the onset is insidious. The principal, but not invariable, clinical findings are anemia, bleeding diathesis, lymphadenopathy, and hepatosplenomegaly. Visual disturbances and a variety of neurologic abnormalities complicate some cases. The disease is similar to multiple myeloma, but it has a more protracted and benign course, and destructive bone lesions do not occur. Amyloidosis has been associated with macroglobulinemia in a few instances. Lymphomatous masses eventually develop in a small percentage (15 per cent or less) of patients, and the transformation to frank lymphosarcoma may be accompanied by a decrease in the macroglobulins.[77]

Diarrhea or steatorrhea is a rare manifestation of Waldenström's macroglobulinemia, and affected patients have significant roentgen abnormalities of the small bowel.[78-80] There is diffuse, rather uniform thickening of the valvulae conniventes, and the mucosal surface has a granular character created by a myriad of punctate filling defects (Fig. 22-27). The appearance is identical to certain cases of Whipple's disease and the single case of histoplasmosis referred to previously.

Pathologically, there is edema of the mucosa and submucosa and lymphangiectasis. The lymphatics are filled with an eosinophilic proteinaceous material, and inspissation of this material is believed to cause the lymphatic distention. The punctate surface defects are greatly distended lacteals in the

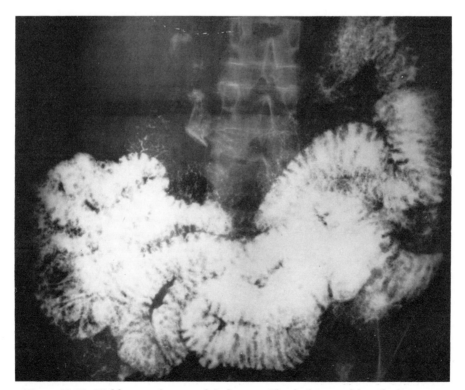

Figure 22-27 *Waldenström's macroglobulinemia.* The thickening of the valvulae conniventes is characteristic of a mucosal infiltrative lesion. The granular appearance is the result of myriads of tiny punctate filling defects which represent greatly enlarged abnormal individual villi.

tips of some villi. Large macrophages in the lamina propria contain eosinophilic material which shows a variable reaction to PAS stains. Mesenteric lymph nodes are enlarged and contain cystic spaces filled with the proteinaceous material. Infiltration by lymphocytoid plasma cells is variable, perhaps due to modification of the abnormal cell population by treatment with alkylating agents or steroids.

NONSPECIFIC ULCERS AND STRICTURES IN SPRUE—CHRONIC ULCERATIVE JEJUNITIS

Nonspecific ulceration of the distal duodenum and jejunum is a well-documented but very rare complication of nontropical sprue.[81-83] The cause is unknown. The ulcers may heal and leave residual strictures which can cause partial intestinal obstruction. In some cases perforation of the ulcers has led to death.[81] Most of the ulcers and strictures occur in the proximal small bowel, although they have been noted in the ileum[81] and even in the colon.[83]

In a typical case the ulcerations and/or strictures occur in the duodenum and jejunum, and the bowel distal to these areas shows the dilatation characteristic of nontropical sprue (Fig. 22-28). Although these complications are

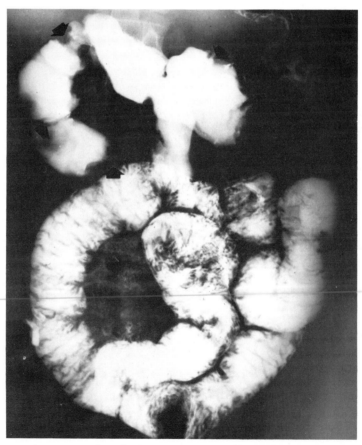

Figure 22-28 Sprue with multiple strictures in the duodenum and proximal jejunum (arrows). An earlier examination demonstrated a large ulcer at one of the stricture sites in the duodenum. Distal to the strictures there is dilatation of the small bowel characteristic of sprue. (Courtesy of Dr. Richard Wolfe, San Francisco, California.)

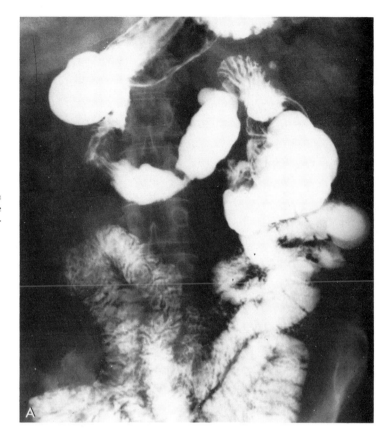

Figure 22-29 *Sprue with multiple strictures in the distal duodenum and proximal jejunum. A,* The initial small bowel series on this patient being evaluated for abdominal pain was rather confusing.

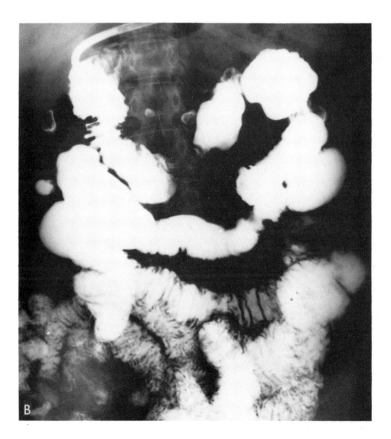

Figure 22-29 *B,* Small bowel enema confirmed the presence of multiple pliable strictures in the distal duodenum and proximal jejunum. Distally the small bowel was slightly dilated. A careful history then revealed symptoms consistent with sprue for 9 years with periods of remission on a gluten-free diet. Laboratory studies indicated malabsorption and small bowel biopsy revealed villous atrophy with a marked inflammatory cell infiltrate in the lamina propria.

potentially serious and often occur in severe cases of sprue, they also may occur in rather mild cases of long duration (Fig. 22-29).

The strictures have been successfully managed in some cases by surgical resection.[84] Once the ulcerative lesions have occurred, many patients who previously were responsive to a gluten-free diet become refractory to this form of therapy. This inflammatory component of sprue may respond to steroid therapy.[85]

The relationship of this unusual complication of sprue to the entity called chronic ulcerative jejunitis is uncertain. The patients reported with the latter diagnosis have had an illness characterized by severe diarrhea, abdominal pain, low grade fever, steatorrhea, and hypoproteinemia.[86–88] Multiple mucosal ulcerations, some associated with stenosis, have been the most consistent pathological findings. Some patients have villous atrophy consistent with sprue, but in many cases this has been patchy in character or even absent.[87]

Because of the atypical mucosal changes and an incomplete or absent response to a gluten-free diet several authorities have been unwilling to accept chronic ulcerative jejunitis as a complication of nontropical sprue,[86–88] even though several cases have been listed both ways in the literature.[84] The relationship of these two entities, therefore, remains speculative. The nosologic problem is well illustrated by the patient described in Fig. 22-30.

It has been suggested that chronic ulcerative jejunitis is an atypical variant of Crohn's disease.[89] There are numerous criticisms of this view. Chronic ulcerative jejunitis patients are older than the usual patients with regional

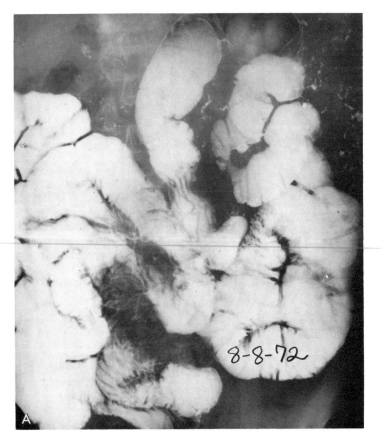

Figure 22-30 This 44 year old man had the onset of diarrhea, abdominal bloating, and weight loss in 1967. Biopsy revealed villous atrophy and mild inflammation. On a gluten-free diet his symptoms subsided and he gained 30 lbs. Symptoms recurred in 1971 when the diet was discontinued and he developed jejunal obstruction and an area of stenosis was bypassed by enteroenterostomy.

Evaluation in mid-1972 revealed malabsorption and small bowel biopsy showed villous atrophy and a dense chronic inflammatory cell infiltrate. Small bowel examination (A) showed a jejunal stricture, the enteroenterostomy and dilatation of the entire small bowel. In November 1972 he was readmitted with nausea, vomiting, and low grade fever.

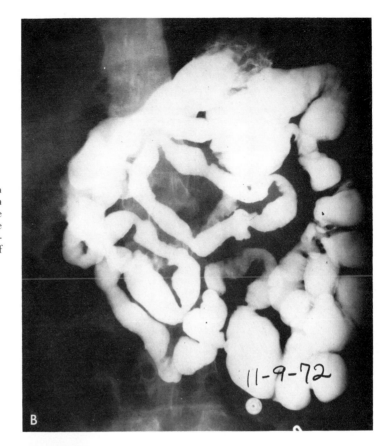

Figure 22-30 Continued B, Examination then revealed thickening of the wall of the proximal jejunum with multiple strictures and ulcers. In January 1973 the blind loop and adjacent jejunum were resected. The specimen showed multiple ulcers, inflammatory infiltrate and villous atrophy. There was no evidence of Crohn's disease.

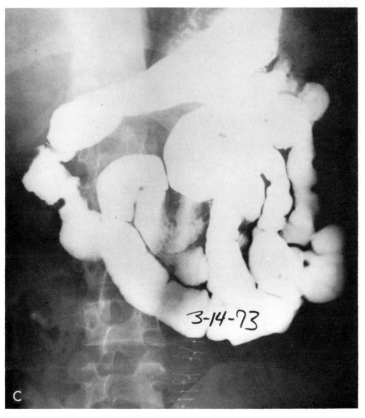

Follow-up examination (C) shows a tubular, slightly dilated bowel. There was symptomatic improvement with steroid therapy in addition to the gluten-free diet and subsequent biopsies revealed some improvement in the villous architecture although evidence of malabsorption continued. The clinical diagnosis in this case remains uncertain; that is, is this sprue complicated by ulcerative jejunitis or just chronic ulcerative jejunitis? (Courtesy of Dr. David Kumpe, Baltimore, Maryland, and Dr. Edward Olinger, Bethesda, Maryland.)

enteritis. Steatorrhea is a prominent symptom. The inflammatory disease is mucosal, not transmural, except at the site of the ulcers, and there is no granulomatous reaction. The gross appearance of the bowel is unlike classic Crohn's disease. The strictures are short and annular. There are no fistulas or other stigmata of Crohn's disease. Distal to the ulcerative stenosing lesions most illustrated cases show the usual radiological features of nontropical sprue.

References

1. Becroft, D. M. O., Costello, J. M., and Scott, P. J.: A-Beta-lipoproteinemia (Bassen-Kornzweig syndrome): Report of a case. *Arch. Dis. Child.,* 40:40–46, 1965.
2. Van Buchem, F. S. P., Pol, G., DeGier, J., Bottcher, C. J. F., and Pries, C.: Congenital beta-lipoprotein deficiency. *Amer. J. Med.,* 40:794–804, 1966.
3. Salt, H. B., Wolff, O. H., Lloyd, J. D., Fosbrooke, A. S., Cameron, A. H., and Hubble, D. V.: On having no beta-lipoprotein: Syndrome comprising a-beta-lipoproteinemia, acanthocytosis and steatorrhea. *Lancet,* 2:325–329, 1960.
4. Isselbacher, K. J., Scheig, R., Plotkin, G. R., and Caulfield, J. B.: Congenital beta-lipoprotein deficiency, an hereditary disorder involving a defect in the absorption and transport of lipids. *Medicine,* 43:347–361, 1964.
5. Sperling, M. A., Hengstenberg, F., Yunis, E., Kenny, F. M., and Drash, A. L.: Abetalipoproteinemia: Metabolic, endocrine, and electron-microscopic investigations. *Pediatrics,* 48:91–102, 1971.
6. Lamy, M., Frezal, J., Polonovski, J., Druez, G., and Rey, J.: Congenital absence of beta-lipoproteins. *Pediatrics,* 31:277–289, 1963.
7. Stacy, G. S., and Loop, J. W.: Unusual small bowel diseases: Methods and observations. *Amer. J. Roentgen.,* 92:1072–1079, 1964.
8. Weinstein, M. A., Pearson, K. D., and Agus, S. G.: Abetalipoproteinemia. *Radiology,* 108:269–273, 1973.
9. Mullins, F., Talamo, R., and diSant'Agnese, P. A.: Late intestinal complications of cystic fibrosis. *J.A.M.A.* 192:741–746, 1965.
10. Jensen, K. G.: Meconium-ileus equivalent in a 15 year old patient with mucoviscidosis. *Acta Paediat.,* 51:344–348, 1962.
11. Seliger, G., Firooznia, H., and Genieser, N. B.: Intestinal obstruction in an adult with cystic fibrosis. *Am. J. Dig. Dis.,* 17:934–938, 1972.
12. Snyder, W. H., Gwinn, J. L., Landing, B. H., and Asay, L. D.: Fecal retention in children with cystic fibrosis: Report of three cases. *Pediatrics,* 34:72–77, 1964.
13. Berk, R. N., and Lee, F. A.: The late gastrointestinal manifestations of cystic fibrosis of the pancreas. *Radiology,* 106:377–381, 1973.
14. Beck, A. R., and Aterman, K.: Intestinal obstruction and mucoviscidosis. *Gastroenterologia,* 106:84–96, 1966.
15. Holsclaw, D. S., Rocmans, C., and Shwachman, H.: Intussusception in patients with cystic fibrosis. *Pediatrics,* 48:51–58, 1971.
16. Grossman, H., Berdon, W. E., and Baker, D. H.: Gastrointestinal findings in cystic fibrosis. *Amer. J. Roentgen.,* 97:227–238, 1966.
17. Thomaidis, T. S., and Arey, J. B.: Intestinal lesions in cystic fibrosis of the pancreas. *J. Pediat.,* 63:444–453, 1963.
18. Djurhuus, M. J., Lykkegaard, E., and Pock-Steen, O. C.: Gastrointestinal radiological findings in cystic fibrosis. *Pediat. Radiol.,* 1:113–118, 1973.
19. Jabro, I. H., and Gibbs, G. E.: Rectal mucosal biopsies as a diagnostic aid in cystic fibrosis. *Lancet,* 86:385–388, 1966.
20. Taussig, L. M., Saldino, R. M., and diSant'Agnese, P. A.: Radiographic abnormalities of the duodenum and small bowel in cystic fibrosis of the pancreas (Mucoviscidosis). *Radiology,* 106:369–376, 1973.
21. Weinstein, L. D., Clemett, A. R., and Herskovic, T.: Morphologic and radiologic findings in the intestines in cystic fibrosis (abstr.). *Gastroenterology,* 54:1282, 1968.
22. Naylor, D., Mullins, J. F., and Gilmore, J. F.: Papulosis atrophicans maligna (Degos' disease); report of the first United States' case and review of literature. *Arch. Dermat.* 81:189–197, 1960.
23. Nomland, R., and Layton, J. M.: Malignant papulosis with atrophy (Degos): fatal cutaneointestinal syndrome. *Arch. Dermat.,* 81:181–188, 1960.
24. Hall-Smith, P.: Malignant atrophic papulosis (Degos' disease); two cases occurring in the same family. *Brit. J. Dermat.,* 81:817, 1969.
25. Durie, B. G. M., Dytouf, J. D., and Kahn, J. A.: Progressive systemic sclerosis with malignant atrophic papulosis. *Arch. Dermat.,* 100:575–581, 1969.
26. Roenigk, H. H., and Farmer, R. G.: Degos' disease (malignant papulosis); report of three cases with clues to etiology. *J.A.M.A.,* 206:1508–1514, 1968.
27. Hall-Smith, S. P.: Malignant atrophic papulosis. *Proc. Roy. Soc. Med.,* 57:519–521, 1964.

28. Strole, W. E., Jr., Clark, W. H., Jr., and Isselbacher, K. J.: Progressive arterial occlusive disease (Kohlmeier-Degos): A frequently fatal cutaneosystemic disorder. *New Eng. J. Med.,* 276:195–201, 1967.

29. Edelman, M. J., and March, T. L.: Eosinophilic gastroenteritis. *Amer. J. Roentgen.,* 91:773–778, 1964.

30. Goldberg, H. I., O'Kieffe, D., Jenis, E. H., and Boyce, H. W.: Diffuse eosinophilic gastroenteritis. *Amer. J. Roentgen.,* 119:342–351, 1973.

31. Heddle, S. B., Parrott, K. B., Paloschi, G. P. G., Prentice, R. S. A., Perysko, L., and Beck, I. T.: Diffuse eosinophilic gastroenteritis. *Canad. Med. Assoc. J.,* 100:554–559, 1969.

32. Kaplan, S. M., Goldstein, F., and Kowlessar, O. D.: Eosinophilic gastroenteritis. Report of a case with malabsorption and protein-losing enteropathy. *Gastroenterology,* 58:540–545, 1970.

33. Gregg, J. A., and Luna, L.: Eosinophilic gastroenteritis. *Amer. J. Gastroent.,* 59:41–47, 1973.

34. Jacobsen, L. B.: Diffuse eosinophilic gastroenteritis: An adult form of allergic gastroenteropathy. *Amer. J. Gastroent.,* 54:580–588, 1970.

35. Waldmann, T. A., Wochner, R. D., Laster, L., and Gordon, R. S.: Allergic gastroenteropathy. A cause of excessive gastrointestinal protein loss. *New Eng. J. Med.,* 276:761–769, 1967.

36. Higgins, G. A., Lamm, E. R., and Yutzy, C. V.: Eosinophilic gastroenteritis. *Arch. Surg.,* 92:476–483, 1966.

37. Dalinka, M. K., and Masters, C. J.: Eosinophilic enteritis. Report of case without gastric involvement. *Radiology,* 96:543–544, 1970.

38. Sivasankar, R., Lane, O. G., and Hjertaas, O. K.: Eosinophilic enteritis of the ileum: A case report. *Canad. J. Surg.,* 15:1–4, 1972.

39. Burhenne, H. J., and Carbone, J. V.: Eosinophilic (allergic) gastroenteritis. *Amer. J. Roentgen.,* 96:332–338, 1966.

40. Landerman, N. S.: Hereditary angioneurotic edema. *J. Allergy,* 33:316–329, 1963.

41. Dennehy, J. J.: Hereditary angioneurotic edema. *Ann. Intern. Med.,* 73:55–59, 1970.

42. Blohme, G., Ysander, L., Korsan-Bengtsen, K., and Laurell, A. B.: Hereditary angioneurotic oedema in three families. *Acta Med. Scand.,* 191:209–219, 1972.

43. Love, R. J. M.: Gastro-intestinal crisis of angioneurotic oedema. *Brit. J. Surg.,* 20:170–172, 1932.

44. Trigg, J. W.: Hereditary angioneurotic edema. *New Eng. J. Med.,* 264:761–763, 1961.

45. Ellis, K., and McConnell, D. J.: Hereditary angioneurotic edema involving small intestine. *Radiology,* 92:518–519, 1969.

46. Biering, A.: Abdominal pains in angioneurotic edema. *Acta Med. Scand.,* 153:373–382, 1956.

47. Pearson, K. D., Buchignani, J. S., Shimkin, P. M., and Frank, M. M.: Hereditary angioneurotic edema of the gastrointestinal tract. *Am. J. Roentgen.,* 116:256–261, 1972.

48. Henderson, R. G., Pinkerton, H., and Moore, L. T.: Histoplasma capsulatum as a cause of chronic ulcerative enteritis. *J.A.M.A.,* 118:885–889, 1942.

49. Kirk, M. E., Lough, J., and Warner, H. A.: Histoplasma colitis: An electron microscopic study. *Gastroenterology,* 61:46–53, 1971.

50. Shull, H. J.: Human histoplasmosis: a disease with protean manifestations often with digestive system involvement. *Gastroenterology,* 25:582–595, 1953.

51. Perez, C. A., Sturim, H. S., Kouchoukos, N. T., and Kamberg, S.: Some clinical and radiographic features of gastrointestinal histoplasmosis. *Radiology,* 86:482–487, 1966.

52. Dietz, M. W.: Ileocecal histoplasmosis. *Radiology,* 91:285–289, 1968.

53. Bersack, S. R., Howe, J. S., and Rabson, A. S.: Inflammatory pseudopolyposis of the small and large intestines with the Peutz-Jeghers syndrome in a case of diffuse histoplasmosis. *Amer. J. Roentgen.,* 80:73–78, 1958.

54. Bank, S., Trey, C., Gans, I., Marks, I. N., and Groll, A.: Histoplasmosis of the small bowel with "giant" intestinal villi and secondary protein-losing enteropathy. *Amer. J. Med.,* 39:492–501, 1965.

55. Bank, S., and Marks, I. N.: Malabsorption in systemic mast cell disease. *Gastroenterology,* 45:535–549, 1963.

56. Jarnum, S., and Zachariae, H.: Mastocytosis (urticaria pigmentosa) of skin, stomach, and gut with malabsorption. *Gut,* 8:64–68, 1967.

57. Robbins, A. H., Schimmel, E. M., and Rao, K. C. V. G.: Gastrointestinal mastocytosis: Radiologic alterations after ethanol ingestion. *Amer. J. Roentgen.,* 115:297–299, 1972.

58. Clemett, A. R., Fishbone, G., Levine, R. J., James, A. E., and Janower, M. L.: Gastrointestinal lesions in mastocytosis. *Amer. J. Roentgen.,* 103:405–412, 1968.

59. Janower, M. L.: Mastocytosis of gastrointestinal tract: Report of a case. *Acta Radiol.,* 57:489–493, 1962.

60. Aach, R. D., Kahn, L. I., and Frech, R. S.: Obstruction of the small intestine due to retractile mesenteritis. *Gastroenterology,* 54:594–598, 1968.

61. Tedeschi, C. G., and Botta, G. C.: Retractile mesenteritis. *New Eng. J. Med.,* 266:1035–1040, 1962.

62. Grossman, L. A., Kaplan, H. J., Preuss, H. J., and Herrington, J. L.: Mesenteric panniculitis. *J.A.M.A.,* 183:318–323, 1963.

63. Handelsman, J. C., and Shelley, W. M.: Mesenteric panniculitis. *Arch. Surg.,* 91:842–850, 1965.

64. Ogden, W. W., Bradburn, D. M., and Rives, J. D.: Mesenteric panniculitis: Review of 27 cases. *Ann. Surg.,* 161:864–875, 1965.

65. Crane, J. T., Aguilar, M. J., and Grimes, O. F.: Isolated lipodystrophy, a form of mesenteric tumor. *Amer. J. Surg.*, 90:169–179, 1955.
66. Kipfer, R. E., Moertel, C. G., and Dahlin, D. C.: Mesenteric lipodystrophy. *Ann. Intern. Med.*, 80:582–588, 1974.
67. Rogers, C. E., Demetrakopoulos, N. J., and Hyamns, V.: Isolated lipodystrophy affecting the mesentery, the retroperitoneal area, and the small intestine. *Ann. Surg.*, 153:277–282, 1961.
68. Carillo, F. J., Ruzicka, F. F., and Clemett, A. R.: Value of angiography in the diagnosis of retractile mesenteritis. *Amer. J. Roentgenol.*, 115:396–398, 1972.
69. Diamond, A. B., Meng, C. H., and Goldin, R. R.: Arteriography of unusual mass lesions of the mesentery. *Radiology*, 110:547–552, 1974.
70. Chanco, A. G., and Rose, E. F.: Mesenteric fibromatosis following colectomy for familial polyposis. *Arch. Surg.*, 104:851–852, 1972.
71. Koren, E., Lazarovitch, A., Baratz, M., Loewenthal, M., and Solowiejczyk, M.: Gardner's syndrome: Report of a family. *Ann. Surg.*, 180:198–202, 1974.
72. McAdam, W. A. F., and Goligher, J. C.: The occurrence of desmoids in patients with familial polyposis coli. *Brit. J. Surg.*, 57:618–631, 1970.
73. Simpson, R. D., Harrison, E. G., Jr., and Mayo, C. W.: Mesenteric fibromatosis in familial polyposis. *Cancer*, 17:526–534, 1964.
74. Roberts, F. M., and Nielsen, O. F.: Retractile mesenteritis. *Amer. J. Dig. Dis.*, 9:231–235, 1964.
75. Dietz, M. W.: Roentgen evaluation of mesenteric panniculitis. *Radiology*, 92:838–842, 1969.
76. Cohen, R. J., Bohannon, R. A., and Wallerstein, R. O.: Waldenström's macroglobulinemia. *Amer. J. Med.*, 41:274–284, 1966.
77. Wood, T. A., and Frenkel, E. P.: An unusual case of macroglobulinemia. *Arch. Intern. Med.*, 119:631–637, 1967.
78. Bedine, M. S., Yardley, J. H., Elliott, H. L., Banwell, G., and Hendrix, T. R.: Intestinal involvement in Waldenström's macroglobulinemia. *Gastroenterology*, 65:308–315, 1973.
79. Cabrera, A., de la Pava, S., and Pickren, J. W.: Intestinal localization of Waldenström's disease. *Arch. Intern. Med.*, 114:399–407, 1964.
80. Khilnani, M. T., Keller, R. J., and Cuttner, J.: Macroglobulinemia and steatorrhea: Roentgen and pathologic findings in the intestinal tract. *Radiol. Clin. N. Amer.*, 7:43–55, 1969.
81. Bayless, T. M., Kapelowitz, R. F., Shelley, W. M., Ballinger, W. F., and Hendrix, T. R.: Intestinal ulceration—A complication of celiac disease. *New Eng. J. Med.*, 276:995–1001, 1967.
82. Seliger, G., Goldman, A. B., Firooznia, H., and Lawrence, L. R.: Ulceration of the small intestine complicating celiac disease. *Amer. J. Dig. Dis.*, 18:820–824, 1973.
83. Stuber, J. L., Wiegman, H., Crosby, I., and Gonzalez, G.: Ulcers of the colon and jejunum in celiac disease. *Radiology*, 99:339–340, 1971.
84. Moritz, M., Moran, J. M., and Patterson, J. F.: Chronic ulcerative jejunitis. *Gastroenterology*, 60:96–101, 1971.
85. Pink, I. J., and Creamer, B.: Response to a gluten-free diet of patients with the coeliac syndrome. *Lancet*, pp. 300–304, February 11, 1967.
86. Corlin, R. F., and Pops, M. A.: Nongranulomatous ulcerative jejunoileitis with hypogammaglobulinemia. *Gastroenterology*, 62:473–477, 1972.
87. Karz, S., Guth, P. H., and Polonsky, L.: Chronic ulcerative jejunoileitis. *Amer. J. Gastroenterology*, 56:61–67, 1971.
88. Jeffries, G. H., Steinberg, H., and Sleisenger, M. H.: Chronic ulcerative (nongranulomatous) jejunitis. *Amer. J. Med.*, 44:47–59, 1968.
89. Aubrey, D. A.: Stenosing jejunitis. *Brit. J. Surg.*, 58:633–635, 1971.

23

Miscellaneous Lesions

INTERNAL HERNIAS*

Internal hernias of the congenital variety are rare lesions. They are the result of various defects which occur in the developing peritoneum and mesenteries. These potential fossae are enlarged as a portion of the developing small bowel elongates within them. The sacculation may contain a few loops or virtually the entire small intestine. In an unusual case, obstruction or strangulation may supervene. In isolated instances the small bowel may herniate into postsurgical or posttraumatic defects. The most frequent sites for congenital internal hernias are:

1. Duodenal-jejunal flexures (paraduodenal hernias)
2. Paracecal or ileocolic junction
3. Small bowel mesentery
4. Foramen of Winslow (lesser sac hernias)
5. Broad ligament (pelvic hernias)
6. Sigmoid mesentery

Paraduodenal hernias outnumber the other types of internal hernias taken together, as seen clinically or at autopsy. These hernias result from a failure of the mesentery to fuse with the parietal peritoneum at the ligament of Treitz. Thus they are also known as mesentericoparietal hernias. Two types occur, either left or right, depending on the relationship to the duodenum as it emerges from its retroperitoneal position, and the direction in which the opening of the fossa faces (Fig. 23-1). Left hernias occur three times more frequently than right hernias.

The preoperative diagnosis depends on the recognition of characteristic changes produced in intestinal pattern seen on small bowel series. The principal finding is that of displaced, bunched loops of small bowel which appear to be contained within a sac (Figs. 23-2 through 23-4). Afferent and efferent loops may

(*Text continued on page 545.*)

*Courtesy of Dr. Robert J. Blahut, Burlingame, California.

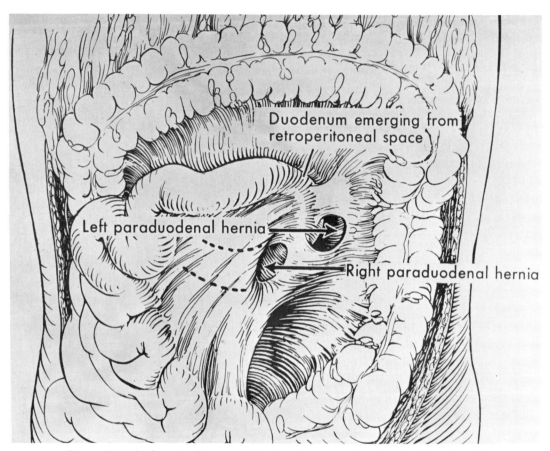

Figure 23-1 *Schematic diagram of the development of paraduodenal hernias. (Figures 23-1 through 23-4, courtesy Dr. Robert J. Blahut, Burlingame, California.)

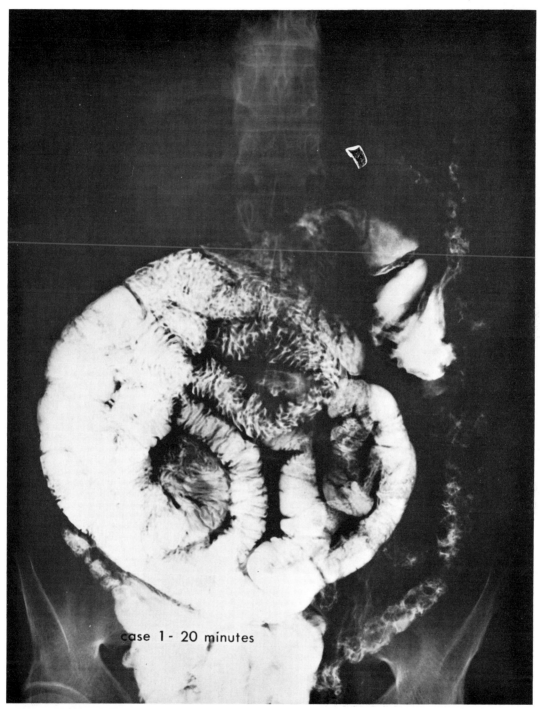

Figure 23-2 *Right paraduodenal hernia.* The small bowel is contained within an oval sac and the stomach is displaced to the left. Nonrotation of the colon is present, but the large bowel is shown to the left of the mass on this film.

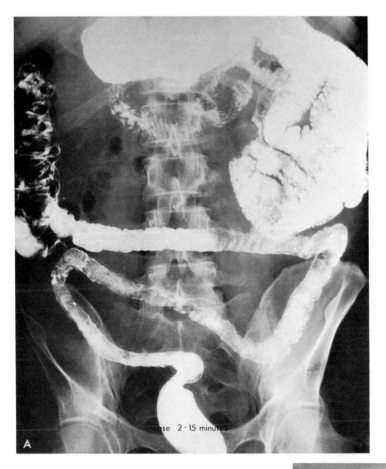

Figure 23-3 **A,** *Left paraduodenal hernia* containing most of the small bowel. In this patient a barium enema preceded the small bowel study, and on this 15 minute film residual barium is present in the colon.

Figure 23-3 *B,* In the same patient, the transverse colon is obviously depressed. At 3½ hours the entire small bowel is revealed and there is a straight line demarcation of the hernia sac where it impinges on the transverse colon. The stomach is elevated and displaced to the right.

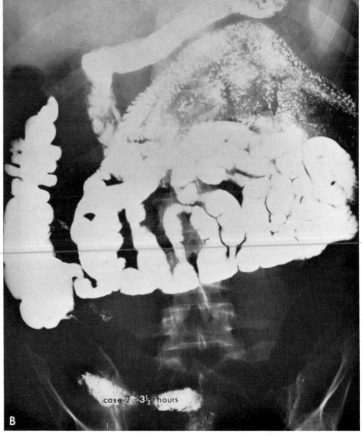

be present. If all, or virtually all, of the small intestine is encapsulated, no loops will be seen to project into the pelvis. If partial obstruction is present, dilatation and delay in transit may be recognized (Fig. 23-4).

Certain features can be utilized to distinguish left and right paraduodenal hernias. These features depend upon the relationship of the hernia mass to the stomach and colon. The colon is generally situated anterior to the left hernia, but in certain instances may be depressed inferiorly by the mass. The stomach sits high over the sac and may be pushed to the right. A right hernia displaces the stomach to the left. Malrotation of the colon frequently accompanies a right lesion, and in such an instance the ascending colon appears displaced to the left.

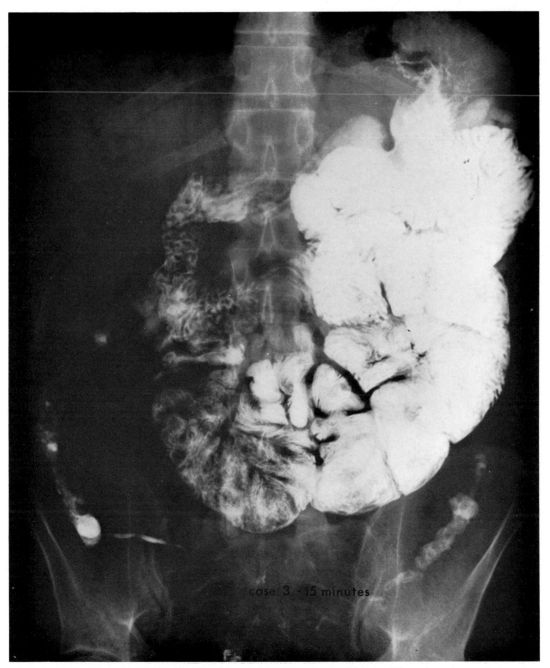

Figure 23-4 *Left paraduodenal hernia* containing most of the small bowel. No loops project over the pelvis and the lobulated sac contour persists on serial films. The bowel loops within the hernia are dilated. This patient had a history indicative of recurrent partial obstruction.

SPIGELIAN HERNIA

A Spigelian hernia is a spontaneous defect of the abdominal wall arising lateral to the rectus muscle. The protrusion passes through the Spigelian line (linea semilunaris). This line may be located on physical examination as a curved tendinous line just lateral to the outer border of the rectus abdominis muscle from the tip of the ninth costal cartilage to the pubic spine. It is formed by the aponeurosis of the internal oblique at the point of its division to enclose the rectus muscle. Posteriorly the linea semilunaris is reenforced in the upper three quarters of its length by the transversus abdominus. As more and more of the fibers of the transversus abdominus join the anterior sheath, the posterior sheath becomes thinner and thinner, and finally it ends midway between navel and pubis as a thin, curved line, the semi-circular line of Douglas. The latter marks an anatomic transition point below which all of the aponeurotic layers of the abdominal muscles pass anterior to the rectus.

The hernial orifice may be placed anywhere along the length of the semi-lunar line. The usual position is at the outer edge of the rectus muscle at the level of the line of Douglas. The hernia may enlarge intramurally deep to the external oblique to form the so-called "masked hernia," then continue to dissect laterally to appear most prominently in the region of the anterior-superior iliac spine. Later the hernia may penetrate the external oblique and appear sub-

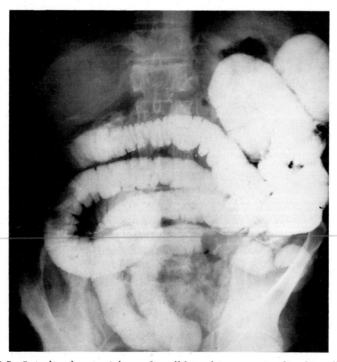

Figure 23-5 *Spigelian hernia.* A loop of small bowel is seen extending laterally into a hernial sac in the left lower quadrant. (Courtesy of Dr. Peter Som, New York City.)

cutaneously. The term Spigelian hernia thus excludes midline, epigastric, umbilical, traumatic, or postoperative herniations of the abdominal wall.

The roentgen findings in each case of Spigelian hernia will depend upon the specific contents and location of the hernial sac. The pertinent radiographic findings (Figs. 23-5 and 23-6) include air- or contrast-filled bowel seen laterally outside the confines of the peritoneal cavity, a sharp constriction of the herniated loop, and the intermittent nature of the hernia.

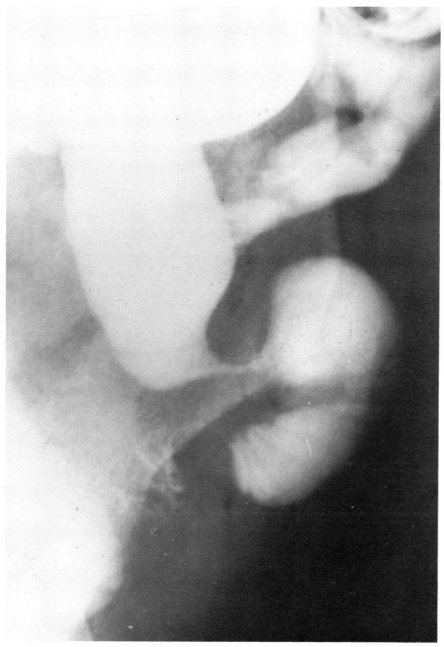

Figure 23-6 *Spigelian hernia.* Same patient as in Figure 23-5, magnified oblique view. There is narrowing of the herniated loop of bowel at the entrance and exit to the sac.

COMMON MESENTERY

In this condition the cecum and ascending colon fail to rotate into the right side of the abdomen and remain in the midline, sharing a mesentery with the small bowel. Because of the long mesentery, volvulus of the small bowel or cecum may occur. If the small bowel is not visualized during a barium enema examination, and the cecum is not identified, a mistaken diagnosis of colonic obstruction may be made (Fig. 23-7). In association with this condition, abnormal peritoneal bands are frequently present, producing obstruction, especially at the ligament of Treitz.

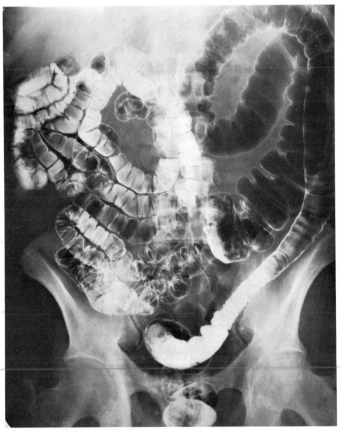

Figure 23-7 Common mesentery. The cecum is visualized to the left of the midline, and the small bowel occupies the right side of the abdomen. The patient had no complaints referable to this finding.

RADIATION ENTERITIS

Following irradiation, especially to the pelvic organs, damage to the small intestine and colon may occur. The effects are similar to those of ischemia. There is a selective destruction of the coats of the bowel, of which the mucosa is the most sensitive. Edema, ulceration, and stenosis are the usual sequelae.

Microscopically, necrosis of the smooth muscle and arteries is observed as well as ulceration of the mucosa.

The roentgen findings reflect the pathological changes and depend upon the stage of evolution of the lesion. Without a history, differential diagnosis from ischemia and regional enteritis may be difficult (Figs. 23-8, and 14-79).

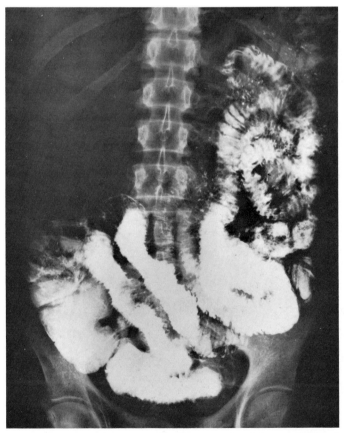

Figure 23-8 Radiation enteritis. The distal two-thirds of the small bowel is moderately rigid and fixed. The folds are hazy, thickened, and edematous. At this stage no strictures are identified.

CRONKHITE-CANADA SYNDROME[2, 3]

Extensive polyposis of many portions of the gastrointestinal tract is rare. When this entity is associated with malabsorption and ectodermal changes, the eponym Cronkhite-Canada Syndrome is applied. The ectodermal changes consist of alopecia, nail atrophy, and hyperpigmentation. Intestinal features include malabsorption, severe diarrhea, and protein loss.

Pathological findings, which are variable, include benign polyps, hypertrophic folds in stomach and colon, and either villous atrophy or thickened folds in the small bowel. On microscopic examination, cyst-like dilatation of the glands, as is seen in Menetrier's disease, is common.

On roentgen examination polypoid lesions are seen distributed throughout the gastrointestinal tract. These are most prominent in the stomach and colon. They can also be recognized in the small bowel as tiny punctate eminences.

The etiology of the syndrome is obscure. The ectodermal changes appear to be unrelated to malabsorption (Figs. 23-9 to 23-11).

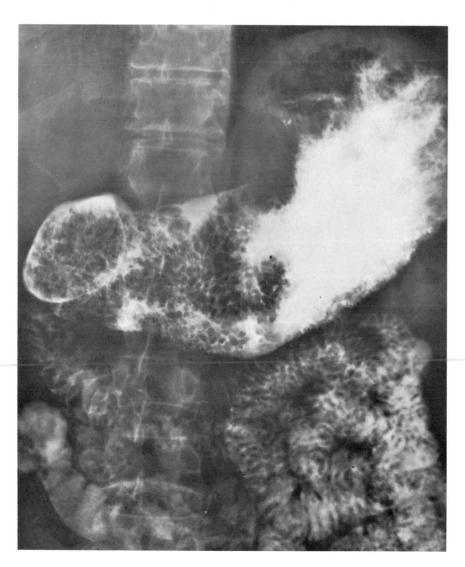

Figure 23-9 Cronkhite-Canada syndrome. Diffuse polyposis involving the entire stomach and duodenal bulb. These lesions disappeared on followup examinations.

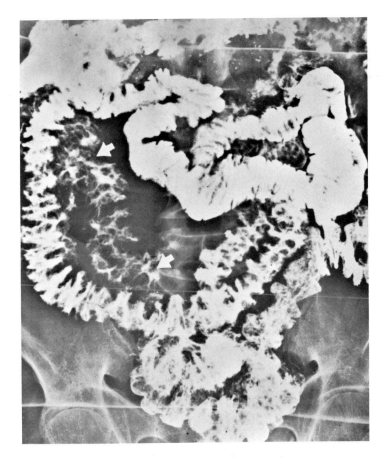

Figure 23-10   Same patient as in Figure 23-7. The folds throughout most of the small bowel are thickened. Tiny radiolucent areas are seen distributed throughout the small intestine. These changes were secondary to hyperplasia of the mucosa.

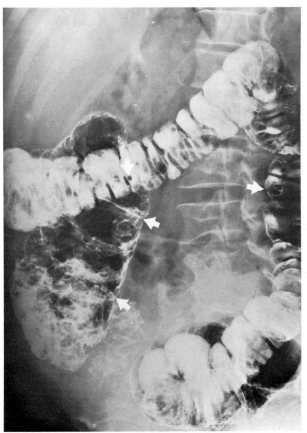

Figure 23-11   Same patient as in Figure 23-7. Numerous polypoid lesions are seen distributed throughout the entire colon. The possibility that there are other lesions in the intestinal tract should always be kept in mind when multiple polyps are seen in the colon.

ENTEROLITHS AND BEZOARS

Most enteroliths are found in patients who have chronic obstruction of the bowel, such as regional enteritis. They may also be found in areas of stasis, such as a Meckel's diverticulum or a blind loop (Fig. 16-35). One of the most frequent types of enteroliths is the ingested prune pit. This has a characteristic configuration with pointed ends and radiolucent center (Figs. 23-12 to 23-15). When a solid material such as a fruit pit remains in the bowel lumen, calcium is added and the foreign body becomes radiopaque (Fig. 23-14). The enterolith may produce ulceration and stenosis (Fig. 23-13), and may be a cause for small bowel obstruction. Occasionally a very large pit is swallowed (Fig. 23-16). Bezoars in the small intestine are uncommon (Figs. 23-17 to 23-19). They are most frequently encountered in patients who have had gastric resections and are edentulous. Repeated episodes of bezoar formation may occur.

(*Text continued on page 558.*)

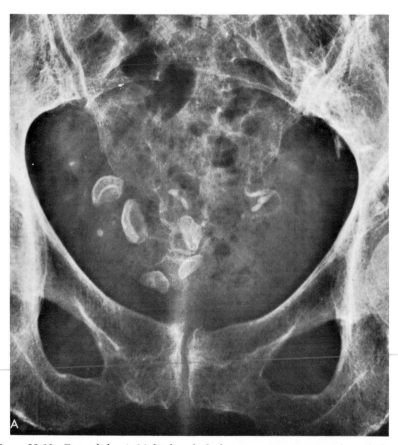

Figure 23-12   Enteroliths. A, Multiple calcified prune pits are seen in the right lower quadrant in a patient with obstructive regional enteritis.

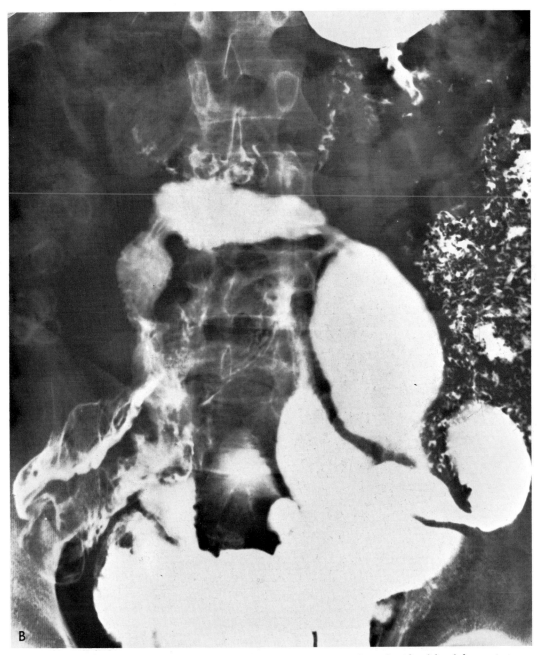

Figure 23-12 Continued *B*, Multiple prune pits are seen in the right side of the abdomen in a patient with regional enteritis. Barium has not yet reached the area of small bowel containing the pits.

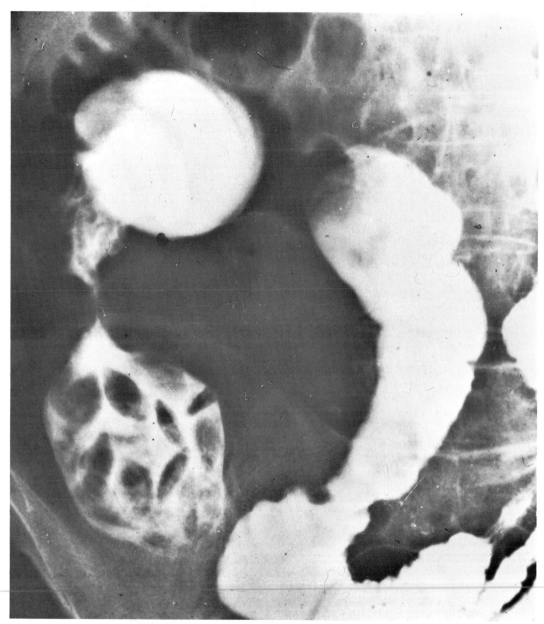

Figure 23-13 Intestinal stenosis produced by multiple prune pits. Note the characteristic configuration of the ingested prune pit with tapering pointed ends and a radiolucent, striated center. In this case there was no other cause for the obstruction except the prune pits.

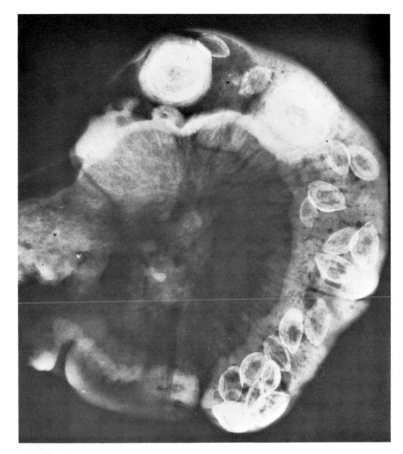

Figure 23-14 Same patient as in Figure 23-13. Photograph of removed specimen. Some of the prune pits are coated with a considerable amount of calcium, producing an appearance suggesting biliary calculi.

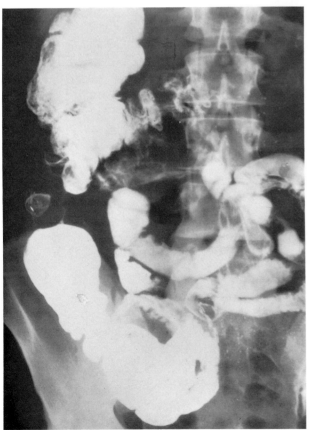

Figure 23-15 *Ileocolitis with obstruction.* The prune pit is seen lateral to the cecal tip.

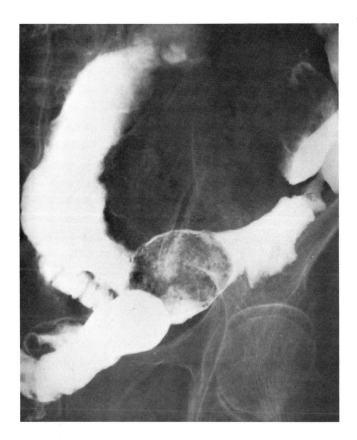

Figure 23-16 This foreign body was the result of an apricot pit.

Figure 23-17 A large bezoar resulting from persimmon seeds is noted in the mid ileum. The mottled appearance of the barium is characteristic of a bezoar.

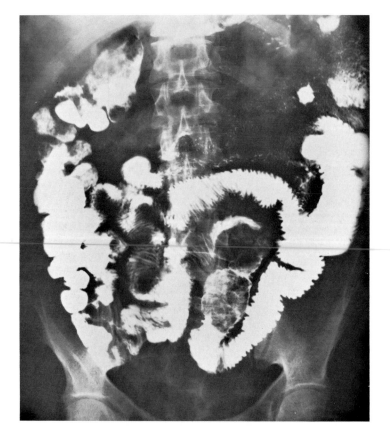

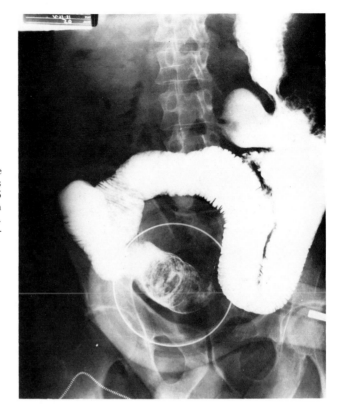

Figure 23-18   Small bowel bezoar. Inspissated vegetable material. This 72 year old man had a gastroenterostomy 25 years before this examination for duodenal ulcer. A circular defect 5 cm. in diameter with numerous overlying flecks of barium is seen in the mid-jejunum. The proximal jejunum is moderately dilated. Minimal intussusception is identified at the site of the obstructing lesion. No barium is seen distal to the defect.

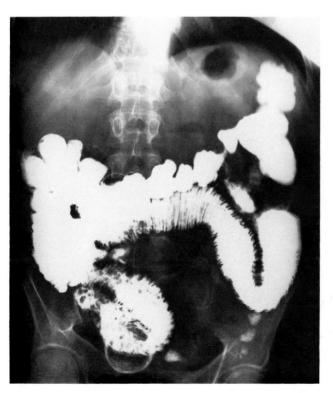

Figure 23-19   Small bowel bezoar. Same patient as Figure 23-18. The defect is again identified. Barium has entered the ileum and colon. At laparotomy the lesion was found to be due to inspissated vegetable matter. Small bowel bezoars are more commonly seen in edentulous and post-gastrojejunostomy patients. They are frequently recurrent. This was the second episode of obstruction in this patient.

GALLSTONE ILEUS

Mechanical obstruction of the intestinal tract by gallstones has been termed gallstone ileus. Often the episode is an acute surgical emergency and only plain films of the abdomen are obtained. Occasionally the obstruction is less dramatic and the cause not obvious, so contrast studies of the bowel are performed (Fig 23-20).

The responsible stone originates in the gallbladder or the duct system and ordinarily enters the bowel by creating a fistula from the biliary tree to adjacent duodenum, colon, or stomach. Usually the offending stone is solitary and rather large, perhaps 2 to 5 cm. in diameter. If the stone enters the gut distal to the pylorus (or having entered the stomach passes through the pylorus) it tends to traverse the small bowel until it becomes impacted in the narrowest portion, the terminal ileum, which is the most common site of gallstone obstruction. In at least half the patients with biliary fistula the stone does not obstruct at all and passes spontaneously from the rectum, and stones which enter the colon directly from the biliary tree do not obstruct.

The clinical features of gallstone ileus are those of distal small bowel obstruction. The great majority of patients are women and are elderly. Only one-half to two-thirds of patients have definite pre-existing symptoms referable to the gallbladder, and symptoms of acute cholecystitis preceding development of ileus are uncommon.

A correct preoperative diagnosis of gallstone ileus can often be made on the basis of radiological criteria: intestinal obstruction with air usually but not

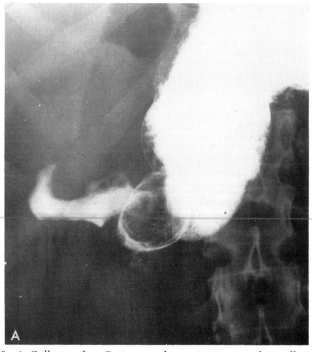

Figure 23-20   A, Gallstone ileus. Barium meal examination reveals an elliptical, smooth filling defect measuring 3 × 4 cm. in the antrum of the stomach. The patient is a 65 year old woman who underwent this study for poorly defined crampy abdominal pain of several months' duration. A broad amorphous patch of barium, not corresponding to the lumen of the intestinal tract, is seen distal to the defect, but the bulb and sweep could not be visualized.

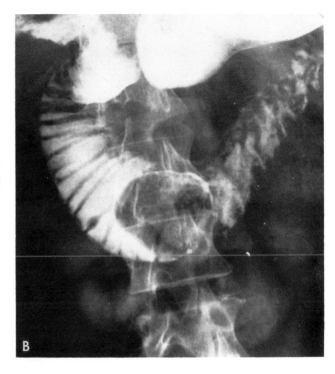

Figure 23-20 Continued B, Gallstone ileus. Same patient as in Figure 23-20A, four hours later. The filling defect is seen in the third portion of the duodenum. A large tract of barium extends laterally from the bulb; this corresponds to the patch of barium seen distal to the filling defect in Figure 23-20A. Migration of a gallstone has been observed from stomach to duodenum during this four hour period.

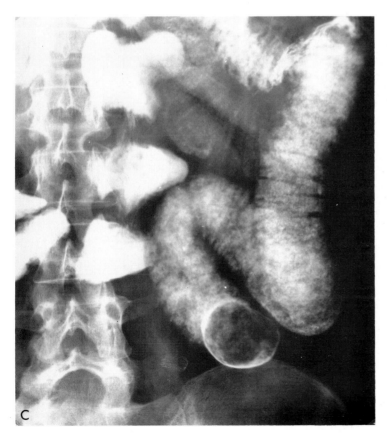

Figure 23-20 C, Gallstone ileus. Same patient as in Figure 23-20A, re-examination the next day. The gallstone is now in mid-jejunum. The stone did not pass spontaneously and at laparotomy a simple lithotomy was performed.

invariably present in the biliary tree; direct or indirect (when contrast studies are feasible) visualization of a stone in the intestine; or change in position of a previously observed gallstone.

Only rarely will a gallstone pass spontaneously once ileus is established, and treatment therefore must be surgical. The usual operation is simple lithotomy, but if the stone is impacted in an inflammatory mass segmental resection of bowel may be required. Chronic gallbladder disease remains after operation, however, to cause subsequent biliary symptoms or recurrent gallstone ileus. Rarely cholangitis may develop via the fistula. Cholecystectomy and closure of the fistula are usually recommended for consideration, either at the time of initial operation or electively thereafter.

CHICKEN POX

Demonstrable involvement of the intestinal tract with viral disease is rare. We have seen one case in which the patient had leukemia and sepsis, and the disease ran a rapid, fatal course. He had no rash. During the illness the patient experienced a severe hemorrhage. X-ray studies revealed multiple small nodules in the stomach and small intestine (Figs. 23-21 to 23-26). Histological examination demonstrated the lesions of varicella. (Case included courtesy of Dr. M. Khilnani, Mt. Sinai Hospital, New York, New York.)

(*Text continued on page 564.*)

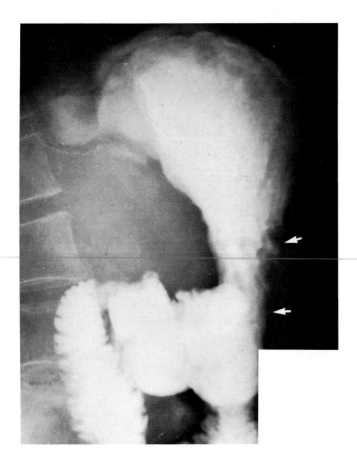

Figure 23-21 Chicken pox in the stomach. Multiple small nodules due to edema, hemorrhage and ulceration are seen in the medial third of the stomach.

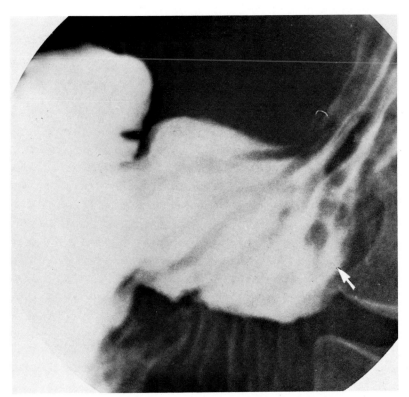

Figure 23-22   Magnified view of Figure 23-21.

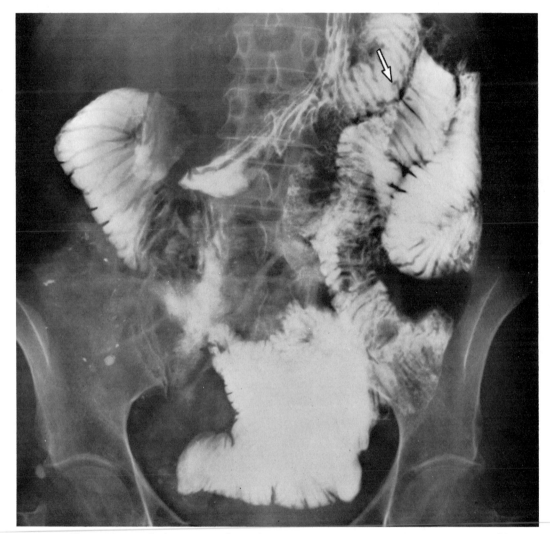

Figure 23-23   *Chicken pox involving the intestine.* Multiple small filling defects caused by edema, ulceration, and hemorrhage are seen in the small bowel.

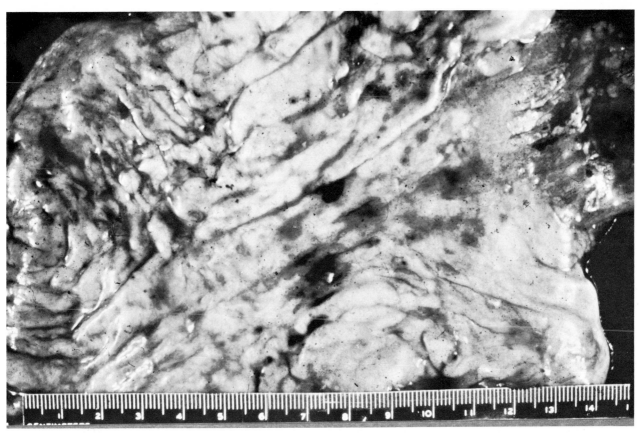

Figure 23-24 *Chicken pox involving the intestine.* Specimen of small bowel obtained at autopsy. Multiple areas of ulceration and hemorrhage are identified.

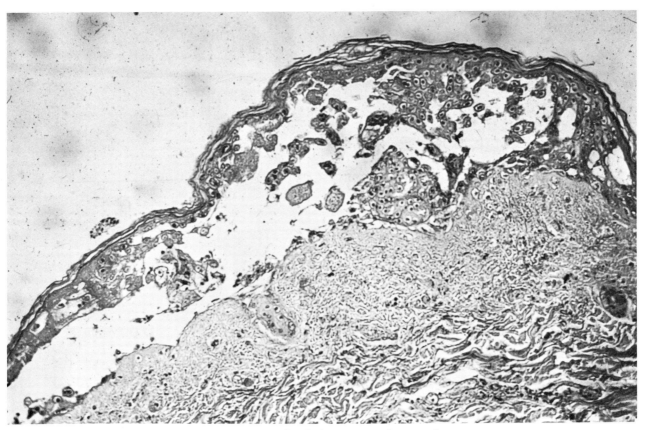

Figure 23-25 The chicken pox vesicle is noted.

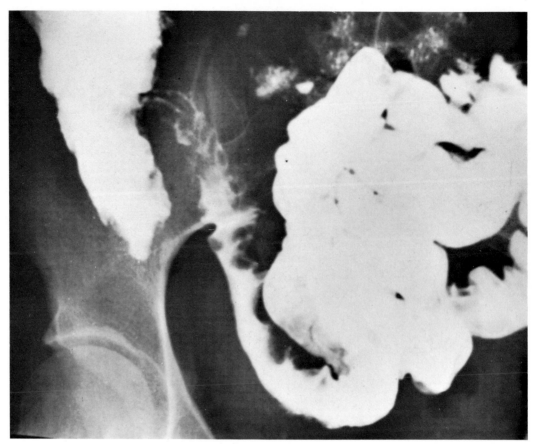

Figure 23-26   *Tuberculosis of small bowel.* A diagnosis of regional enteritis was made in this case. At surgery the findings were found to be the result of tuberculosis.

TUBERCULOSIS[4]

We have not included a separate chapter on intestinal tuberculosis because the disease entity is rare today in the United States and in our own experience. It is difficult, even impossible, to distinguish intestinal tuberculosis from regional enteritis radiologically (Figs. 23-26 and 14-78). Tuberculous peritonitis should be suggested whenever there is ascites with dilated partially obstructed loops of small bowel, angulation, and kinking of the small intestines. As a rule, in tuberculosis there is deeper ulceration, more irregular scarring, and marked stricture formation. Severe deformity of the ileocecal valve and involvement of the cecum and ascending colon are common.

INFLAMMATORY LESIONS OF THE SMALL BOWEL SECONDARY TO COLONIC DIVERTICULITIS[5]

Inflammatory changes in the small bowel secondary to colonic diverticulitis are probably more frequent than is realized (Figs. 23-27 to 23-29). In most of these cases the small bowel is not examined radiographically, and therefore the inflammatory process is not found. Because of the pericolonic inflamma-

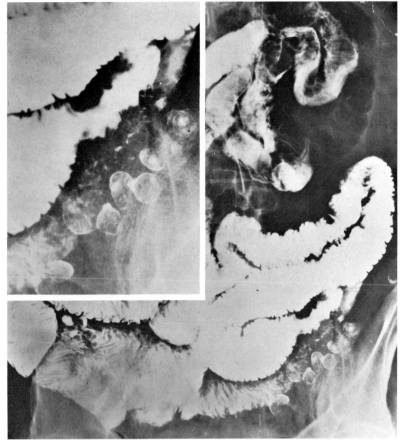

Figure 23-27 *Small bowel inflammation associated with colonic diverticulitis.* Adjacent to the diverticula is seen a segment of jejunum which is fixed in position and shows narrowing and rigidity of the lumen and thickening of the mucosal folds.

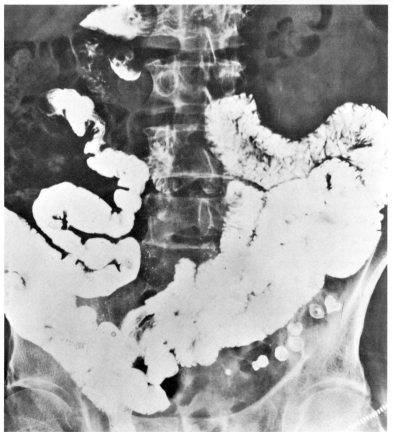

Figure 23-28 Same patient as in Figure 23-27, two weeks later, after antibiotic therapy. The inflammatory process has resolved and the small intestine appears normal.

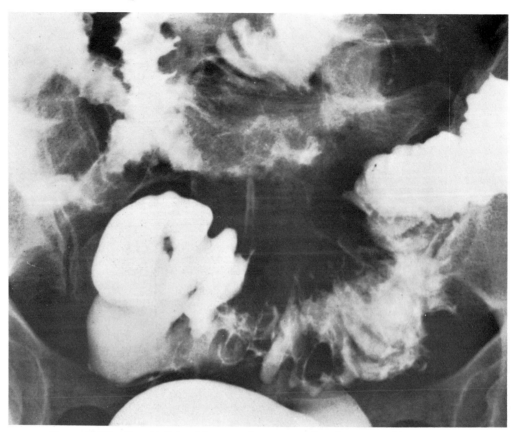

Figure 23-29 *Diverticulitis with a pericolonic mass.* The adjacent small bowel shows spasm, irritability, and thickening and edema of the folds.

tion, however, alterations of the small bowel may be seen which can be confused with intrinsic disease in the small intestine. It should be noted that the formation of a fistula from the colon to the small bowel in diverticulitis is extremely rare. When this occurs the possibility that the diverticulitis is actually granulomatous colitis should be considered.

ILEAL DIVERTICULITIS[6]

Most diverticula of the small bowel are confined to the jejunum. Occasionally only the terminal ileum is affected (Fig. 23-30). Most of these diverticula lie near the ileocecal valve and are located more distal than a Meckel's diverticulum. Acute diverticulitis can occur. The symptoms are generally those of acute appendicitis. Initially only a mass may be identified. With resolution of the process the orifice of the diverticulum may open and subsequently be visualized.

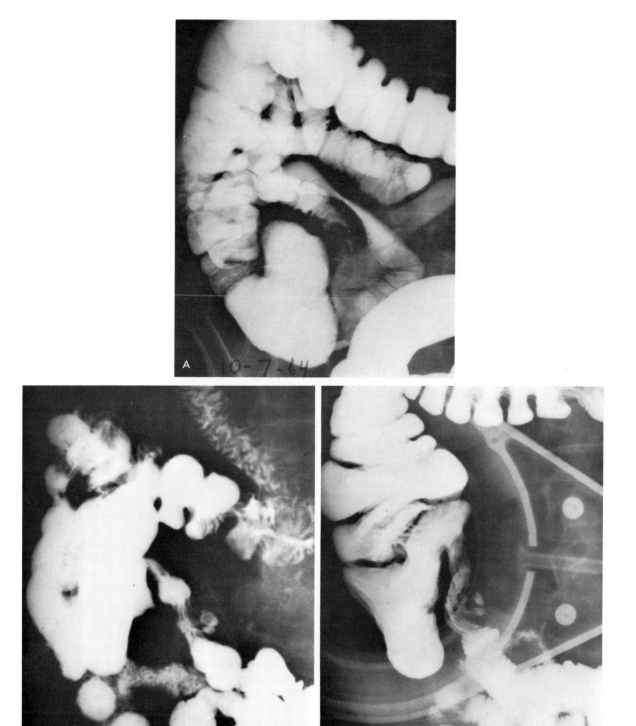

Figure 23-30 A, An extrinsic pressure defect is identified in the region of the terminal ileum. *B* and *C*, Two months later there is minimal extrinsic pressure. At this time two diverticula are identified in this region. (Courtesy of Dr. W. B. Miller and Dr. B. Felson, University of Cincinnati, Cincinnati, Ohio.)

INVERTED DUODENAL DIVERTICULUM

This diverticulum usually originates in the descending duodenum and hangs as a sac-like structure within the duodenal loop. Rarely it extends into the proximal small bowel. A clear zone, which has been called the "comma sign," corresponds to the wall of the diverticulum (Fig. 23-31).

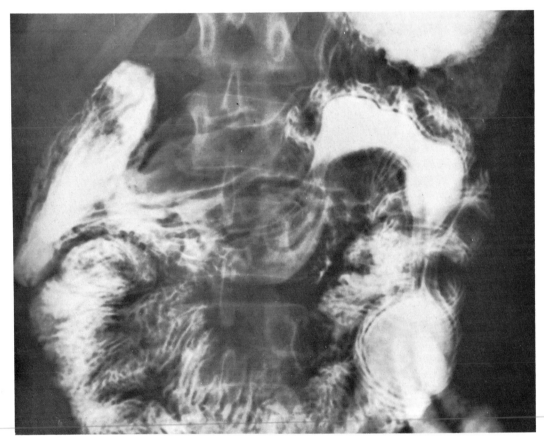

Figure 23-31 Inverted intraluminal duodenal diverticulum, extending into the proximal jejunum. (Courtesy of Dr. James Martin, Bowman-Gray School of Medicine, Winston-Salem, North Carolina.)

CYSTS AND TUMORS OF THE MESENTERY[7]

Mesenteric tumors may be cystic or solid. Many of the solid tumors arise in the intestinal tract, slough, and are mistaken for primary mesenteric tumors. Cysts are more common and can be found in any portion of the mesentery. They are usually benign. The roentgen findings depend on the size of the tumor mass. In most cases they displace the small bowel in a smooth, even fashion, producing a space-occupying mass of variable size (Figs. 23-32 to 23-35). Rarely such lesions as dermoids and desmoids may be seen. Calcification is seldom present.

(*Text continued on page 573.*)

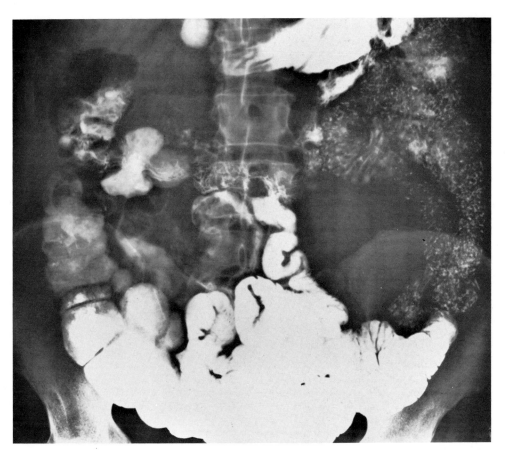

Figure 23-32   A mesenteric cyst is seen in the midportion of the left abdomen, displacing the loops of small bowel.

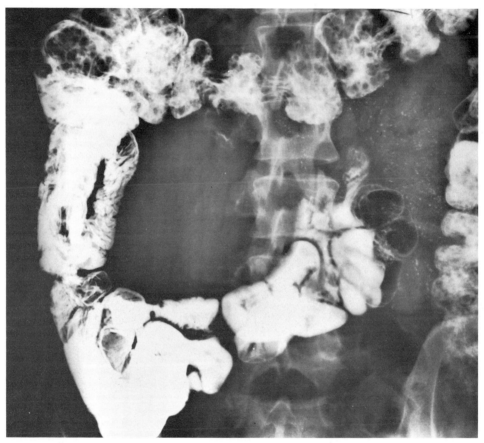

Figure 23-33 *Desmoid tumor of the mesentery.* This is a 29 year old woman who had multiple intestinal polyposis. A large desmoid tumor was removed two years previously. This examination revealed a recurrence of the mass.

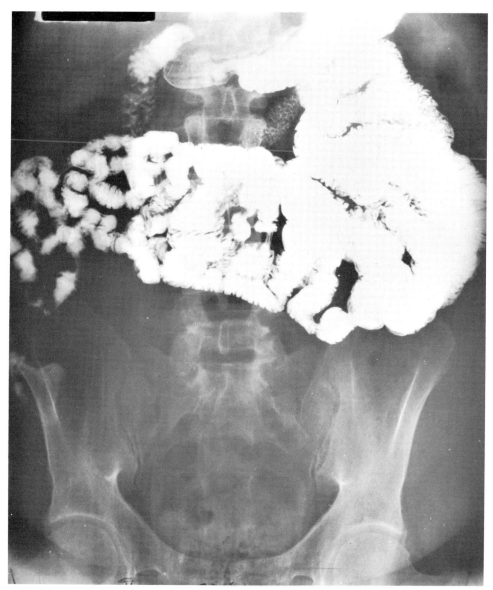

Figure 23-34 Lipoma of the mesentery. A large mass in the lower abdomen displaces the small bowel superiorly. This was a 40 year old male who weighed 275 pounds. The pendulous abdomen is noted.

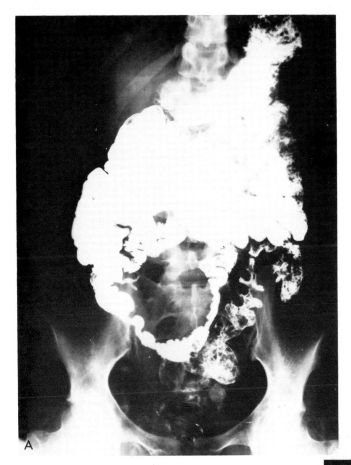

Figure 23-35 A, *Pelvic kidney simulating mesenteric tumor.* There is a well-circumscribed mass in the right lower quadrant displacing adjacent loops of small intestine. The mass causes extreme pressure on the bowel but there is no intrinsic involvement of the gut. The location of the mass suggested the possibility of a pelvic kidney.

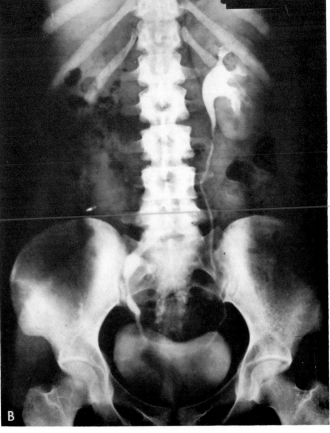

Figure 23-35 B, *Intravenous pyelogram.* Same patient as Figure 23-35A. A small ectopic kidney at the pelvic brim is seen to be the mass noted on small bowel examination.

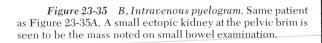

PNEUMATOSIS CYSTOIDES INTESTINALIS[8]

Pneumatosis cystoides intestinalis is an uncommon condition characterized by the presence of multiple gas cysts in segments of the small bowel. It has also been identified in the colon. This condition is usually found in association with other diseases such as mesenteric occlusion, scleroderma, Whipple's disease, and other diarrheal states. Many of the patients have an associated lung condition such as interstitial fibrosis, emphysema, or pneumothorax. The symptoms are nonspecific. They are usually those of the primary disease. Partial intestinal obstruction can be seen.

The roentgen findings are fairly typical and consist of radiolucent areas which follow the contour of the bowel (Fig. 23-36). The gas cysts may protrude into the bowel lumen and at times can be identified in the mesentery. The exact cause of these cysts is not determined. The cysts may disappear spontaneously or persist for prolonged periods of time. In most cases no treatment is available or necessary.

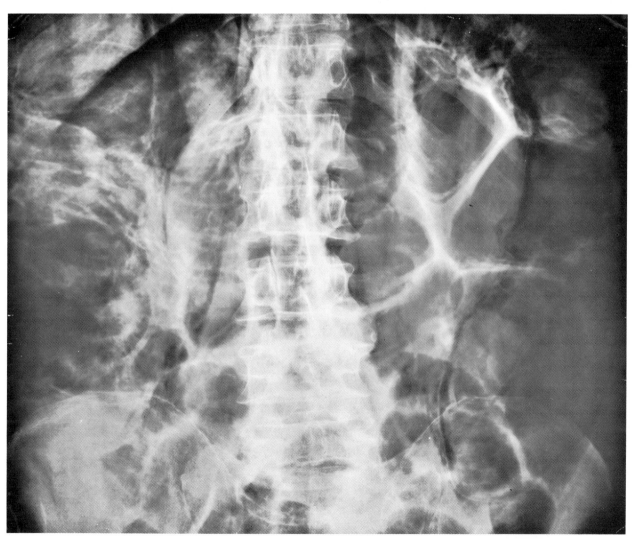

Figure 23-36 Transient pneumatosis intestinalis involving terminal ileum and colon in a patient with Whipple's disease. Death occurred four years later with no intramural gas found at autopsy. Roentgenogram of entire abdomen shows not only intramural gas but also gas in the retroperitoneal area outlining the right kidney. (Courtesy of Dr. W. Seaman, Presbyterian Hospital, New York, New York.)

INTESTINAL PSEUDO-OBSTRUCTION

Apparent chronic mechanical obstruction of the bowel may occasionally occur in clinical situations in which true obstruction cannot be demonstrated. Patients present with abdominal distention, cramps, and hyperactive bowel sounds. Diagnostic studies, even to laparotomy, fail to reveal an obstructing lesion and the entity has been termed pseudo-obstruction.[9] It may occur with infiltrative disease of the bowel wall, such as amyloidosis,[10] in scleroderma, in such neurological diseases as familial autonomic dysfunction, and in myxedema.[11] In some cases the cause cannot be established and the disease must be classified as idiopathic. Treatment is directed to the underlying disease, if it can be identified, and to general supportive measures.

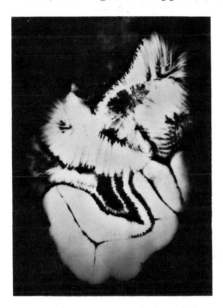

Figure 23-37 *Idiopathic pseudo-obstruction.* This 65 year old woman had clinical findings of intestinal obstruction with no known systemic disease. There is moderate dilatation of most of the small bowel. The collapsed loops of proximal ileum became dilated when the patient was placed in a supine position and do not represent areas of constriction. The terminal ileum is normal. No persistent areas of narrowing were seen in the roentgen examination. At laparotomy, moderate dilatation of the intestine was found, and the bowel was edematous but no obstucting lesion was present. No other intra-abdominal pathology could be identified. Full thickness biopsy of the small bowel was normal. A diagnosis of idiopathic pseudo-obstruction of the small bowel has been made.

References

1. Estrada, R.: Anomalies of Internal Rotation and Fixation. Springfield, Illinois, Charles C Thomas, 1958.
2. Jarnum, S., and Jensen, H.: Diffuse gastrointestinal polyposis with ectodermal change. A case of severe malabsorption and enteric loss of plasma proteins. *Gastroenterology*, 50:107-118, 1966.
3. Cronkhite, L. W., and Canada, W. J.: Generalized gastrointestinal polyposis. An unusual syndrome of polyposis, pigmentation, alopecia and onychotropia. *New Eng. J. Med.*, 252:1011-1015, 1955.
4. Brombart, M., and Massion, J.: Radiologic differences between ileocecal tuberculosis and Crohn's disease. I. Diagnosis of ileocecal tuberculosis. *Amer. J. Dig. Dis.*, 6:589, 1961.
5. Marshak, R. H., and Eliasoph, J.: Inflammatory lesions of the small bowel secondary to colonic diverticulitis. *Amer. J. Dig. Dis.*, 6:423-428, 1961.
6. Miller, W. B., and Felson, B.: Diverticulitis of the terminal ileum. *Amer. J. Roentgenol.*, 96:351-365, 1966.
7. Hardin, W. J., and Hardy, J. D.: Mesenteric cysts. *Amer. J. Surg.*, 119:640-645, 1970.
8. Seaman, W. B., Fleming, R. J., and Baker, D. H.: Pneumatosis intestinalis of the small bowel. *Seminars in Roentgenol.*, 1:234, 1966.
9. Moss, A. A.: Intestinal pseudo-obstruction. *Critical Reviews in Radiological Sciences*, 3:363-387, 1972.
10. Legge, D. A., Wollaeger, E. E., and Carlson, H. C.: Intestinal pseudo-obstruction in systemic amyloidosis. *Gut*, 11:764-767, 1970.
11. Abbasi, A. E., Douglass, R. C., Bissell, G. W., et al.: Myxedema ileus. A form of intestinal pseudo-obstruction. *J.A.M.A.*, 234:181-183, 1975.

24

Small Bowel Angiography

by STANLEY BAUM, M.D.

Detailed step-by-step description of the technique of selective mesenteric arteriography can be found in many standard angiographic textbooks[1,2] and is beyond the scope or purpose of this chapter. The examination is almost always performed under local rather than general anesthesia and unless there are specific contraindications, the femoral artery is used as the site of percutaneous puncture and catheter insertion. Selective catheterization of the celiac, superior, and inferior mesenteric arteries is accomplished by manipulation of the catheter under image intensification fluoroscopy. Following the selective catheterization of the mesenteric artery, contrast material is injected at a constant rate through the use of a pressure injector. In most cases, 40–50 cc. of contrast medium is injected at 5–8 cc. per second. This is followed by serial filming during the arterial, capillary, and venous phases. Most of the examinations are carried out with the patient in the supine anterior-posterior position, although on occasion oblique and lateral films are taken.

NORMAL ANGIOGRAPHIC ANATOMY

Arteries

The superior mesenteric artery (Fig. 24-1) is a ventral branch of the abdominal aorta arising 1 to 2 cm. below the celiac axis at the level of the body of L-1. The very proximal portion of the superior mesenteric runs caudally behind the pancreas. As it exits from the inferior border of the pancreatic neck, it enters

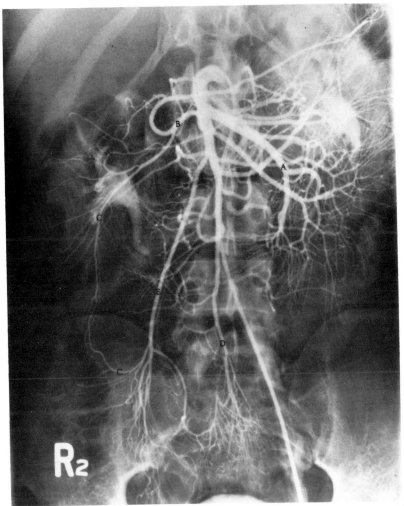

Figure 24-1 *Normal superior mesenteric arteriogram.* (A) Jejunal branches, (B) middle colic, (C) right colic, (D) ileal branches, (E) ileocolic branch.

the root of the mesentery, ventral to the fourth portion of the duodenum. In its course through the mesentery it gives rise to:

(A) Twelve or more jejunal and ileal branches. These vessels form communicating arcades that give origin to the vasa recta of the small bowel.

(B) Colic (middle and right) arteries. These anastomose with the left colic branch of the inferior mesenteric artery to form the arcade of Riolan or marginal anastomosis of Drummond.

(C) The inferior pancreaticoduodenal artery that anastomoses with the superior pancreaticoduodenal branch of the gastroduodenal artery. This anastomosis provides a major collateral route in occlusive disease of either celiac or superior mesenteric arteries.

Many variations occur in the arterial anatomy of the abdominal viscera. Since only about 50%[3] of people fit into the classic textbook description of a three-vessel celiac trunk, etc., it is important to be familiar with the commonly encountered anatomical variations[4] (Fig. 24-2), and if unusual patterns are encountered, one of the detailed anatomical source books[3] should be consulted.

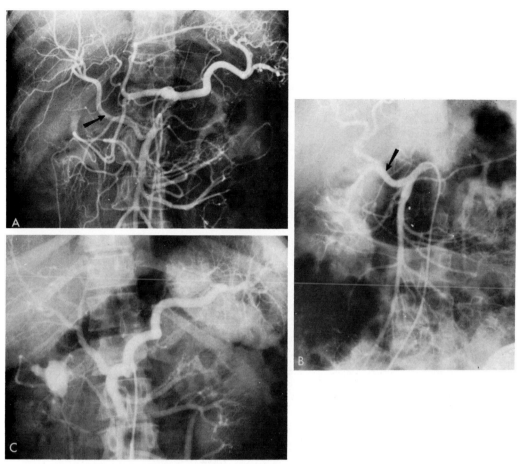

Figure 24-2 Variations of normal celiac and superior mesenteric artery anatomy. *A.* Contrast injected simultaneously into two catheters, one positioned in the celiac axis and the other in the superior mesenteric artery. The right hepatic artery takes origin from superior mesenteric artery (arrow). The celiac axis gives origin to the left and middle hepatic arteries. The gastroduodenal artery takes origin from the left hepatic artery. *B.* Superior mesenteric arteriography shows the entire hepatic artery originating from the superior mesenteric artery. The splenic and left gastric arteries have a common separate origin from the aorta. *C.* The superior mesenteric, hepatic, and splenic arteries originate from the aorta as a common celiaco-mesenteric trunk. The left gastric artery in the same patient came directly from the abdominal aorta.

Veins

All the veins of the gastrointestinal tract drain into the portal venous system. The superior mesenteric vein drains the entire jejunum, ileum, cecum, right colon, and part of the transverse colon. The remaining portion of the transverse, descending, and sigmoid colons drain via the inferior mesenteric vein, which enters the splenic vein to the left of the superior mesenteric vein. The portal vein is formed by the junction of the splenic and superior mesenteric veins.

Developmental Anomalies

Anomalies of fixation and rotation of the intestinal tract are generally not symptomatic. Malrotation of the gut may be discovered unexpectedly during exploratory laparotomy or as an incidental finding of a barium examination. When symptoms exist they are usually those of partial recurrent intestinal obstruction due to midgut volvulus which may or may not be associated with vascular occlusion. Although barium examination of the stomach and the small and large bowel is obviously the easiest way to establish a diagnosis, angiography can on occasion play an important role in demonstrating the presence of the volvulus with co-existing blood vessel traction. Buranasiri[5] has described a very coiled appearance of the superior mesenteric artery and vein that resembled a "barber pole" because of the rotation of the small intestines around the root of the mesentery (Fig. 24-3). The severity of the vascular compromise varies with the number of rotations and the degree of tightness of the mesenteric pedicle.

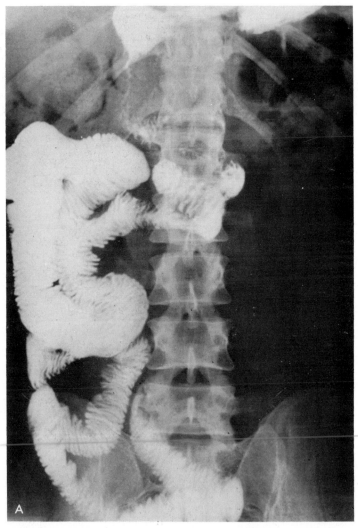

Figure 24-3   Midgut malrotation, with volvulus of the small bowel, in a 26 year old woman who has been complaining of intermittent severe abdominal pain since childhood. A. Upper gastro-intestinal study shows malrotation of the small intestines with the ligament of Treitz in the right side of the abdomen.

Figure 24–3 Continued B. Selective superior mesenteric arteriography during the arterial phase demonstrates marked twisting of the jejunal and ileal branches upon the ileocolic artery, giving the appearance of a "barber pole." There is narrowing of the proximal portion of the midjejunal artery (black arrow) that is probably caused by the volvulus itself. The middle and right colic arteries (open arrows) are in the upper and left portions of the abdomen. *C.* The venous phase of the superior mesenteric arteriogram demonstrates dilatation of the jejunal, ileal, and superior mesenteric veins. The veins themselves are being twisted around the root of the mesentery, presumably as a result of the volvulus. At surgical exploration a congenital band was found attaching the cecum to the left upper quadrant with rotation of the mesentery. This was released and the jejunum and ileum returned to their normal positions. *D.* Superior mesenteric arteriography postoperatively shows that the jejunal and ileal arteries had returned to normal position.

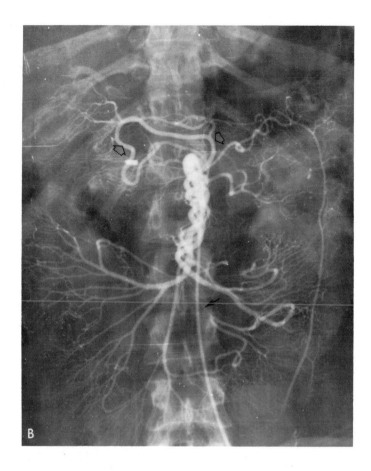

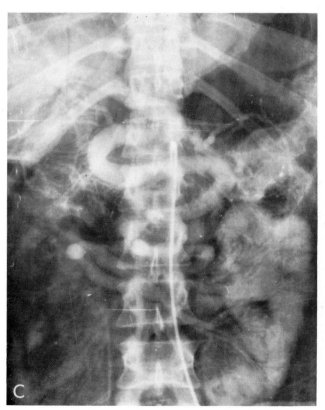

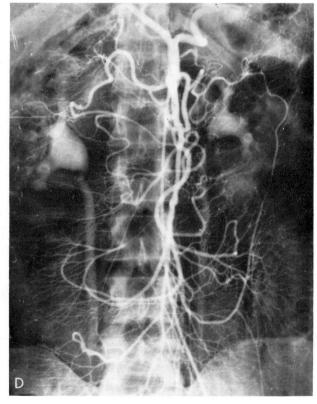

BLEEDING

There are at present only two clinically useful techniques that precisely identify the site of bleeding from the small bowel. One is visualizing the bleeding lesion by endoscopy and the other is demonstration of extravasated contrast material on selective angiography. In small bowel bleeding endoscopy is particularly useful in the proximal duodenum. If bleeding is massive, the endoscopic confirmation of the site of bleeding can be very difficult. Angiography, on the other hand, can identify bleeding lesions throughout the small bowel and the accuracy of the technique is enhanced rather than hindered by increases in bleeding rates. The intermittent nature of the gastrointestinal hemorrhage is the major shortcoming of selective angiography. Although arteriography is capable of showing arterial and/or capillary bleeding of as little as 0.5 ml. per minute,[6] it is necessary to have the patient actively bleeding at the time of the examination.

An outgrowth of the arteriographic diagnosis of gastrointestinal bleeding has been the use of the angiographic catheter as a vehicle for selectively infusing vasoconstricting drugs or selectively embolizing bleeding vessels in an attempt to control the hemorrhage once the diagnosis is established.[7, 8, 9] Because of this potential for therapy in the bleeding patient, selective angiography is performed in many patients even when the cause of bleeding is established by other techniques, such as endoscopy.

Bleeding Duodenal Diverticula

Bleeding from a diverticulum of the duodenum is rare. When severe bleeding does occur, about half the reported cases have involved diverticula arising from the third or fourth portions of the duodenum and are therefore easily detected by selective mesenteric arteriography (Fig. 24-4).

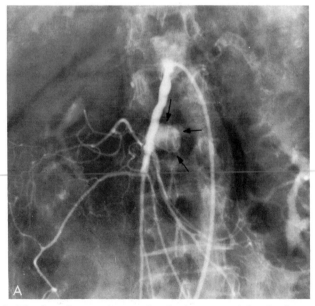

Figure 24-4   Bleeding diverticulum in the third portion of the duodenum in a 78-year-old woman with massive gastrointestinal bleeding. A. Arterial phase of a superior mesenteric arteriogram demonstrates extravasation of contrast material (arrows) from proximal branches of the superior mesenteric artery.

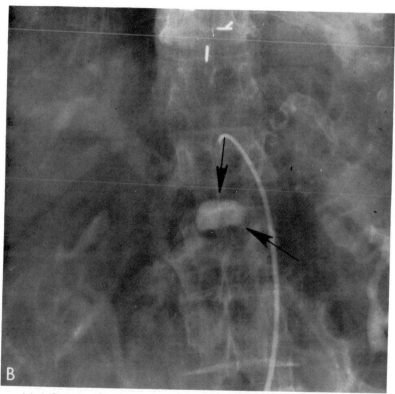

Figure 24-4 Continued *B.* Contrast material persists within a diverticulum in the third portion of the duodenum (arrows).

Anastomotic Ulcers

Bleeding from anastomotic ulcers following gastric surgery is difficult to diagnose. Barium studies and even endoscopy may be unsuccessful in diagnosing these lesions since they are so often shallow and hidden behind edematous gastric or jejunal folds. If they are actively bleeding, selective arteriography can demonstrate the site of extravasation, which is usually from a jejunal branch of the superior mesenteric artery (Fig. 24-5). These lesions can also be arteriographically controlled by the selective infusion of Pitressin.

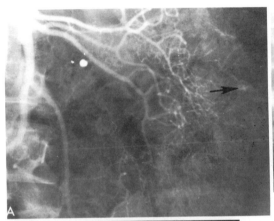
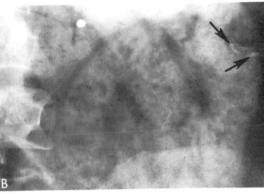
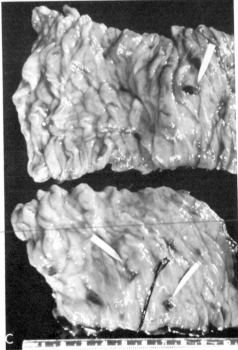

Figure 24-5 Bleeding from an anastomotic ulcer. This patient had undergone gastrectomy, left colectomy, and subsequently right colectomy for chronic gastrointestinal hemorrhage. He was admitted with a hematocrit of 19% and selective arteriography was performed to localize the site of bleeding. *A.* Arterial phase of a superior mesenteric arteriogram shows arterial extravasation in the proximal jejunum (arrow). *B.* Late phase of the superior mesenteric arteriogram demonstrates persistence of extravasation (arrows). The patient underwent surgery, and superficial ulcerations were found on the jejunal side of a gastrojejunostomy. *C.* Arrow points to superficial ulcerations in the resected specimen.

Meckel's Diverticulum

The three most common causes of gastrointestinal hemorrhage in infants and children are peptic ulcer disease, portal hypertension, and ulceration in a Meckel's diverticulum. If bleeding originates from a Meckel's diverticulum it is the result of ulceration secondary to acid secretions from the ectopic gastric mucosa, which is present in approximately one half of all cases. Without the preoperative use of angiography, the diagnosis of the bleeding site is difficult to localize with certainty. Angiography can be used to provide a specific diagnosis as to the site of the bleeding. Also, the extravasated contrast can on occasion fill the diverticulum (Fig. 24-6).

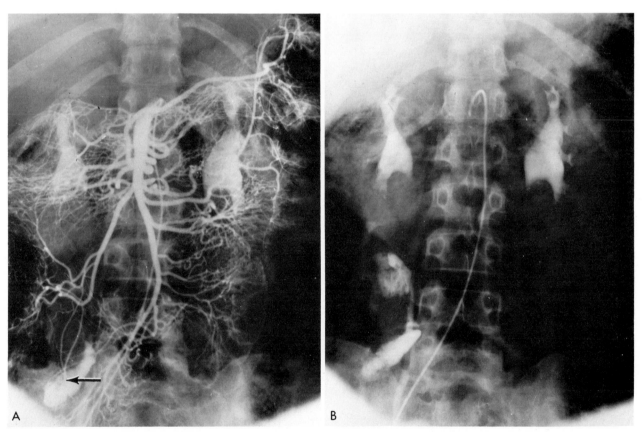

Figure 24-6 Angiographic demonstration of a bleeding Meckel's diverticulum. *A.* During the arterial phase of a selective superior mesenteric arteriogram extravasation is seen originating from a branch of the ileocolic artery (arrow). *B.* Fifteen seconds after the injection, contrast material remains within the bleeding Meckel's diverticulum. (This study is courtesy of Dr. M. Gyepes, UCLA Medical Center, Los Angeles, California.)

Ischemic Ileitis

As has been described in earlier sections of this text, disturbances of the arterial supply to the small bowel or colon may be responsible for a great variety of clinical and roentgenographic findings. Complete occlusion of major mesenteric vessels can result in complete necrosis of the bowel, with resulting peritonitis, shock, and death. At the other end of the spectrum are those patients who have minor occlusions and adequate collateral flow so that symptoms, if they do appear, are very mild. Between these two extremes all variations can be seen in which collateral flow is capable of preventing necrosis of the intestines, yet is not adequate enough to allow complete recovery. Mucosal ulcerations that occur secondary to the initial vascular occlusion occasionally are the cause of massive bleeding. Arteriography performed under these circumstances not only identifies the area that is bleeding but also provides a very accurate arterial road map of the site of occlusion and major sources of collateral flow (Fig. 24-7). If patients are going to have embolectomies or another type of reconstructive surgery of the mesenteric arteries, this preoperative information is obviously indispensible.

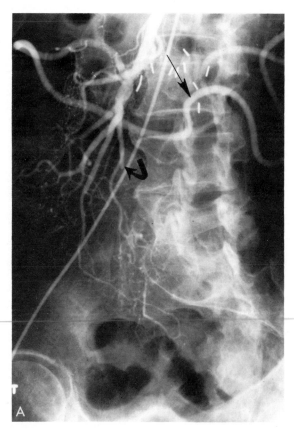

Figure 24-7   Bleeding mucosal ulcerations in the ileum secondary to ischemic ileitis. *A.* Selective superior mesenteric arteriography was performed on a 68-year-old man with lower gastrointestinal bleeding. The patient had a previous resection of an abdominal aortic aneurysm. Multiple occlusions are seen in jejunal branches (curved arrow) and the ileocolic artery cannot be identified. The middle colic–left colic anastomosis is large (straight arrow) since the abdominal aortic aneurysm had occluded the inferior mesenteric artery at its origin.

Figure 24-7 Continued B. A film taken late in the arterial phase of the mesenteric artery injection demonstrates extravasation of contrast material within one of the ileal loops (arrows) in that segment of bowel that is not being supplied by the ileocolic artery.

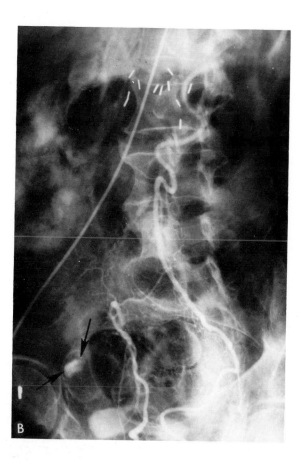

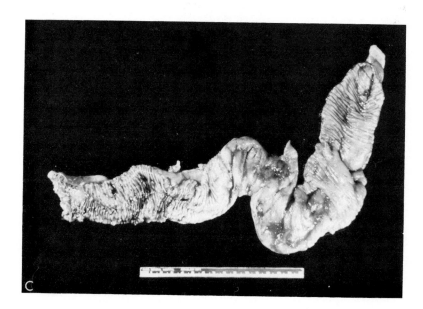

Figure 24-7 C. The resected specimen demonstrates an 8 to 10 cm. long segment of slightly narrowed and ulcerated portion of ileum. This was an area of segmental infarction on the basis of atheromatous occlusion of the ileocolic artery.

Hemorrhagic Telangiectasia

Intestinal telangiectasia as part of hereditary hemorrhagic telangiectasia is well recognized. If the disease is generalized, there is involvement of multiple systems and vascular lesions can be seen in the lips, oral cavity, genitourinary tract, lungs, brain, and other organs. Gastrointestinal lesions, however, can be the only manifestation of the disease (Fig. 24-8), and gastrointestinal hemorrhage may be frequent and very difficult to diagnose.

Although these lesions are referred to as arteriovenous malformations, the primary vascular abnormality is often at the capillary and venous level and therefore selective arteriography can be unrevealing. In most instances, the elastic lamina is absent and therefore angiectasis is a prominent feature. Because these vascular channels have very thin walls, bleeding occurs even after very minimal trauma. Vascular telangiectasia sometimes presents as a progressive disease and resection of one area of the bowel will not result in cure since other areas of the gastrointestinal tract may manifest the same changes months or years later (Fig. 24-9).

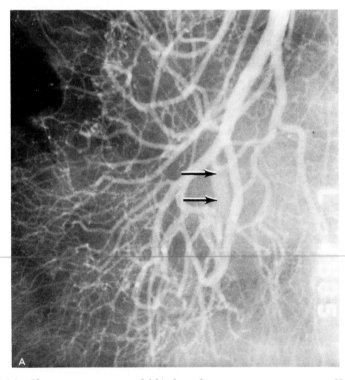

Figure 24-8 Chronic gastrointestinal bleeding due to an arteriovenous malformation of the small bowel. This patient had cutaneous and buccal mucosal changes of diffuse hereditary hemorrhagic telangiectasias. A. Selective superior mesenteric arteriogram demonstrates bleeding in an area corresponding anatomically with the distal ileum (arrows).

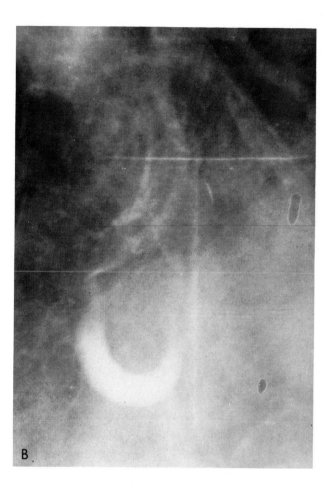

Figure 24-8 Continued   B. A film taken at the end of the serial filming demonstrates persistence of contrast material in the distal ileum.

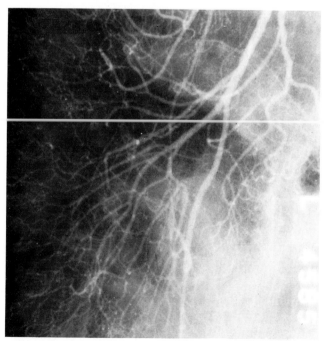

Figure 24-8   C. The selective superior arteriography during infusion of 0.2 units per minute of Pitressin demonstrates complete cessation of bleeding.

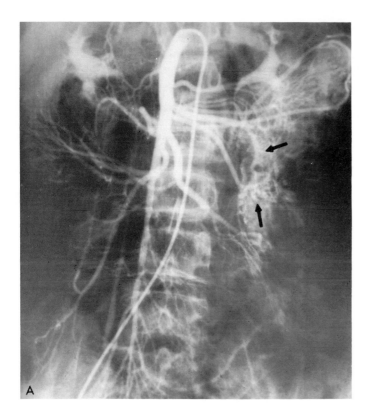

Figure 24-9 *Arteriovenous malformations of the small intestines.* This young adolescent girl had repeated episodes of massive upper gastrointestinal bleeding. Previous conventional barium studies of the stomach, duodenum, and small intestines were all negative. Exploratory laparotomy during one of the episodes of hemorrhage failed to disclose the site of bleeding. A. Selective superior mesenteric arteriography demonstrates marked dilatation of the vessels supplying the proximal jejunum (arrows). Early venous return was apparent in later films on the series. During the next episode of bleeding the patient was re-explored and 10 inches of jejunum were resected and an end-to-end anastomosis performed. Histologic sections of the resected specimen demonstrated marked dilatation of both the intramural arteries and veins consistent with an arteriovenous malformation.

Figure 24-9 *B.* Repeat superior mesenteric arteriography performed five months after the jejunal resection demonstrates marked arterial dilatation and an intense capillary blush in the right upper quadrant loops of the small bowel that were previously noted to be normal preoperatively. This case illustrates rapidly developing arteriovenous malformation that involves several areas of the small bowel.

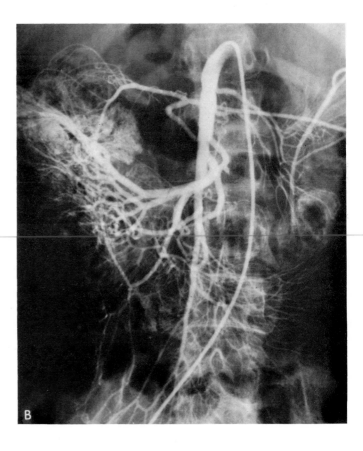

Bleeding Mesenteric Varices

Very fine venous communications exist between the portal tributaries of the mesenteric vein on the parietal surface of the gut and the systemic venous channels in the retroperitoneum and abdominal wall. Although most varices from portal hypertension occur in the esophagus, rectum, and around the umbilicus, some patients have intestinal varices as a result of dilatation of these pre-existing intestinal branches.[10] This is especially true in patients who have had previous laparotomies and develop adhesions between loops of bowel and the abdominal wall. In portal hypertension these varices may become very large and capable of bleeding in a manner similar to esophageal varices.

This same type of collateral communication may grow across adhesions in the pelvis that allow decompression of the mesenteric vein via the gonadal systemic veins (Fig. 24-10). Localized varicosities involving the superior mesenteric vein and its tributaries can also occur secondary to pancreatic malignancy invading the mesenteric vein or to neoplasms of the gastrointestinal tract that secondarily occlude veins within the mesentery.[11] Cases have been described[12] of extensive desmoplastic reaction in the root of the mesentery

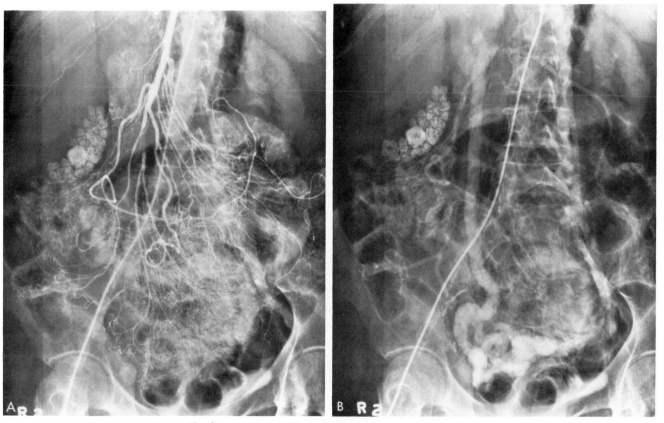

Figure 24-10   Bleeding mesenteric varices. A 68 year old woman known to be cirrhotic presenting with lower gastrointestinal bleeding. *A.* Selective superior mesenteric arteriogram failed to demonstrate any evidence of a site of arterial bleeding. *B.* During the venous phase of the superior mesenteric arteriogram, retrograde flow is seen down the superior mesenteric vein into large varicosities in the pelvis. On later films in the serial study the contrast material was seen draining via the left ovarian vein. This patient had had pelvic surgery many years before. The pelvic varices decompressed the mesenteric vein via the gonadal venous system. At surgery adhesions containing large varicosities were seen between the pelvic organs and ileal loops of small bowel. In the resected specimen of the ileum one of the large veins in the wall of the ileum was bleeding as the result of an overlying area of mucosal ulceration.

secondary to carcinoid tumors that also have resulted in localized mesenteric varices. Angiography obviously plays an important role in documenting the venous obstruction and showing the presence of varices when they exist, and also in excluding other sources of gastrointestinal hemorrhage.

TUMORS

Selective arteriography has had a very limited application in the study of gastrointestinal tumors because of the relative avascular nature of adenomas and adenocarcinomas. This is probably also the result of the ease with which most small bowel tumors can be diagnosed by conventional barium studies. Villous adenomas are notable exceptions since they do exhibit a marked amount of tumor neovascularity, capillary staining, and early venous filling.[13]

Although one would expect that hemangiomas would be easily diagnosed on selective arteriography, our experience has been that since these lesions are so often made up of ectatic venules, even they can be difficult to detect by means of selective arteriography.

The major use of selective arteriography in small bowel tumors has been in cases of leiomyomas and carcinoid tumors.

Leiomyomas

Leiomyomas of the small bowel, unlike those of the stomach, are almost always hypervascular, with evidence of tumor vessels, staining, and early venous filling[14] (Fig. 24-11). Although angiographically the distinction between benign

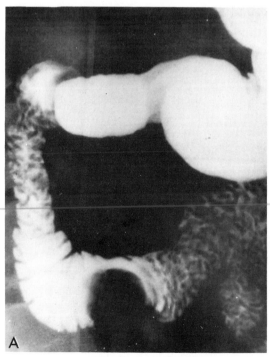

Figure 24-11 *Leiomyoma of the third portion of the duodenum. A.* Spot film of an upper gastrointestinal series shows a mass in the third portion of the duodenum. The patient presented with low grade gastrointestinal bleeding.

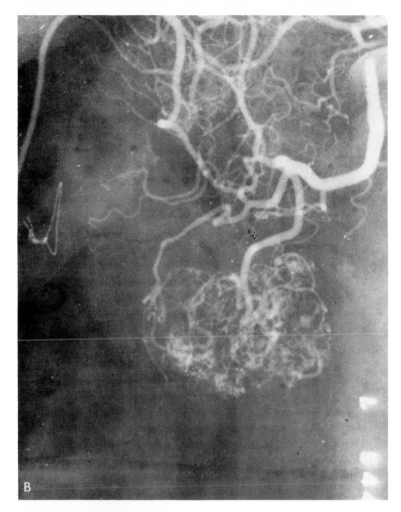

Figure 24-11 Continued B. Selective direct serial magnification arteriography of the gastroduodenal artery shows abundant tumor vessels arising from the inferior pancreatico-duodenal artery, supplying a mass corresponding to the defect noted on the barium examination.

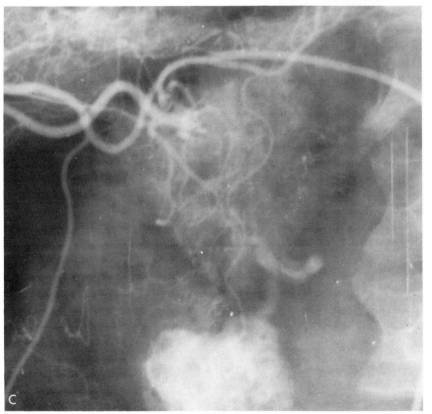

Figure 24-11 C. During the late phase of the same injection there is an intense blush of the tumor. A duodenal leiomyoma was confirmed at surgery.

591

and malignant leiomyomas cannot be made, malignant degeneration can obviously be suspected when the tumors are very large, lack encapsulation, or exhibit evidence of metastases. For reasons that are not at all clear, leiomyomas of the stomach often lack the hypervascular appearance that exhibits when they are in the small bowel.[15]

Tumors of neurogenic origin, such as Schwannomas of the small bowel, are indistinguishable from leiomyoma.[16]

Carcinoid Tumors

Diagnosis of carcinoid tumors is frequently made on the basis of the extreme thickening, fibrosis, and shortening of the mesentery that occurs in association with this tumor. It is thought that the fibrosis associated with this tumor is related to the metabolic breakdown products of serotonin and is analogous to the retroperitoneal fibrosis occurring in some patients taking an antiserotonin drug, methysergide for migraine.[12] The hypervascular appearance of mesenteric vessels in patients with carcinoid tumors therefore may actually represent crowding of the mesenteric arcades owing to the retraction of the mesentery as well as the development of collateral vessels distal to areas of occlusion.[17] The venous structures coursing within the mesentery also are encased by the fibrosis and on occasion patients will present with signs of intestinal ischemia as a result of vascular compromise (Fig. 24-12). Cases also have been seen in which this

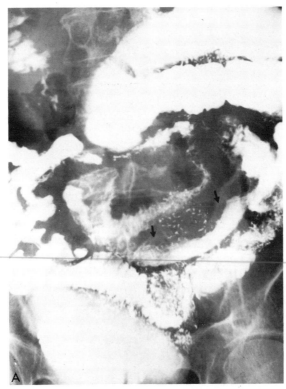

Figure 24-12 Ileal carcinoid tumor with metastases and fibrosis in the root of the mesentery presenting as ischemic enteritis. *A.* Barium meal examination showing a rigid loop of jejunum in the left lower quadrant of the abdomen (arrows).

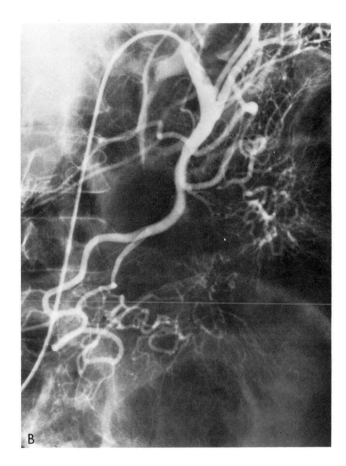

Figure 24-12 Continued *B.* Selective superior mesenteric arteriography demonstrates a lack of filling of many of the jejunal branches in the area of abnormality noted on the barium study.

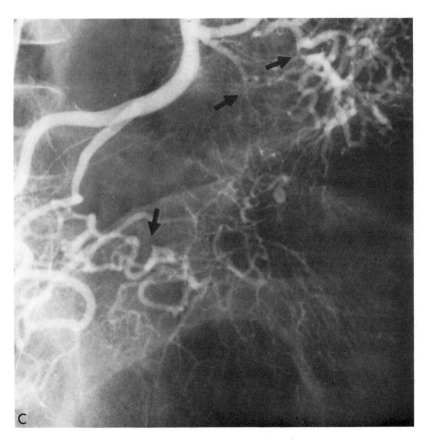

Figure 24-12 *C.* A magnified view of the abnormal area demonstrates encasement resulting in marked narrowing and occlusion of many of the jejunal arteries (upper arrows) as well as attempts at collateral filling of the abnormal jejunal segments (lower arrow). At surgery a carcinoid of the ileum was found with metastases and fibrosis in the mesenteric lymph nodes and mesentery, resulting in encasement of the mesenteric arteries.

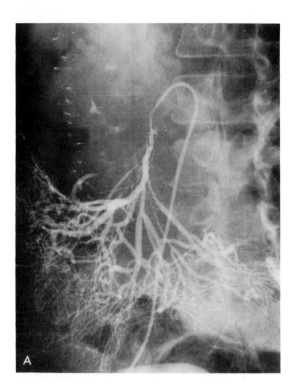

Figure 24-13 Desmoplastic reaction in the root of the mesentery from an ileal carcinoid, resulting in gangrene of the small bowel. A. Selective superior mesenteric arteriography demonstrates marked narrowing of the proximal 5 cm. of the superior mesenteric artery in a patient complaining of severe abdominal pain.

lesion has progressed to cause complete obstruction of the superior mesenteric artery (Fig. 24-13), resulting in gangrene of the small bowel. Other lesions that mimic the mesenteric changes of carcinoid are lymphomatous involvement of the mesentery and retractile mesenteritis.[18] The latter condition is thought by many to represent an extension of retroperitoneal fibrosis.

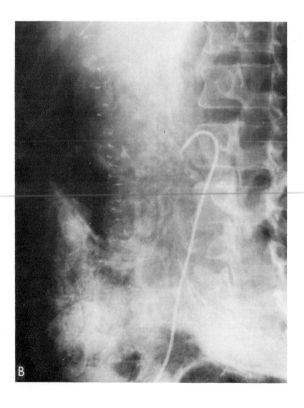

Figure 24-13 B. The venous phase of the study demonstrates the superior mesenteric vein completely occluded with intrahepatic branches of the portal vein filling via collaterals. This patient died of mesenteric infarction and at post mortem examination the changes in the root of the mesentery were seen to be caused by an extreme desmoplastic reaction. There was no evidence of metastatic tumor.

INFLAMMATORY DISEASE OF THE GUT

The angiographic findings of acute enteritis or colitis, regardless of cause, are hypervascularity of the involved segment of the gut, with an increase in the size of the vasa recta, intense capillary blush of the bowel, and early appearing and densely opacified veins.

As the inflammatory process subsides, the vascular pattern becomes normal, and if fibrosis and scarring are sequellae the vasa recta may even be decreased in number as well as in calibre. The discrepancies in the angiographic literature describing the findings of inflammatory disease of the bowel[19, 20] are almost certainly the result of different angiographers looking at different stages of the same disease.

Regional Enteritis

In most cases of regional enteritis selective arteriography demonstrates a marked increase in the blood supply of the affected area of the bowel similar to the changes seen in any inflammatory process.[19] The peripheral segmental arteries to the involved area, however, show dilated, tortuous, and markedly disorganized vasa recta as they enter the bowel wall. During the capillary phase of the study the thickened bowel wall exhibits an intense parenchymal blush. This angiographic picture (Fig. 24-14) is in contrast to the very organized,

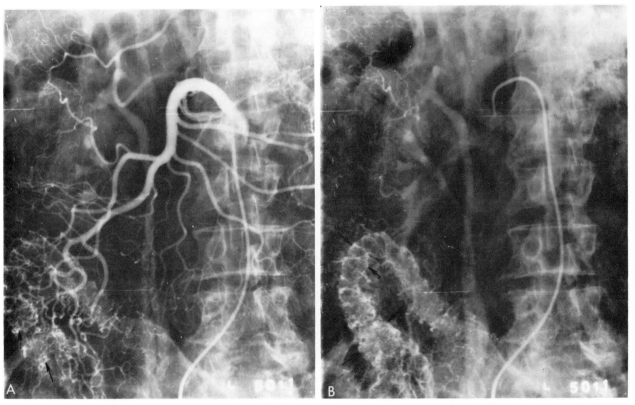

Figure 24-14 *Regional enteritis, active. A.* Selective superior mesenteric arteriography demonstrates moderate enlargement and marked tortuosity of the segmental branches (arrows) to a loop of the distal ileum. The remainder of the small bowel branches appear normal. *B.* During the capillary phase of the examination there is an intense stain of that segment of the ileum (arrows) supplied by the tortuous dilated vessels. This segment of bowel also had early draining and moderately enlarged ileal veins.

nontapered, stepladder appearance of the vasa recta as seen in ulcerative colitis.

When regional enteritis subsides, the mesenteric vessels return to a normal appearance. Because of the marked mesenteric thickening and fibrosis in patients with progressive disease, small bowel arterial branches within the mesentery become irregular, stenotic, and occasionally occluded.[1]

VASCULAR DISEASE

Disorders of the arterial or venous supply to the small bowel may occur on the basis of either large or small vessel disease. The ease with which these conditions can be diagnosed *in vivo* by selective arteriography depends greatly on the size of the affected vessels. Large vessel disease generally causes no difficulty in diagnosis; however, abnormalities involving small vessels can be exceedingly difficult to detect. This is further complicated by the fact that small vessel disease is often functional in the form of intense vasoconstriction rather than occlusive on an organic basis. For these reasons, in this text large vessel disease is described separately from those diseases primarily affecting smaller vessels.

Large Vessel Disease

ATHEROMATOUS OCCLUSIVE DISEASE

The most common site of atheromatous stenosis and occlusion of the celiac, superior, and inferior mesenteric arteries is at their origin at the abdominal aorta. The lesions usually result from plaque formation and are circumferential. If the stenotic area is hemodynamically significant and causes a drop in pressure distal to the narrowing, and if the peripheral resistance in the mesenteric bed is low, collateral flow occurs in a very predictable pattern.

Collateral Pathways

In the 17th century Jean Riolon pointed out that communications exist between the superior mesenteric and inferior mesenteric arteries. In 1913 Drummond[21] demonstrated that the right, middle, and left colic arteries as well as the sigmoid arteries communicate with each other, so that if the ileocolic artery were injected with dye all three vessels filled. Examination of the specimen demonstrated filling of both a central anastomotic artery in the mesentery and a "marginal" artery adjacent to the medial aspect of the colon. This anastomotic complex has been called the marginal artery of Drummond. Drummond also showed communications between the superior hemorrhoidal branch of the inferior mesenteric artery and the middle hemorrhoidal branch of the internal iliac artery.

The angiographic visualization of dilated collateral vessels indicates occlusive disease.[22, 23] If one therefore is familiar with the normal collateral pathways, the site of stenosis or occlusion can be inferred by the pattern and direction of collateral flow.

Collateral Flow Between the Superior
Mesenteric and Inferior Mesenteric Arteries

If the superior mesenteric artery is stenotic or occluded, collateral flow is almost entirely through the pancreaticoduodenal arcades and the marginal anastomotic artery of the colon. Occasionally, the dorsal pancreatic-superior mesenteric artery anastomosis is functional.

In most occlusions of the superior mesenteric artery, the marginal or meandering branch of the inferior mesenteric artery courses parallel to the colon and eventually terminates in the middle or right colic branch of the superior mesenteric artery (Fig. 24-15). The superior mesenteric artery is then reconstituted and the flow to the small bowel and right colon is supplied in a normal manner. If, in addition, the celiac axis is occluded, the anastomotic artery will reconstitute the celiac as well through the pancreaticoduodenal anastomosis (Fig. 24-16). If the superior mesenteric artery is occluded distal to the origin of the middle colic artery, neither the marginal artery nor the pancreaticoduodenal arcades are functional. In these instances small mesenteric collaterals that attempt to bridge the occlusion are generally not adequate enough to maintain viability of the bowel.

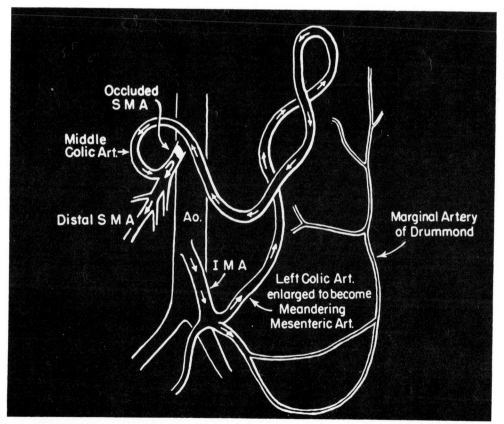

Figure 24-15 Schematic representation of the direction of flow within the marginal anastomotic complex from the left to middle colic arteries in cases of superior mesenteric artery occlusion.

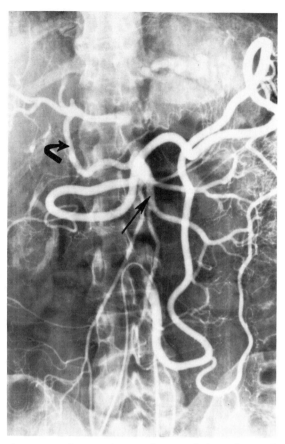

Figure 24–16 Asymptomatic, complete occlusion of the celiac and superior mesenteric arteries with excellent collateral filling via the inferior mesenteric artery. Selective inferior mesenteric arteriography demonstrates collateral filling of the superior mesenteric artery (straight arrow) via the marginal anastomotic artery of the colon extending from the left colic to middle colic arteries. The celiac axis fills via the inferior pancreaticoduodenal artery (curved arrow).

Collateral Flow to an Occluded Inferior Mesenteric Artery

Of the three major mesenteric arteries, the inferior mesenteric artery is probably occluded most often. This tends to be the rule in abdominal aortic aneurysms; and in these patients the marginal vessels can be seen extending from the middle colic to left colic, and the inferior mesenteric artery is reformed in a retrograde direction. The superior hemorrhoidal branch of the inferior mesenteric artery also forms anastomosis with the middle hemorrhoidal branch of the hypogastric artery, and there are many instances of patients who have severe atherosclerotic occlusive disease of the distal aortoiliac vessels that perfuse both lower extremities via the communication of the hypogastric with the inferior mesenteric artery.

Because of the abundant collateralization that has been described, symptomatic occlusive disease of the large vessels is a relatively uncommon condition (Fig. 24-17). All angiographers can recall studying many asymptomatic patients who had a complete occlusion of either the celiac, superior, or inferior mesenteric arteries. Cases also exist in which patients had two or even three of these vessels completely occluded at their origins, and yet were asymptomatic because of excellent perfusion of their gut through collateral channels.

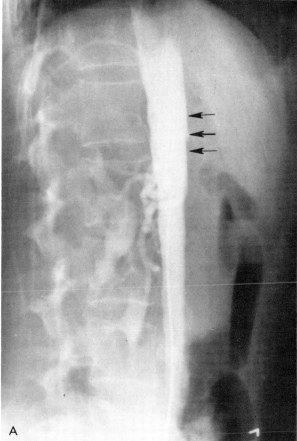

Figure 24-17 A 56 year old woman with abdominal pain secondary to atherosclerotic occlusions at the origins of the celiac and superior mesenteric arteries. *A.* A lateral abdominal aortogram fails to demonstrate filling of either the celiac or superior mesenteric arteries (arrows).

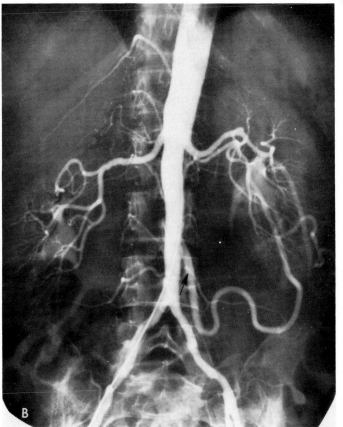

Figure 24-17 *B.* In the A-P projection both renal arteries are filled without any evidence of either the celiac or superior mesenteric artery. The inferior mesenteric artery (arrows) is large and serves as the major collateral vessel.

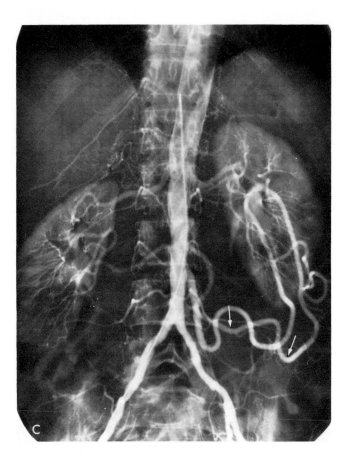

Figure 24-17 Continued   *C.* Several seconds after the injection of contrast material into the abdominal aorta the marginal anastomotic artery of the colon is identified (arrows) coursing in a retrograde direction from the inferior mesenteric artery.

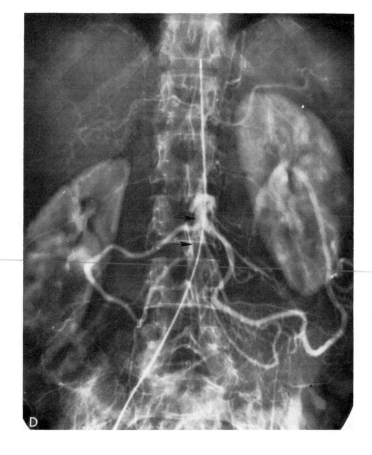

Figure 24-17   *D.* Ten seconds after the injection of contrast material the superior mesenteric artery (arrows) reconstitutes via the marginal anastomotic artery. The celiac axis has reconstituted through collaterals from the lumbar, intercostal, and inferior phrenic arteries.

ANEURYSMS

Aortic Aneurysms

Most aneurysms of the abdominal aorta are atherosclerotic and begin below the origin of the renal arteries, sparing the celiac and superior mesenteric artery, but almost always occluding the inferior mesenteric artery. In approximately 5 per cent[24] of cases, the aneurysms extend above the renal arteries and in these instances the superior mesenteric artery may be involved.

Dissecting aneurysms, although rarely originating in the abdomen, frequently extend from the thoracic aorta so as to compromise arterial flow to the kidney and viscera. Occasionally the presenting symptom of a patient with an aortic dissection is an acute abdomen secondary to mesenteric arterial occlusion[25] (Fig. 24-18). The importance of making this diagnosis preoperatively is obvious.

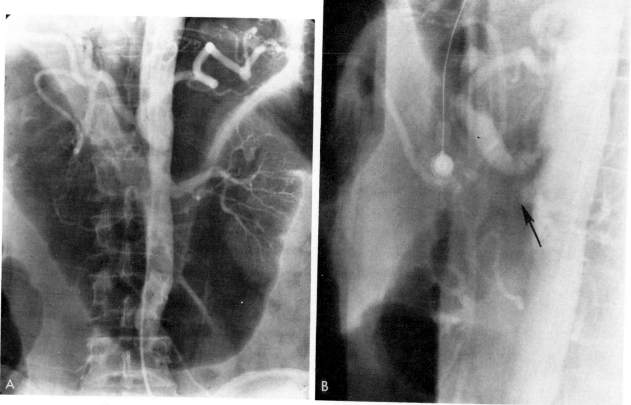

Figure 24-18 Dissecting aneurysm of the thoracic aorta extending into the abdomen and occluding the right renal and superior mesenteric artery. This 55-year-old man was brought to the hospital after being found unconscious. On physical examination the abdomen was distended and no bowel sounds could be heard. *A.* Abdominal aortography demonstrates a dissection of the abdominal aorta with occlusion of the right renal and superior mesenteric arteries. *B.* A lateral film of the abdomen shows with better definition the complete occlusion of the superior mesenteric artery immediately distal to its origin (arrow).

Branch Aneurysms

With the exception of the splenic artery, atheromatous aneurysms of the celiac and superior mesenteric artery branches are rare. Most of these aneurysms are traumatic (Fig. 24-19), mycotic, or a result of digestion of the arterial wall by leaking pancreatic enzymes from pancreatitis. Because of the high incidence of intramural dissection associated with fibromuscular disease, aneurysm formation may be the dominant arteriographic finding in this disease.

The complications of celiac and mesenteric artery aneurysms are gastro-intestinal or intra-abdominal bleeding and occlusion of major branches.

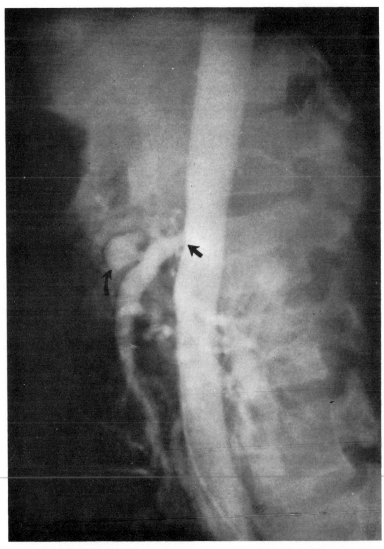

Figure 24-19 Traumatic aneurysm of the superior mesenteric artery following an automobile accident. A lateral film of an abdominal aortogram demonstrates slight narrowing at the origin of the superior mesenteric artery (straight arrow) and an aneurysm on the superior aspect of the proximal superior mesenteric artery (curved arrow). The etiology of the aneurysm presumably is based on trauma.

Embolization

Emboli of the larger branches of the superior mesenteric artery are frequently caused by cardiac disease (Fig. 24-20). Small emboli present as filling defects, generally lodged at the divisions of the mesenteric artery into its branches. Because the emboli frequently are peripheral, collateral flow is usually not adequate.

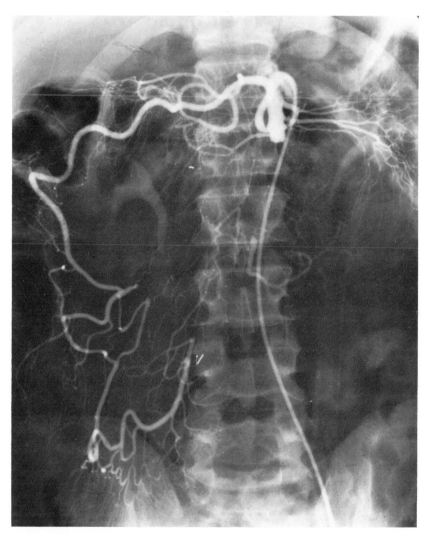

Figure 24-20 Embolus to the superior mesenteric artery from a thrombus in an akinetic segment of the left ventricle in a 36-year-old man. The embolus is lodged immediately distal to the origin of the middle colic artery. Collateral flow to the remainder of the small bowel occurs through the middle colic–right colic anastomosis.

Small Vessel Disease

The arteriographic evaluation of the small vessels of the gut presents unique problems that are generally not encountered in studying other vascular beds. One of the major limitations in attempting to evaluate small vessels of the intestines is related to the superimposition caused by the crowding together of more than 20 feet of intestines into a relatively closed space such as the abdomen. It is virtually impossible, therefore, to attempt to evaluate the distribution of blood flow to specific segments of the bowel, such as the mucosa and submucosa.[26]

These small vessels are exceedingly important when one considers the autoregulatory control of intestinal blood flow. These are the vessels that have been referred to as the resistance vessels of the peripheral mesenteric bed, and they probably experience the greatest pressure changes. The large and small arteries probably do not make very significant contributions to blood flow regulation and therefore the radiographic appearance of these vessels merely represents changes resulting from increased or decreased flow. These arteries can be compared to conduits that reflect the regulation of flow occurring in the smaller vessels. It has been estimated that 70 per cent of the true regulatory vessels of the gut are at precapillary levels and are probably in the order of 100 microns in diameter.[27] The size of this regulatory system can best be appreciated when one considers that the splanchnic bed is capable of siphoning off all of man's blood volume and is probably the largest regional circulatory system in the body.

If angiography is to play a useful role in evaluating mesenteric blood flow it must be concerned with small vessel angiography. It is obvious from the preceding statements that the vascular changes caused by the regional adjustments in flow are well beyond the scope of conventional, clinically performed angiograms. Attempts at trying to evaluate these smaller vessels require changing the conventional means of performing angiography. To date the only successful approach to this problem has been the technique of direct serial magnification, using fractional focal spots having effective size of 0.3 mm. or less.

It is convenient to consider the diseases of the small vessels of the intestines under the separate categories of inflammatory changes, degenerative changes, and structural changes.[28]

INFLAMMATION. Vasculitis of the mesenteric vessels can be conveniently classified as follows:

Primary Vasculitis. These are primary changes within the blood vessels themselves and are usually part of systemic diseases. Necrotizing arteritis of small or medium-sized vessels with perivascular inflammation and fibrinoid necrosis is seen in several diseases. In addition to polyarteritis nodosa, these changes can also be identified in other collagen disorders such as lupus erythymatosis, scleroderma, rheumatoid arthritis, and dermatomyositis.[29] The arterial involvement may be segmental, with only a small portion of the wall being involved. This is especially true in polyarteritis nodosa. The end result of the arterial injury may be rupture, aneurysm formation, fibrosis, and/or thrombosis.

If medium or large-sized vessels such as the middle colic artery are involved, the arteriographic diagnosis is not difficult (Fig. 24-21). If, however, the involvement is limited to the smaller vessels, the diagnosis can be difficult to

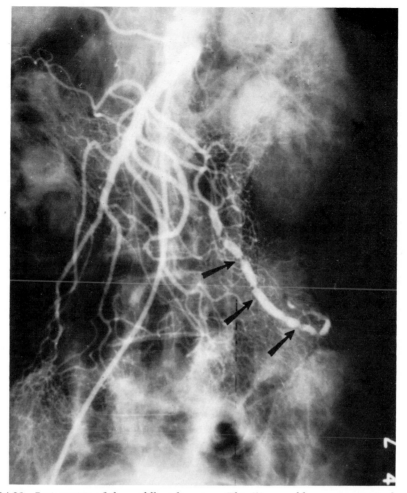

Figure 24-21 *Periarteritis of the middle colic artery.* This 56-year-old woman presented with intra-abdominal bleeding caused by rupture of the middle colic artery into the transverse mesocolon. Selective superior mesenteric arteriography demonstrates marked irregularity, tortuosity, and beading of the middle colic artery in its distal portion (arrows).

establish by means of conventional techniques and direct magnification studies are needed (Fig. 24-22).

An unusual feature of periarteritis nodosa has been the involvement of the middle and left colic arteries.[30] Necrosis of the wall of the vessel produces aneurysmal dilatation associated with areas of intramural dissection, giving a very characteristic nodularity and beaded appearance (Fig. 24-21). This can lead to intra-abdominal or retroperitoneal hemorrhage, mesenteric infarction, and occasionally intestinal perforation.

Local Vasculitis. As vessels pass through areas of inflammation, necrosis occurs in the walls of the vessels, which can result in obliteration of the smaller veins and arteries. An example of these secondary changes can be found in most cases of ileocolitis, as well as vascular changes occurring at the base of a peptic ulcer. This also is seen following radiation and may occur in malignant or benign masses that produce an extreme desmoplastic reaction. Another example of a local vasculitis is the digestion of the wall and subsequent aneurysm formation of arteries adjacent to areas of pancreatitis.[31]

DEGENERATIVE DISEASE. Degenerative diseases of the small vessels include those lesions that bear no resemblance to atherosclerosis, yet the lumen of

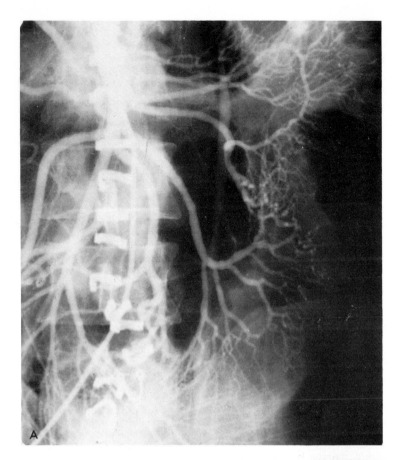

A

Figure 24-22 *Periarteritis of the midjejunal arterial branches resulting in infarction of four feet of small bowel.* A. Selective superior mesenteric arteriography demonstrates marginal irregularity of the vessels going to the midjejunum.

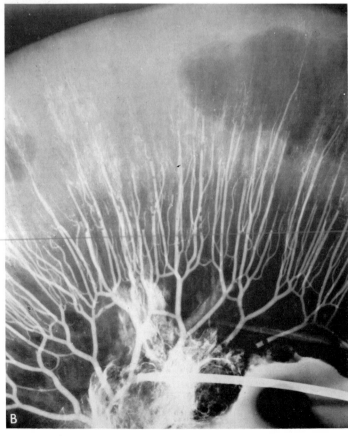

B

Figure 24-22 B. Injection specimen using 0.05 mm. focal spot demonstrates occlusion of almost all of the intramural peripheral arterial branches in the involved segment of bowel. The occlusions themselves are probably in branches measuring less than 100 microns in diameter.

the arteries is moderately to highly narrowed owing to marked thickening and fibrosis of the intima and media.

STRUCTURAL DISEASES OF THE SMALL VESSELS. This is the category where hereditary hemorrhagic telangiectasia is placed as well as pseudoxanthoma elasticum.

NONOCCLUSIVE MESENTERIC ISCHEMIA

Nonocclusive mesenteric ischemia has been reported to represent 20 to 50 per cent of all cases of ischemic bowel disease.[32, 33] Because of the lack of early clinical and radiological findings, the disease is usually not considered until irreversible intestinal necrosis occurs, and at this stage of disease the mortality rate approaches 100 per cent. The basic initiating mechanism of nonocclusive mesenteric ischemia is thought to be an intense peripheral vasoconstriction and redistribution of the splanchnic blood flow second to low cardiac output states, such as congestive heart failure and cardiac arrythmias. The disease is also associated with digitalis ingestion and is probably related to the severe splanchnic vasoconstrictor effect of digitalis preparations.

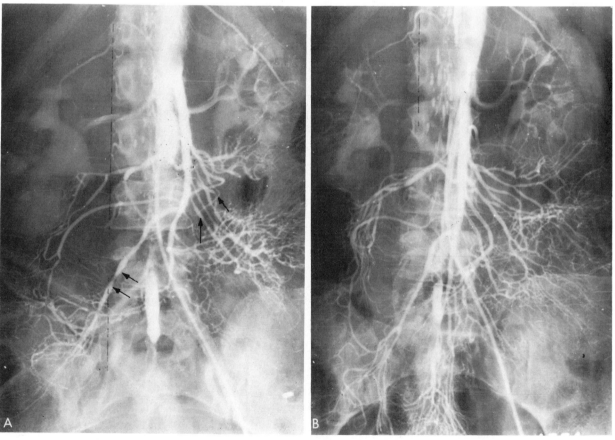

Figure 24-23 Treatment of nonocclusive mesenteric ischemic disease by the selective arterial infusion of vasodilating agents. *A.* Selective superior mesenteric arteriography demonstrates multiple narrowed segments of both the small and medium sized vessels (arrows) as well as a marked decrease in the peripheral filling of the small mesenteric branches. *B.* Repeat superior mesenteric arteriography after the injection of 25 mg. of priscoline demonstrates an increase in the amount of peripheral arterial filling, less reflux in the abdominal aorta indicating a decrease in peripheral resistance, and dilatation in many of the segments of narrowing noted on the pre-priscoline arteriogram.

Even brief lowering of the superior mesenteric artery flow initiates persistent vasoconstriction which may last for hours despite correction of the primary cause of the mesenteric ischemia.[34] Once nonocclusive mesenteric ischemia is thought of as a diagnostic possibility, the intra-arterial infusion of vasodilating drugs such as papaverine or Priscoline can be used in an attempt to reverse the potentially lethal vasoconstriction (Fig. 24-23).[35, 36] Experience with these procedures is presently still very limited and it is obvious that much more work needs to be done in this statistically common yet uncommonly diagnosed disease.

The angiographic features of nonocclusive mesenteric ischemia are mainly those of intense peripheral resistance within the splanchnic bed. As a result, injections made into the superior mesenteric artery tend to equal mesenteric blood flow very quickly so that even at injection rates of 5 cc. per second, spill-over occurs into the abdominal aorta. The most peripheral branches of the superior mesenteric artery are very slow to fill and some areas of the gut do not appear to be perfused. Because of the intense peripheral vasoconstriction concentric areas of narrowing are seen in many of the major branches of the mesenteric artery, especially at their origins. This may also be associated with irregularities in the intestinal branches, narrowing of certain segments of the arteries, and abnormal tapering patterns.[35]

ANGIODYSPLASIA

Angiodysplasia or vascular ectasias involving the cecum and right colon are often seen in elderly patients presenting with chronic gastrointestinal bleeding.[37, 38] Although these lesions are usually not in the small bowel, they have been included in this discussion because they derive all of their blood supply from the superior mesenteric artery and are detected on superior mesenteric arteriography.

Although angiodysplasias are visible on conventional nonmagnified superior mesenteric arteriography, they are seen to much better advantage when direct serial magnification techniques are used. The angiographic findings consist of an increase in the number of small vessels in the cecum and right colon that are usually toward the antimesenteric surface of the bowel, a blush of the area during the capillary phase of the study, and early venous drainage of the involved segment of the bowel (Fig. 24-24).

Even with advanced knowledge of their exact location, the surgeon cannot detect the lesions at the operating room table. Since the lesions are discrete and focal in distribution, the pathologist has great difficulty in identifying them histologically. For this reason we have recently started injecting the arteries of the resected specimen with a silicone rubber compound[39] and, following formaldehyde fixation, subjecting the specimen to tissue clearing techniques and viewing under a dissecting microscope (Fig. 24-25). Since no tissue has been destroyed in the process, the abnormal area is identified and sent to pathology for histologic section. Pathologically these lesions are primarily in the submucosa and consist of dilated submucosal arteries and veins associated with areas of overlying mucosal thinning and occasionally ulceration. Under the

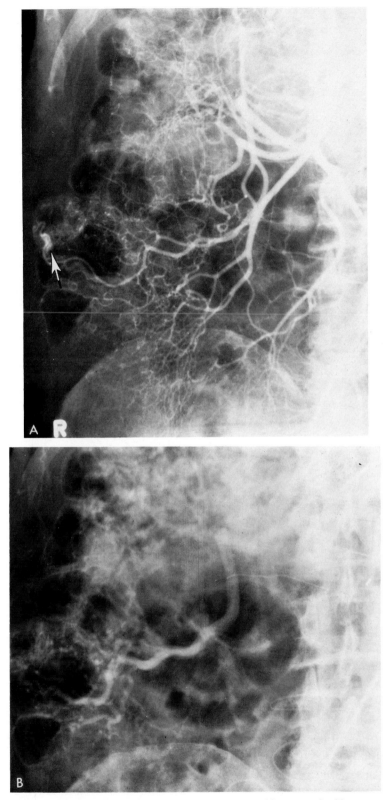

Figure 24-24 Angiodysplasia in the cecum in a 75-year-old man studied because of recurrent melena. *A.* Selective superior mesenteric arteriography, early arterial phase demonstrating a cluster of abnormally dilated arteries (arrow) on the antimesenteric border of the cecum. *B.* During the late capillary phase of examination early filling, large draining veins can be seen coming from the cecum. This patient underwent a right colectomy and histologically several angiodysplasias were found in the cecum and proximal ascending colon.

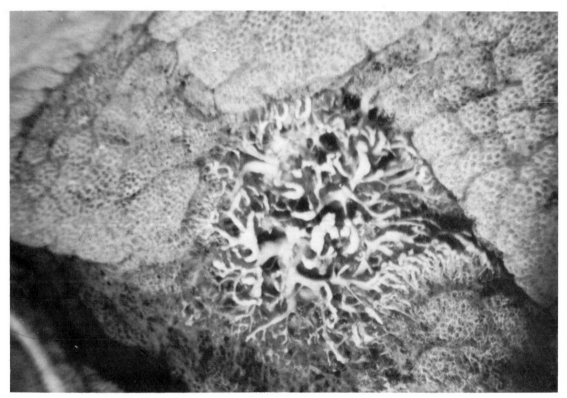

Figure 24-25 Angiodysplasia of the right colon after silicone-rubber injection and clearing, demonstrating a cluster of tortuous vessels surrounded by otherwise normal mucosal vasculature (×20). This photograph was taken under a dissecting microscope.

dissecting microscope the lesions look very much alike, from specimen to specimen, and resemble a lace coral.

Patients having these lesions are generally over the age of 50. It is very unlikely that these angiodysplasias are congenital AV malformations since histologically they do not resemble congenital AV malformations in other parts of the body and they are seen almost exclusively in the older age group.

The etiology of these lesions as well as explanation for their propensity for the cecum and right colon remain obscure. Many of these patients have evidence of decreased perfusion of the gut on the basis of valvular heart disease, congestive heart failure, atheromatous aortic disease, cholesterol embolization, or other disorders of this type.

Increasing intraluminal pressure has been shown to cause mucosal ischemia and arteriovenous shunting within the submucosa. It is therefore possible that the submucosal angiodysplasias are actually a result of chronic submucosal shunting. For all of these reasons, it is thought that the lesions represent a chronic form of ischemic bowel disease.

The almost exclusive location of the lesions in the right colon is difficult to explain. It may, however, be related to the increased transmural pressure in the wall of the cecum and ascending colon as a function of its increased diameter in keeping with Laplace's Law.

References

1. Reuter, S. R., and Redman, H. C.: *Gastrointestinal Angiography*. Philadelphia, W. B. Saunders Co., 1972.
2. Hanafee, W. N., et al.: *Golden's Diagnostic Radiology: Section 18: Selective Angiography*. Baltimore, The Williams & Wilkins Co., 1972.
3. Michels, N. A.: *Blood Supply and Anatomy of Upper Abdominal Organs with Descriptive Atlas*. Philadelphia, J. B. Lippincott Co., 1955.
4. Nebesar, R. A., Kornblith, P. L., Pollard, J. J., and Michels, N. A.: *A Correlation of Angiograms and Dissections*. Boston, Little Brown & Co., 1969.
5. Buranasiri, S., Baum, S., Nusbaum, M., and Tumen, H.: The angiographic diagnosis of midgut malrotation with volvulus in adults. *Radiology*, 109:555–556, Dec. 1973.
6. Nusbaum, M., and Baum, S.: Radiographic demonstration of unknown sites of gastrointestinal bleeding. *S. Forum*, 14:374, 1963.
7. Baum, S., and Nusbaum, M.: The control of gastrointestinal hemorrhage by selective mesenteric arterial infusion of vasopressin. *Radiology*, 98:497, 1971.
8. Baum, S., Athanasoulis, C. A., Waltman, A., and Ring, E.: Angiographic diagnosis and control of gastrointestinal bleeding. *In* Advances in Surgery, C. Welch (ed.), Yearbook Medical Publishers, Chicago (Jan) 1974, Vol. 7, pp. 149–198.
9. Rösch, J., Dotter, C. T., and Brown, M. J.: Selective arterial embolization: A new method for control of acute gastrointestinal bleeding. *Radiology*, 102:303, 1972.
10. Gray, R., and Grollman, J. H., Jr.: Acute lower gastrointestinal bleeding secondary to varices of the superior mesenteric venous system: angiographic demonstration. *Radiology*, 111:559, 1974.
11. Case Records of the Massachusetts General Hospital (Case 31–1974). *New Engl. J. Med.*, 291:295–301, 1974.
12. Case Records of the Massachusetts General Hospital (Case 1–1973). *New Engl. J. Med.*, 288:36–43, 1973.
13. Abrams, H. L.: Inferior mesenteric arteriography. *In* Angiography, Vol. II, H. L. Abrams (ed.), Boston, Little, Brown & Company, pp. 1143–1165, 1971.
14. Boijsen, E., and Reuter, S. R.: Mesenteric angiography in the evaluation of inflammatory and neoplastic disease of the intestine. *Radiology*, 87:1028, 1966.
15. Baum, S.: Angiography of localized gastric lesions. *Seminars in Roentgenology*, 6:207–219, April 1971.
16. Capdeville, R., Bennett, J., Dubois, F., and Toulet, J.: L'Arteriographie des Tumeurs du Grele: A Propos de 3 Cas de Schwannomes, *Arch. Franc. Mal. Appar. Dig.*, 59:453, 1970.
17. Reuter, S. R., and Boijsen, E.: Angiographic findings in two ileal carcinoid tumors. *Radiology*, 87:836, 1966.
18. Case Records of the Massachusetts General Hospital (Case 27–1972). *New Engl. J. Med.*, 287:35–40, 1972.
19. Boijsen, E., and Reuter, S. R.: Mesenteric angiography in the evaluation of inflammatory and neoplastic disease of the intestine. *Radiology*, 87:1028–1036, 1966.
20. Brahme, F.: Mesenteric angiography in regional enterocolitis. *Radiology*, 87:1037–1042.
21. Drummond, H.: Some points relating to the surgical anatomy of the arterial supply of the large intestine. *Proc. Roy. Soc. Med.*, 7:185, 1913.
22. Kahn, P., and Abrams, H. L.: Inferior mesenteric arterial patterns: angiographic study. *Radiology*, 82:429, 1964.
23. Moskowitz, M., Zimmerman, H., and Felson, B.: The meandering mesenteric artery of the colon. *Amer. J. Roentgen.*, 92:1088, 1964.
24. Brewster, D. C., Retana, A., Waltman, A. C., and Darling, C.: Angiography in the management of abdominal aortic aneurysms: its value and safety. *New Engl. J. Med.*, 292:822, 1975.
25. Case Records of the Massachusetts General Hospital (Case 32–1974). *New Engl. J. Med.*, 291:350–358, 1974.
26. Baum, S.: Small vessel angiography of the gut. *In* Hilal, S. K. (ed.), *Small Vessel Angiography. Imaging, Morphology, Physiology, and Clinical Applications*, St. Louis, C. V. Mosby Co. 1973, pp. 454–478.
27. Landis, E. M.: The capillary pressure in mammalian mesentery as determined by the micro-injection method. *Amer. J. Physiol.*, 93:353, 1930.
28. Feller, E., Richet, R., and Spiro, N. M.: Small vessel disease of the gut. *In* Boley, S. J. (ed.), *Vascular Disorders of the Intestine*, New York, Appleton-Century-Crofts, Inc., 1971, p. 483.
29. Case Records of the Massachusetts General Hospital (Case 45–1974). *New Engl. J. Med.*, 291:1073–1080, 1974.
30. Buranasiri, S., Baum, S., Nusbaum, M., and Finkelstein, D.: Periarteritis of the middle colic artery: arteriographic, surgical, and pathologic correlation. *Amer. J. Gastroent.*, 59:73–76, 1973.
31. Baum, S., and Athanasoulis, C. A.: Angiography of the duodenum and pancreas. *In* Eaton, S. B., and Ferrucci, J. T., Jr. (eds.), *Radiology of the Pancreas and Duodenum*, Philadelphia, W. B. Saunders Co., pp. 227–260, 1973.
32. Williams, L. F., Jr., and Kim, J. P.: Non-occlusive mesenteric ischemia. *In* Boley, S. J. (ed.), *Vascular Disorders of the Intestine*. New York, Appleton-Century-Crofts, Inc., 1971, p. 519.

33. Ottinger, L. W., and Austen, W. G.: A study of 136 patients with mesenteric infarction. *Surg., Gynec., Obstet.*, 124:251, 1967.
34. Boley, S. J., and Siegelman, S. S.: Experimental and clinical nonocclusive mesenteric ischemia: pathophysiology, diagnosis and management. *In* Hilal, S. K. (ed.), *Small Vessel Angiography Imaging, Morphology, Physiology, and Clinical Applications.* St. Louis, C. V. Mosby Co., 1973, pp. 438–453.
35. Siegelman, S. S., Sprayregen, S., and Boley, S. J.: Angiographic diagnosis of mesenteric arterial vasoconstriction. *Radiology*, 112:533–542, 1974.
36. Habboushe, F., Wallace, H. W., Nusbaum, N., Baum, S., Dratch, P., and Blakemore, W. S.: Nonocclusive mesenteric vascular insufficiency. *Ann. Surg.*, 180:819–822, 1974.
37. Baum, S., Athanasoulis, C. A., and Waltman, A. C.: Acquired vascular ectasias of the cecum and right colon as a cause of chronic gastrointestinal bleeding. Abstract No. 181, Presented at the 58th Scientific Assembly and Annual Meeting of the Radiological Society of North America, Chicago, Illinois, Nov. 26–Dec. 1, 1972.
38. Galloway, S. J., Casarella, W. J. and Shimkin, P. M.: Vascular malformations of the right colon as a cause of bleeding in patients with aortic stenosis. *Radiology*, 113:11–15, 1974.
39. Reynolds, D. G.: Injection techniques in the study of intestinal vasculature under normal conditions and in ulcerative colitis. *In* S. J. Boley (ed.), *Vascular Disorders of the Intestine,* Appleton-Century-Crofts, Inc., New York, 1971, pp. 383–395.

Index

Note: Page numbers in *italic* indicate a figure; numbers followed by a t indicate a table.

613